Infection in the Neonate:
A Comprehensive Guide to Assessment, Management, and Nursing Care

Debbie Fraser Askin, RNC, MN

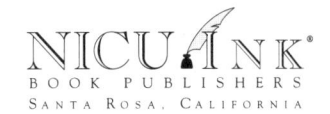

NICU Ink®
BOOK PUBLISHERS
SANTA ROSA, CALIFORNIA

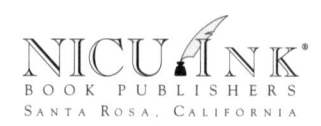

NICU INK®
BOOK PUBLISHERS
SANTA ROSA, CALIFORNIA

2270 Northpoint Parkway
Santa Rosa, CA 95407-7398

Copyright © 2004 by NICU INK®

All rights reserved. No part of this publication may be reproduced, stored in a retrieval system, or transmitted in any form or by any means: electronic, mechanical, photocopying, or otherwise, without prior written permission from the publisher.

Trademarks: Throughout this book we use trademarked names. Instead of using a trademark symbol with each occurrence, we state that we are using the names in an editorial fashion to the benefit of the trademark owner, with no intention of infringement of the trademark.

EDITOR-IN-CHIEF: Charles Rait, RN, MSEd, PNC

MANAGING EDITOR: Suzanne G. Rait, RN

EDITORIAL COORDINATOR: Tabitha Parker

CONTINUING EDUCATION COURSE CONTENT: Debbie Fraser Askin, RNC, MN

REVIEWERS:	EDITORS:
Mary Klawitter, RNC, MSN	Beverley DeWitt, BA
Maria Lofgren MSN, ARNP, APN	Sylvia Stein Wright, BA
Janice Thape, RNC, MSN	Carol Trotter, PhD, NNP
Laurel Vessey, RN, BSN	

PROOFREADER: Joanne Gosnell, BA

INDEXER: Gerry Lynn Messner, BSN, MBA

MEDICAL ILLUSTRATOR: Elizabeth Weadon Massari, MSMI, CMI

BOOK DESIGN AND COMPOSITION: Marsha Godfrey Graphics

LIBRARY OF CONGRESS CATALOGING-IN-PUBLICATION DATA
Askin, Debbie Fraser, 1959–
Infection in the neonate : a comprehensive guide to assessment, management, and nursing care / Debbie Fraser Askin.
    p. ;   cm.
    Includes bibliographical references and index.
    ISBN 1-887571-11-6
    1. Neonatal infections. 2. Infants (Newborn)—Diseases—Nursing. I. Title.
    [DNLM: 1. Bacterial Infections—Infant, Newborn. 2. Infection—Infant, Newborn. 3. Mycoses—Infant, Newborn. 4. Nursing Care—methods. 5. Virus Diseases—nursing—Infant, Newborn. WC 200 A835i 2003]
RJ275.A856 2003
618.92'01—dc22

2003070248

Table of Contents

Introduction v

Acknowledgments vii

1 Introduction to Microbiology 1

2 The Immune System 13

3 Intrauterine Infections 37

4 Bacterial Infections 61

5 Neonatal Viral and Fungal Infections 83

6 Clinical and Laboratory Evaluation of Neonatal Infection 129

7 Management of Neonatal Infection, Sepsis, and Complications 143

8 Pharmacologic Management of Neonatal Infection 163

Appendices

A Normal Laboratory Values for Evaluation of Infection and CSF Findings in Term and Premature Infants 181

B White Cell and Differential Counts in Premature Infants 185

C Leukocyte Values and Neutrophil Counts in Term and Premature Infants 187

D Antimicrobial Agents Used to Treat Neonatal Infection 189

E Recommendations for Immunizations for Communicable Diseases 199

F Therapeutic Serum Peak and Trough Levels for Antimicrobial Agents 203

G Calculations for Evaluating White Blood Cell Count 205

   Glossary 209

   Index 215

   Continuing Education Test 231

Contributing Authors

Debbie Fraser Askin, RNC, MN
   University of Manitoba
   St. Boniface General Hospital
   Winnipeg, Manitoba

Terri A. Cavaliere, RNC, MS, NNP
   North Shore University Hospital
   Manhasset, New York
   State University of New York
   Stony Brook, New York

Susan Givens Bell, MS, RNC
   All Children's Hospital
   St. Petersburg, Florida

Ellen Tappero, RNC, MN, NNP
   Neonatology Associates, Ltd.
   Phoenix, Arizona

Catherine Witt, RNC, MS, NNP
   Presbyterian/St. Luke's Medical Center
   Denver, Colorado

Debra Sansoucie, EdD, RNC, NNP
   Stony Brook University
   School of Nursing
   Health Sciences Center
   Stony Brook, New York

INTRODUCTION

Congenital and acquired infections continue to pose a serious threat to the newborn infant. The survival of smaller and sicker neonates has resulted in an increased rate of nosocomial infections, particularly line-related coagulase negative staphylococcal infections. Preventive measures and early recognition of the signs of infections are critical to the well-being of very low birth weight infants.

This book was compiled with the goal of providing a comprehensive overview of neonatal infection for neonatal staff nurses, advanced practice nurses, medical residents, and other health care providers. The book addresses congenital and acquired infections caused by bacteria, viruses, fungi, and protozoa, with an emphasis on the most common causes of neonatal infection. This information will provide a basis for the recognition and treatment of neonates at risk.

We begin with a discussion of basic microbiology designed to provide a refresher for those who may not have regular contact with the world of bacteria, viruses, fungi, and protozoa. The complexities of the immune system are addressed from both embryologic and functional perspectives with special emphasis on the deficits and challenges faced by neonates. Enhanced knowledge of microbiology and the workings of the immune system will facilitate an understanding of the assessment, diagnosis, and treatment of infection.

The growing number of antibiotic-resistant strains of bacteria is cause for great concern in the NICU. The development of new and more powerful drugs is only part of the answer. The judicious use of antibiotics and the development of new strategies to recognize and appropriately treat neonates are of the utmost urgency. Careful attention to prevention of infection is also critical in avoiding unnecessary antibiotic exposure. The information in this text is intended to familiarize care providers with the assessment, diagnosis, and management of common neonatal infections in order to minimize the risk and provide quality care to our patients and their families.

Debbie Fraser Askin, RNC, MN

Acknowledgments

This book is dedicated to our smallest, most vulnerable patients and those who provide their daily care.

My thanks go to the dedicated authors, reviewers, and editorial staff who persevered through the lengthy process of seeing a book from conception to publication. Chuck, Suzanne, and Tabby never lost faith in our ability to get this done! I am grateful to my colleagues at St. Boniface General Hospital NICU and the University of Manitoba faculty of nursing for their continued support.

Special thanks to my parents, Bill and Viona Fraser, for instilling in me a healthy work ethic and to my family, Cayly, Nicole, Anna, Liam, and Bill.

Debbie Fraser Askin

CHAPTER 1

Introduction to Microbiology

DEBBIE FRASER ASKIN, RNC, MN

There are four common classifications of microorganisms: bacteria, viruses, fungi, and parasites, which include protozoa. In neonates, the types of organisms most often responsible for infection are bacteria, followed by viruses and fungi. In the developed world, very few neonatal infections are associated with protozoa. This chapter provides an overview of the morphology and nomenclature of these four types of microorganisms. It also contains a brief discussion of medical microbiology principles and normal flora of the human body.

In the eighteenth century, Carolus Linnaeus derived the first system, or taxonomy, for categorizing microorganisms. Linnaeus assigned each organism two names, a genus label and a second, more specific, epithet, which together were referred to as species. For example, Staphylococcus is the genus and aureus is the specific epithet. Together *Staphylococcus aureus* is the species. Organisms were then classified into larger groups based on similarities and differences.[1]

Many subsequent attempts have been made to develop a taxonomic classification that is both clear and comprehensive. In 1984, the classification system for bacteria was reorganized, and 3,000 different bacteria were described.[2] This number was thought to represent about 1 percent of the total number of bacteria present in nature.[1]

BACTERIA

Cells are the fundamental building blocks of all living organisms. Ranging in size from 0.1 to 20 µm or longer, bacteria are the smallest of cells.[3] Classified as prokaryotic (from the Greek for "primitive nucleus") organisms, bacteria are simple in structure—unicellular organisms that do not contain a nuclear membrane, mitochondria, or Golgi bodies and that reproduce by asexual division. Each cell contains the DNA needed for reproduction and the essentials for energy production (Figure 1-1). Bacteria are capable of surviving and even growing in very hostile environments, such as extreme temperatures or dryness, environments in which plant and animal cells would die.

Some bacteria have the ability to exchange small packets of genetic information with diverse organisms. It is speculated that this information

FIGURE 1-1 ♦ Prokaryotic cell.

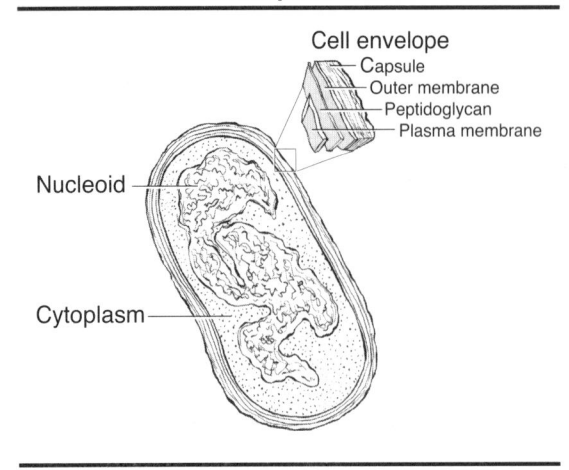

may be carried on plasmids, small genetic elements that replicate independent of the bacterial chromosome. Information carried by plasmids may include drug resistance, rendering diverse bacteria resistant to antibiotic treatment.[4]

Many characteristics of a bacterium are examined to determine its classification. They include morphology, staining, movement, growth, atmospheric and nutrient requirements, biochemical and metabolic activities, pathogenicity, sequencing of proteins, and genetic composition.

Morphology

The shape, or morphology, of a bacterium was the primary characteristic used in the early classifications and remains an important aspect to this day. There are three basic bacterial shapes: spherical or coccoid (referred to as cocci), rod shaped (referred to as bacilli), and curved or spiral. The presence of appendages such as flagella (axial filaments) can also play an important role in typing. Shape can be further described as outlined in Table 1-1.

Staining

The application of various stains is a relatively easy and inexpensive test that facilitates rapid identification of the two major classifications of bacteria: Gram-positive and Gram-negative organisms. The thickness and chemical composition of the bacterium's cell wall determine the color at the end of the staining process. To perform a Gram's stain, bacteria are dried on a slide and then stained with an application of crystal violet followed by Gram iodine. Excess stain is washed away, and a counterstain of safranin is applied. Gram-positive bacteria, with their thick cell walls, retain the violet stain, whereas Gram-negative bacteria, which have thin cell walls, accept the counterstain and appear red.[3]

Another type of stain, called acid-fast, is used to identify mycobacteria, which have a waxy outer shell. Mycoplasma, which has no cell wall, is not identified with routine Gram's staining. Therefore, if Mycoplasma is part of the differential diagnosis for neonatal infection, the laboratory needs to be notified so that additional tests may be performed for proper identification.

TABLE 1-1 ♦ Bacterial Shapes

Shape	Arrangement	Description	Shape
Cocci (spherical)	Pairs	Diplococci	
	Chains	Streptococci	
	Clusters	Staphylococci	
Bacilli (rod shaped)	Short or long, thick or thin, single or in pairs	Streptobacilli	
	Chains	Coccobacilli	
	Very short		
Spirals (curved)	Usually single; may form chains and are described according to the presence of rigid or flexible walls	Spirillum	

FIGURE 1-2 ♦ Flagellated bacteria.

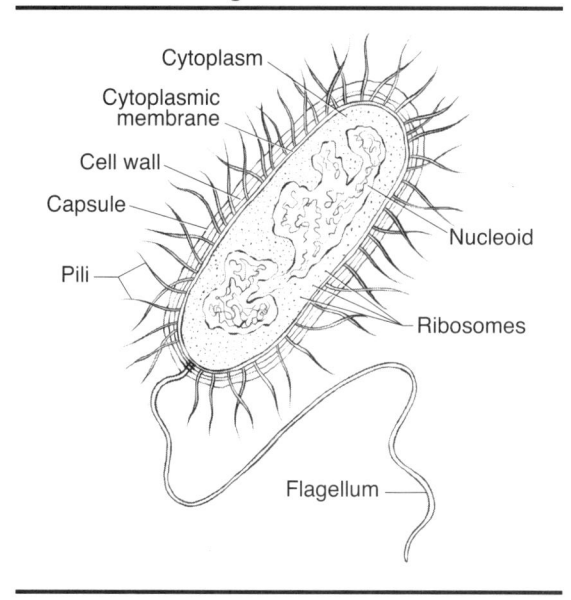

Movement

Some bacteria have the ability to move, usually by way of flagella or hairlike structures called pili. The characteristic whiplike movement of the flagellum is visible under a microscope. Many varieties of bacteria have flagella or pili, including proteus, salmonella, and pseudomonas (Figure 1-2). Flagella allow bacteria to reach areas of the body that nonmotile organisms cannot.

Growth

The size, color, and shape of a bacterial colony growing on a plate are distinguishing characteristics. The rate of growth (or bacterial cell multiplication) is determined in part by temperature, pH, moisture content, and available nutrients and is also important in determining the type of bacteria present. When bacteria are added to growth medium in a laboratory, a period of adaptation occurs before growth begins. This is known as lag time. Once growth begins, a bacterium divides at a doubling time characteristic of its strain. Changes in bacterial population over an extended period of time can be plotted on a graph and compared to known patterns.[1]

Atmospheric and Nutrient Requirements

The relationship between bacteria and oxygen provides both a classification mechanism and a tool for understanding a bacterium's pathogenicity. Organisms that must have oxygen to grow, such as *Mycobacterium tuberculosis*, are termed obligate aerobes. Those that cannot survive in oxygen, such as *Clostridium perfringens*, are referred to as obligate anaerobes. Most bacteria can grow with or without oxygen and are called facultative anaerobes. The temperature range within which bacteria can grow provides another clue as to their identity, as do optimal pH and pH ranges.

Nutritionally, all bacteria require certain basic elements: carbon, hydrogen, nitrogen, and a source of water. Some bacteria require special elements, such as copper, manganese, magnesium, or iron. A few organisms, such as *Treponema pallidum*, have such complex nutritional requirements that laboratory media capable of supporting their growth have not been developed.[3]

Biochemical and Metabolic Activities

All bacteria produce waste products and secretions as a result of metabolism. Products of bacterial metabolism include enzymes that enhance the organism's ability to invade its host and cause illness. These secretions can be used to identify some organisms, such as Staphylococcus and Streptococcus. In the laboratory, bacteria can be inoculated into certain substrates such as blood agar, carbohydrates, or amino acids to see if they possess the enzymes needed to break these substances down.

Pathogenicity

As part of their protective mechanisms, some bacteria are enclosed in capsules, which serve to protect them against the body's defenses. Others, such as those in the family Enterobacteriaceae, produce characteristic protective endotoxins. These endotoxins are powerful stimuli for the human body's immune response and are

FIGURE 1-3 ◆ Enveloped virus.

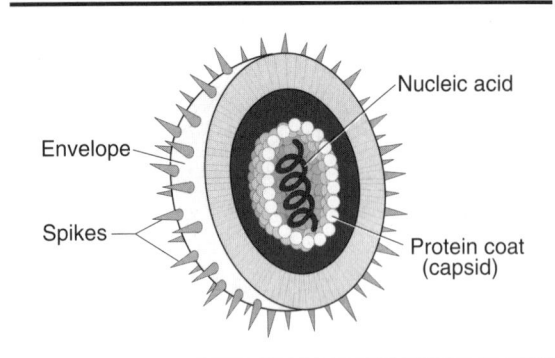

FIGURE 1-4 ◆ Virus with capsule.

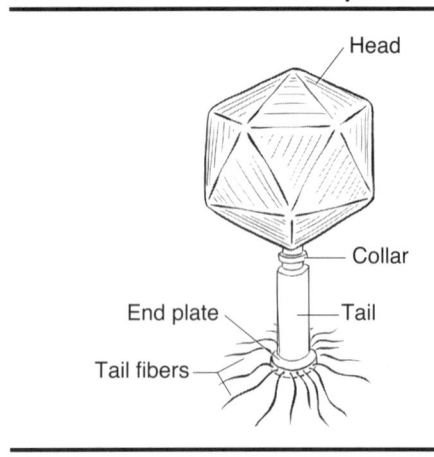

responsible for a number of toxic effects, such as hypotension, shock, and disseminated intravascular coagulation (DIC) seen in Gram-negative sepsis. Pathogenicity is further discussed in "Virulence Factors."

Protein Sequencing and Genetic Composition

By comparing the protein sequencing in bacteria, one can determine the relationship between bacterial species. The most accurate method of classifying bacteria is through analysis of DNA. DNA from two or more isolates can be compared to determine if the isolates are from the same genus or species. This is particularly useful in identifying epidemic outbreaks such as necrotizing enterocolitis. It is now possible to rapidly identify bacteria using DNA probes. This approach is particularly valuable for the identification of slow-growing or difficult-to-grow organisms.

VIRUSES

Viruses, ranging in size from 18 to 300 nm, are the smallest known infectious particles. They are classified as obligate intracellular parasites dependent on their host for survival. These particles lack the ability to produce their own energy or proteins.

Viruses consist of a nucleic acid molecule, either RNA or DNA, enclosed in either an envelope or a protein coat known as a capsid (Figures 1-3 and 1-4). The enclosure protects the nucleic acid and helps the virus attach to and penetrate the host cell. Removal or disruption of the envelope or capsid inactivates the virus.

The type of protein in the envelope or capsid determines the interaction of the virus with the host cell. The type of outer coat protecting the virus also determines some of its other characteristics, such as its mode of transmission. The capsid is a rigid protein structure resistant to drying, acids, and detergents. It is capable of surviving in the human gastrointestinal (GI) tract as well as in sewage. Viruses with capsids are often transmitted by the fecal-oral route, but may also be transmitted in dust particles, on contaminated objects (fomites), or hand to hand. Enveloped viruses have an outer membrane composed of lipids, proteins, and glycoproteins that is easily disrupted by drying, acid conditions, detergents, and solvents. This type of virus must remain wet and is usually transmitted in a fluid vector, such as blood, tissue, or respiratory secretions.

Viral taxonomy may describe physical characteristics, the geographic location where the virus was identified, the disease with which it is associated, or the part of the body in which it was first isolated. Viruses are grouped according to the following characteristics: type and form of nucleic acid, size, shape, substructure, and form of replication. Within groups, viruses are further divided into genera and species. The definitive work on naming and classifying viruses comes from the International Committee on the Taxonomy of Viruses (ICTV).[5] The ICTV has approved 73 families and groups of viruses, some of which are listed in Table 1-2.

Viral Replication

Viruses begin the process of replication by first recognizing and attaching to an appropriate host cell. The virus penetrates the cell and releases its genetic material into either the cytoplasm or the nucleus of that cell. The host cell replicates the virus's genetic material, assembles it into new viral particles, and releases them. In some cases, the host cell is killed in the process of viral replication; in other cases, it is not. Each infected cell produces as many as 100,000 new viral particles, but because of mutations and assembly errors, only 1–10 percent of these new particles are infectious.[3]

DNA versus RNA Viruses

Some significant differences exist between viruses containing DNA and those based on RNA. These dissimilarities play a role in the virulence of the virus as well as in its identification and treatment.

Unlike RNA, DNA is not transient; viral DNA remains in the host cell and is often associated with persistent or latent infections such as herpes zoster or shingles caused by varicella. Most RNA viruses replicate in the cell cytoplasm, whereas DNA viruses replicate in the cell nucleus. RNA viruses are more prone to mutation and assembly errors than are DNA viruses. Discussions of viral infections common to neonates are found in Chapters 3 and 5.

Laboratory Identification

Viral identification can be accomplished by a variety of means, depending on the structure and characteristics of the virus and its effects on the host cells. In many cases, viral material is difficult to culture under laboratory conditions, and other means of identification must be used. These can include observation of the cytopathologic effects of the virus on its host cell, such as

TABLE 1-2 ◆ Classification of Viruses

Family	Members
RNA Viruses	
Paramyxoviridae	Parainfluenza virus, Sendai virus, measles virus, mumps virus, respiratory syncytial virus
Orthomyxoviridae	Influenza virus types A, B, and C
Coronaviridae	Coronavirus
Arenaviridae	Lassa virus, Tacaribe virus complex (Junin and Machupo viruses), lymphocytic choriomeningitis virus
Rhabdoviridae	Rabies virus, vesicular stomatitis virus
Filoviridae	Ebola virus, Marburg virus
Bunyaviridae	California encephalitis virus, La Crosse virus, sandfly fever virus, hemorrhagic fever virus, Hantavirus
Retroviridae	Human T-cell leukemia virus types I and II, human immunodeficiency virus, animal oncoviruses
Reoviridae	Rotavirus, Colorado tick fever virus
Picornaviridae	Rhinoviruses, poliovirus, echoviruses, Coxsackie virus, encephalomyocarditis virus
Togaviridae	Rubella virus; western, eastern, and Venezuelan equine encephalitis virus; Ross River virus; Sindbis virus; Semliki Forest virus
DNA Viruses	
Poxviridae	Smallpox virus, vaccinia virus
Herpesviridae	Herpes simplex virus types 1 and 2, varicella zoster virus, Epstein-Barr virus, cytomegalovirus, human herpesviruses 6, 7, and 8
Adenoviridae	Adenovirus
Hepadnaviridae	Hepatitis B virus
Papovaviridae	JC virus, BK virus, SV40, papilloma virus
Parvoviridae	Parvovirus B19, adeno-associated virus

Adapted from: Murray PR, et al. 1998. *Medical Microbiology*, 3rd ed. St. Louis: Mosby-Year Book, 44–45. Reprinted by permission.

FIGURE 1-5 ♦ Budding yeast.

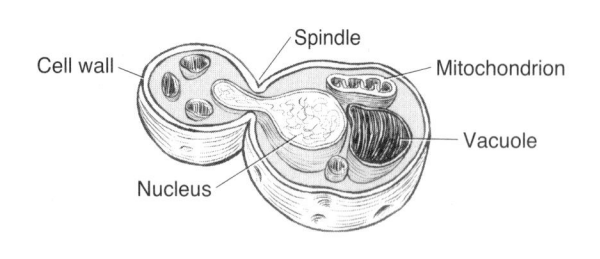

FIGURE 1-6 ♦ Cellular structure of fungi.

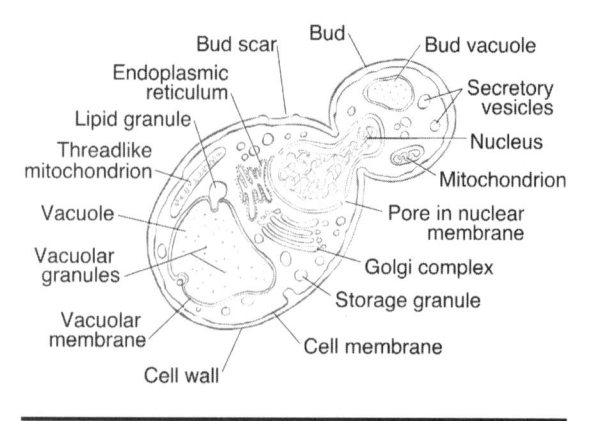

cell lysis or the presence of inclusion bodies; identification of viral particles with an electron microscope; identification of viral components such as proteins or nucleic acids; and evaluation of the neonate's serologic response to the virus (i.e., immunoglobulin—IgM or IgG). Cytologic examination of specimens yields information that can allow for rapid identification of certain viruses with characteristic cellular effects. For example, owl-eye or nuclear inclusion bodies can be found in the sediment of urine in infants with cytomegalovirus (CMV). Cells infected with herpes simplex virus may appear fused and contain Cowdry type A inclusions.

Electron microscopy is not routinely used to examine clinical specimens, but may be particularly useful in cases where an infection with an enteric virus is suspected. In other cases where viral growth is difficult, special techniques can be used to look for specific viral components. For example, cells infected with influenza or parainfluenza virus release proteins that cause agglutination of erythrocytes, a process known as hemagglutination. Detection of viral material is also accomplished through polymerase chain reaction (PCR) testing, which is becoming increasingly available. With this test, specific chemical primers can be used to amplify the presence of viral material in a specimen, making it easier to detect. Blot tests (Western, Northern, and Southern) are other specialized tests used to detect viral RNA or DNA.[3]

Viral serology is a commonly ordered test in the NICU. Because IgM does not cross the placenta, its presence in the neonate's blood signifies that he has been exposed to the virus being tested for. However, elevated levels of IgG may represent maternal infection and are less helpful.

FUNGI

Fungi are classified as eukaryotic organisms possessing a nucleus enclosed by a nuclear membrane. Fungi cannot independently synthesize energy and therefore live either on dead or decaying material (saprobes) or in coexistence with another organism (symbionts or commensals). Although thousands of species of fungi have been identified, fewer than 100 routinely cause disease in humans.[3]

Fungi also play a role in food spoilage, wood rot, and deterioration of cloth goods. As beneficial organisms, fungi break down organic matter in the soil and are used in the manufacture of products such as antibiotics, steroids, baked goods, and alcohol.

Fungi may be unicellular or multicellular and are grouped into three categories: mushrooms, yeasts, and molds. Yeasts, usually unicellular, are defined as cells that reproduce by budding (Figure 1-5). Molds are multicelled organisms with threadlike filaments termed hyphae.[6] Some fungi exist in both yeast and mold forms and are known as dimorphic. Histoplasma and blastomyces, both of which can cause

TABLE 1-3 ◆ Classification of Fungi

Classification	Sexual Characteristics	Medically Important Genera
Phylum Zygomycota	Sexual reproduction occurs through fusion of compatible gametangia to produce a zygote. Asexual reproduction is characterized by production of sporangiospores.	Agents causing zygomycosis
Phylum Dikaryomycota	Dikaryotic life cycle includes extended dikaryotic phase after sexual conjugation (i.e., haploid nuclei do not fuse immediately).	
Subphylum Ascomycotina	Sexual reproduction occurs through fusion of two compatible nuclei to form a diploid nucleus, followed by meiosis to yield haploid progeny. Entire process occurs within a sac called an ascus, and resulting spores are called ascospores.	Agents causing ringworm, histoplasmosis, and blastomycosis
Subphylum Basidiomycotina	Sexual reproduction takes place in a sac called a basidium, where two compatible nuclei fuse to form a diploid nucleus, followed by meiosis to yield haploid progeny. Haploid progeny are called basidiospores.	Agent causing cryptococcosis
Form-class Deuteromycotina	Sexual stage has not been observed in fungi classified in this category.	Candida, Trichosporon, Torulopsis, Pityrosporum, Epidermophyton, Coccidioides, and Paracoccidioides species

Adapted from: Murray PR, et al. 1998. *Medical Microbiology*, 3rd ed. St. Louis: Mosby-Year Book, 60. Reprinted by permission.

disease in pregnant women and their offspring, are examples of dimorphic fungi.

Fungi reproduce by budding, hyphal extension, or forming spores. Fungi are classified according to the type of sexual spore they produce or the structure on which they produce it.[1]

As do human cells, the cells of a fungus contain ribosomes, mitochondria, Golgi apparatus, and other structures (Figure 1-6). Fungal cells differ from human cells in their cell wall, however, which is rigid and multilayered. The inner layer of the cell wall, the plasmalemma, contains ergosterol rather than cholesterol. This difference forms the basis of most antifungal treatments.[3]

Fungi have adapted well to the hostile environment found in human tissues. Those that invade the hair and nails or that colonize the skin metabolize keratin as a source of nutrition. Other fungi have altered their preferred temperature range to survive at human body temperature rather than at the cooler temperatures in the environment.

The best known fungal infection in neonates is caused by the yeast *Candida albicans*, a commensal that usually grows harmlessly on the skin and mucous membranes in humans. The immature immune system common to neonates results in a state of immunosuppression that provides the opportunity for Candida to flourish and cause infection. Candida infections are discussed in Chapter 5.

Classification

Because fungi were originally classified with plants, the International Code of Botanical Nomenclature governs their nomenclature.[6] Table 1-3 illustrates the classification of some of

FIGURE 1-7 ◆ Structure of a paramecium.

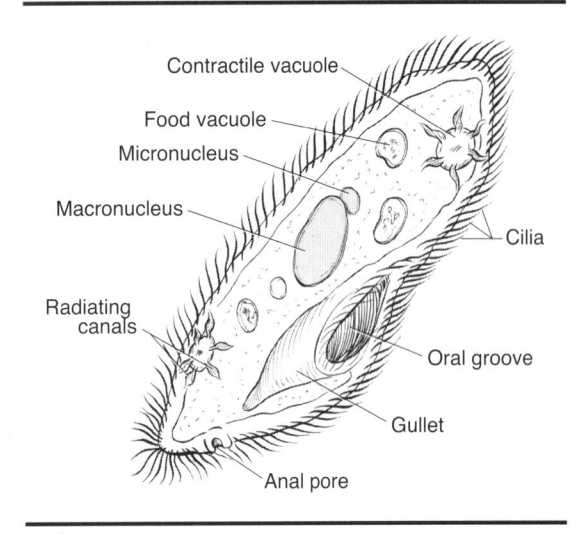

Labels: Contractile vacuole, Food vacuole, Micronucleus, Macronucleus, Radiating canals, Cilia, Oral groove, Gullet, Anal pore

the clinically significant members of the fungi family.

Laboratory Identification

The diagnosis of fungal infection is usually made by culturing the pathogen from tissues taken from the lesion or from the blood. Because some fungi such as Candida are part of the body's normal flora, recognition of a skin infection may be based on clinical characteristics rather than culture findings.

PROTOZOA

Classified as part of the group of human parasites, protozoa represent the most complex category of microbes. Protozoa are usually unicellular organisms that range in size from 2 to 2,000 µm.[1] Like fungi, protozoa have a membrane-enclosed nucleus and cytoplasm, which contains numerous organelles. Parasitic protozoa break down nutrients from their host. Some protozoa have mechanisms such as flagella or cilia that allow them to move (Figure 1-7). Many protozoa can develop cysts surrounded by thick cell walls that protect the organism from harsh environmental conditions. The cyst is often the mechanism by which the organism is transferred from host to host.

Classification

Protozoa are divided into seven phyla, four of which have medical significance to humans. Diseases caused by protozoa in older children and adults include malaria, giardiasis, and amebic dysentery. For neonates in North America, the protozoon of concern is *Toxoplasma gondii*, one of the Coccidia subclass. For more information on this protozoon, see the discussion in Chapter 3.

Laboratory Identification

Diagnosis of an acute Toxoplasmosis infection is through serial serologic testing, which demonstrates increasing antibody titers. Repeated titers are needed to distinguish active infections from previous asymptomatic or chronic infections.[3] The presence of cysts in body fluids or tissue represents a definitive diagnosis.

MICROBES AND THE HUMAN BODY

The human body is home to thousands of microorganisms, particularly bacteria. These usually exist in harmony with their human host, causing no ill effects and in fact providing many beneficial functions. These organisms are referred to as commensals, or normal flora. A pathogen is defined as an organism that can produce disease. Pathogens may exist in the human body without causing disease, a state referred to as colonization. Colonization may be transient or permanent. Someone who is colonized with an organism has no symptoms of disease, but may be able to transmit the organism to others. A few organisms are strict pathogens—that is, when they are present, they always cause disease.

Both commensals and pathogens are capable of producing infection, a state in which a microbe successfully multiplies within a host, causing damage to it. When commensals are introduced into areas of the body where they are not normally found, such as the bloodstream or tissue, or when the normal balance of commensal organisms is upset, such as occurs following a course of antibiotics, these organisms may become opportunistic pathogens, resulting in the development of an infection.[3]

Virulence Factors

The ability of an organism to invade the human body and cause damage is dependent in part on its virulence—that is, how well it is able to infect the host and protect itself from the body's defenses, as well as how severe the resulting disease is for the host. Several characteristics contribute to an organism's virulence or pathogenicity.

In bacteria, the presence of certain structural characteristics, enzymes, toxins, or other chemicals collectively known as virulence factors is responsible for the microorganism's ability to invade host cells and tissues, to adhere to cells, and to produce substances that damage or break down host tissue.

Structural Factors

Those bacteria with flagella or pili are better equipped to invade aqueous areas of the body because of their motility. In addition to facilitating movement, pili enable bacteria to anchor themselves to tissue, enhancing the organism's ability to cause infection. For example, pilated strains of *E. coli* are able to cause cystitis, whereas nonpilated strains are flushed away during urination. The pili of some strains of bacteria, such as *Streptococcus pyogenes*, contain a protein (M protein) that functions as an antiphagocytic, protecting the organisms from being destroyed by the body's phagocytes.[1]

Most pathogenic bacteria have an outer coating or capsule, which may consist of a slimy polysaccharide layer or contain proteins. The capsule protects the bacterium from phagocytosis (ingestion/digestion by other cells) and improves its ability to adhere to tissues. Several proteins found in bacterial capsules have been shown to have a specific role in helping bacteria penetrate host cells. These include M protein, internalin, and opacity-associated proteins (Opa).[4]

Enzymes

Several bacterial enzymes have also been shown to play a role in facilitating bacterial invasion of host cells. Coagulase is produced by organisms such as *Staphylococcus aureus* and causes formation of clots in plasma. The *S. aureus* bacteria then surround themselves with a fibrin coat to protect themselves from the body's defense systems. Kinases have the opposite effect, in that they dissolve clots and allow bacteria such as *S. pyogenes* and *S. aureus* to spread through the body tissues.

Several genera of bacteria, including Staphylococcus, Streptococcus, and Clostridium, produce hyaluronidase, which loosens the bond that holds tissue together and facilitates the spread of the bacteria. *C. perfringens*, the organism responsible for gas gangrene, is able to secrete collagenase, which, as the name suggests, breaks down the collagen found in tendons, cartilage, and bones, causing tissue destruction.[1]

Hemolysin is produced by members of the hemolytic Streptococcus family and is responsible for the breakdown of red blood cells that is characteristic of these organisms. Red blood cell breakdown releases iron needed by the bacteria for growth.

Toxins

Exotoxins, proteins secreted by many Gram-positive and Gram-negative organisms, are often named for the target organ they affect. Neurotoxins are responsible for the characteristic nerve destruction and spasmodic muscle contractions seen with botulism, diphtheria, and tetanus. Many enteric pathogens secrete enterotoxins, which affect the vomiting center of the brain and also cause diarrhea.[4] Leukocidin, which causes the destruction of white blood cells, is secreted by some species of Staphylococcus and Streptococcus.[1] Exfoliative toxins produced by *S. aureus* are responsible for the skin sloughing seen in scalded skin disease (see Chapter 4).

The cell walls of Gram-negative organisms contain lipopolysaccharide (LPS), an endotoxin.

TABLE 1-4 ♦ Common Commensal Organisms in the Human Body

Skin
- *Staphylococcus epidermidis*
- *Staphylococcus aureus* (in small numbers)
- Micrococcus species
- Nonpathogenic Neisseria species
- α-hemolytic and nonhemolytic streptococci
- Diphtheroids
- Propionibacterium species
- Small numbers of other organisms (e.g., Candida species, Acinetobacter species)

Nasopharynx
- Any amount of the following: diphtheroids, nonpathogenic Neisseria species, α-hemolytic streptococci, anaerobes (too many species to list; include varying amounts of Prevotella species, anaerobic cocci, diphtheroids, and Fusobacterium species)
- Lesser amounts of the following when accompanied by organisms just listed: yeasts, Haemophilus species, pneumococci, *S. aureus*, Gram-negative rods, *Neisseria meningitidis*

Gastrointestinal Tract and Rectum
- Various members of the Enterobacteriaceae family except Salmonella, Shigella, Yersinia, Vibrio, and Campylobacter species
- Nondextrose-fermenting Gram-negative rods
- Enterococci
- *S. epidermidis*
- α-hemolytic and nonhemolytic streptococci
- Diphtheroids
- *S. aureus* in small numbers
- Yeasts in small numbers
- Anaerobes in large numbers (too many species to list)

Genitalia
- Any amount of the following: Corynebacterium species, Lactobacillus species, α-hemolytic and nonhemolytic streptococci, nonpathogenic Neisseria species
- The following when mixed and not predominant: enterococci, members of the Enterobacteriaceae family and other Gram-negative rods, *S. epidermidis*, *Candida albicans* and other yeasts
- Anaerobes (too many to list); the following may be important when in pure growth or clearly predominant: Prevotella, Clostridium, and Peptostreptococcus species

From: Brooks GF, Butel JS, and Morse SA. 2001. *Jawetz, Melnick and Adelberg's Medical Microbiology*, 22nd ed. New York: McGraw-Hill, 178. Reprinted by permission.

Endotoxins—unique to Gram-negative organisms—are not actively secreted, but are often released upon cell death. LPS has been shown to cause fever, leukopenia, hypotension, and hypoglycemia in the host. In addition, LPS activates the clotting cascade as well as plasminogen, resulting in the development of DIC. LPS may activate the alternative pathway of the complement cascade (see Chapter 2), resulting in cell membrane damage and chemotactic responses.[4]

Colonization of the Human Body

The fetus exists, for the most part, in a sterile environment. Beginning with rupture of the amniotic membranes and subsequent passage through the birth canal, the neonate is immediately exposed to a multitude of organisms that colonize first the skin, followed by the oropharynx, and then the GI tract and other mucous membranes. In most neonates, these organisms proliferate without causing illness. Factors such as prematurity, low birth weight, trauma at delivery, prolonged rupture of membranes, maternal infection, and fetal hypoxia place the newborn at increased risk of developing an infection as a result of contact with microorganisms of the maternal genital tract.

Many kinds of microorganisms are generally in permanent residence on the human skin and mucous membranes. Table 1-4 outlines the most common human commensal organisms. They are usually found in certain anatomic locations and, if removed, soon re-establish residence.

There is also a transient population of microorganisms that seems to be just passing through the human host. These nonpathogenic or potentially pathogenic microorganisms come from the environment and temporarily inhabit the skin and mucous membranes, but do not generally produce disease. They may remain for hours to weeks, but they do not take up permanent residence. If the resident microorganisms are in normal balance, these transient microorganisms are of little concern because the resident floras prevent them from proliferating and causing infection. If the resident floras are diminished, however, these transient microorganisms may colonize, proliferate, and produce disease.

Temperature, moisture, and the presence of nutrients and inhibitory substances determine the resident flora population. These microorganisms do more than protect against invasion by other bacteria; they are also involved in some of the body's functions. For example, resident floras of the GI tract synthesize vitamin K, help convert bile pigments and bile acids, and facilitate the absorption of some nutrients. Under certain circumstances, the normal resident floras can become pathogenic. One such circumstance is traumatic injury, which could introduce a resident microorganism from the skin into a formerly sterile body cavity. Another such situation involves use of antibiotics, which may eliminate one type of normal flora and allow another to become overgrown and cause disease. Candida infection frequently occurs for this reason.

The types of organisms that take up residence in the neonate's body depend on the flora of the maternal vaginal tract and the types of organisms present in the environment. A premature or ill newborn will become colonized with a very different group of organisms than will a healthy newborn who spends only a short time in the hospital environment.

Neonates are exposed to noncommensal, or pathogenic, organisms in a variety of ways. The source of a pathogenic bacterium—known as a reservoir, or a site where a bacterium can survive until it is transferred to a host—depends on the organism. Some bacteria survive in noninfected humans (known as carriers), others, in animals, birds, insects, or inanimate objects. Transfer to, or between, human hosts may occur through direct contact with infected particles: The contact may be skin to skin or via mucous membranes (as in kissing or sexual contact). Infection can also occur through indirect contact, from inhalation of airborne droplets from respiratory secretions. Bacteria can also be acquired through ingestion of contaminated food or water. Finally, bacterial transmission can occur through contact with fomites (contaminated objects). These include respiratory equipment, bedding, articles of clothing, and hospital equipment that might be contaminated with blood, urine, stool, or respiratory secretions.[1]

Summary

The four types of microorganisms responsible for infection in neonates—bacteria, viruses, fungi, and protozoa—represent a diverse group with very different characteristics and tools for penetrating human hosts. Recognition of the differing patterns of disease caused by these organisms will aid the clinician both in recognizing illness in the neonate and in preventing exposure to potential pathogens.

Increasingly sophisticated mechanisms for identifying and characterizing microorganisms have resulted in an ever-changing classification system and an enhanced understanding of the role of these organisms in both health and disease. Further work remains in increasing our understanding of the mechanisms by which disease-causing microorganisms enter the body and evade detection and destruction. The development of new techniques for rapidly identifying organisms responsible for infection, coupled with expansion of mechanisms to prevent infection and to enhance the neonate's ability to fight infection, will be key.

REFERENCES

1. Burton GRW, and Engelkirk PG. 2000. *Microbiology for the Health Sciences*, 6th ed. Philadelphia: Lippincott Williams & Wilkins.
2. Holt JG, and Bergey DH. 1984. *Bergey's Manual of Systematic Bacteriology.* Philadelphia: Lippincott Williams & Wilkins.
3. Murray PR, et al. 1998. *Medical Microbiology*, 3rd ed. St Louis: Mosby-Year Book, 6–22.
4. Brooks GF, Butel JS, and Morse SA. 2001. *Jawetz, Melnick and Adelberg's Medical Microbiology*, 22nd ed. New York: McGraw-Hill.
5. Melnick JL. 1999. Taxonomy and classification of viruses. In *Manual of Clinical Microbiology*, 7th ed., Murray PR, et al., eds. Washington, DC: ASM Press, 835–842.
6. Dixon DM, Rhodes JC, and Fromtling RA. 1999. Taxonomy, classification, and morphology of the fungi. In *Manual of Clinical Microbiology*, 7th ed., Murray PR, et al., eds. Washington, DC: ASM Press, 1161–1166.

NOTES

Chapter 2

The Immune System

Terri Cavaliere, RNC, MS, NNP

The immune system plays a vital role in the detection, destruction, and elimination of material perceived as foreign to the body. Its components include hematopoietic cells, substances secreted by these cells, and other humoral factors produced by nonhematopoietic cells. These various elements, operating synergistically, give the immune system the capability of responding to a seemingly unlimited variety of substances that are alien to the self.[1] Immunologic responses serve three host functions: resistance against infection (defense), removal of incapacitated host cells (homeostasis), and perception and destruction of foreign or mutant cells (surveillance).[2]

Immunity, the characteristic of being resistant, develops as the result of the complementary work of two interdependent parts of the immune system, innate or nonspecific immunity and adaptive or specific immunity.[2] The responses of the two systems differ both in the degree of selectivity and in the timing of the response.[3] An individual achieves mature immunologic status through adaptive changes that are stimulated by exposure to a vast array of antigens.

During gestation, the fetus normally is isolated from encounters with pathogens. Neonates, therefore, have an immature host defense system in that it lacks prior experience with antigens. They are thus especially susceptible to infection and disruption of homeostasis.[2] This chapter reviews the development of the immune system and how it functions to protect the neonate from infection. Comparisons are drawn between the immune defense mechanisms of the neonate and the adult to highlight differences in the former.

The Immune Response

The immune response is comprised of two functional phases: recognition and reaction. Initially, substances are recognized as being foreign, or nonself. This is accomplished through either nonspecific (innate) mechanisms based on differences such as a pathogen's surface charge or specific antibody/antigen interactions (acquired or adaptive immunity). Cells and humoral (soluble) mediators are then mobilized to react to and eliminate or neutralize nonself substances. These are listed in Table 2-1.[1,4]

Innate (Nonspecific) Immunity

Innate immunity involves host defense mechanisms that are nonspecific to a particular

TABLE 2-1 ◆ Categories of Immune Response[1,4,11]

Category	Provided By
Innate	
Anatomic barriers	Skin
	Mucous membranes
Physiologic barriers	Temperature
	pH
	Oxygen tension
	Soluble factors
	Lysozyme
	Interferon
	Kinins
	Histamine
Inflammatory barriers	Platelets
	Basophils
	Eosinophils
	Mast cells
Phagocytes	Neutrophils (PMNs)
	Monocytes/macrophages
Complement	Serum proteins
Adaptive	
Cell-mediated factors	T lymphocytes
	Helper cells
	Cytotoxic cells
	Suppressor cells
Humoral factors	B lymphocytes
	IgG
	IgD
	IgM
	IgE
	IgA

microorganism. This type of immunity is the host's primary line of defense against pathogenic invasion, becoming active immediately upon exposure to a foreign agent. Innate immunity includes anatomic and physiologic barriers, the inflammatory response, phagocytic cells, and complement. Innate mechanisms make use of generic recognition mechanisms that allow interaction with components of the invading pathogen. These function well during the first encounter with an invading organism. The infant's immune system does not require prior exposure to a foreign substance to recognize it as such.

Anatomic and Physiologic Barriers

Anatomic barriers, skin and mucous membranes, are the body's first defense against the entry of pathogens. Physiologic barriers, such as temperature, pH, oxygen tension, and various soluble factors (such as lysozyme and interferon), act to destroy or neutralize microorganisms that penetrate the anatomic barriers. For example, the low pH of the skin, low oxygen tension, and both normal body temperature and fever serve to inhibit the growth of certain bacteria. Chemical mediators, such as lysozyme, interferon, and complement, destroy or inactivate organisms and facilitate phagocytosis.

Inflammatory Response

Tissue injury secondary to a wound or entry of a pathogenic organism initiates a complex sequence of events. Activation of nonspecific immunity may involve the inflammatory response during which basophils, eosinophils, and mast cells are activated to respond to foreign pathogens or to tissue damage. Chemical mediators are involved in the inflammatory process. These substances are derived from (1) the invading pathogens themselves, (2) damaged host cells responding to tissue injury (acute-phase proteins), (3) plasma enzyme systems (kinins, coagulation factors), and (4) white blood cells (WBCs) (histamine). To concentrate cells of the immune system at the site of infection, vasoactive substances released in response to pathogen invasion increase blood supply to the area while vasoconstriction decreases venous drainage away from the area, creating engorgement of the capillary network. Inflammatory mediators diffuse to the vessel walls, causing phagocytes to adhere to the endothelium. Capillary permeability is increased, causing cellular and soluble mediators of immunity to move into the surrounding tissues.[1,5]

Phagocytic Cells

Phagocytic WBCs initially migrate to the site of infection, or damage, where they engulf and break down foreign particles and tissue debris. Polymorphonuclear leukocytes (PMNs) are the most prevalent phagocytic cell in the early stages of the inflammatory process; they

FIGURE 2-1 ◆ Summary of events in the inflammatory process.

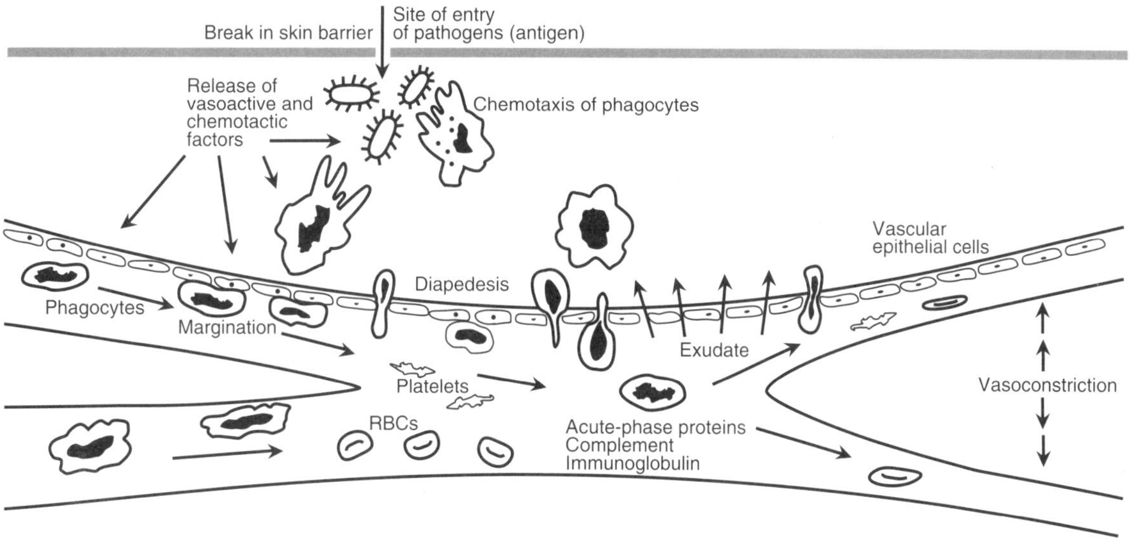

are joined later by macrophages, monocytes, and lymphocytes. Phagocytic cells recognize foreign and abnormal cells because of surface abnormalities such as roughness occurring due to injury, because of the presence of molecules commonly found on the surface of foreign cells, or because foreign cells are deliberately marked for phagocytosis by chemical mediators from the immune system known as opsonins.

Phagocytes adhere to the endothelial walls (margination); squeeze between the capillary endothelial cells (diapedesis); and, under the influence of chemoattractants, move in a directed fashion to the site of the inflammatory process (chemotaxis).[1] Once stimulated, phagocytes also release chemical mediators, which further induce a range of immune activities. Figure 2-1 summarizes the steps in the inflammatory process.

Complement

The complement system is comprised of inactive serum proteins that serve to augment the immune response.[1,2,6,7] Activation of complement pathways by infectious agents results in destruction of foreign cells and also causes the release of inflammatory mediators.[1,5]

Adaptive (Specific) Immunity

Adaptive immunity relies on specific immune responses targeted against recognized foreign material and involves the cell-mediated and humoral systems. These elements are critical to adaptive immune responses because they provide for recognition of individual pathogens. Specific immune mechanisms display the attributes of specificity, memory, and diversity.[1,4]

Specificity

Specificity is based on the recognition and binding of specific antibodies with unique antigens. Although antibodies have certain generic properties, heterogenicity or variation in these serum proteins enables them to respond to very specific amino acid sequences in foreign proteins. Essentially, for every protein or antigen that is recognized as nonself, there is a unique antibody that binds to it. During the initial exposure of antibody to antigen, specific B cells that produce these antibodies are stimulated to produce more of themselves. This accounts for the ability of the acquired immune system to "remember" previous exposures to antigens.[5]

TABLE 2-2 ◆ Immune System Development Timetable[2,9,11,13]

Gestational Age (weeks)	Developmental Milestone	Location
3	First blood cells appear	Yolk sac
4–5	Synthesis of complement occurs	Liver
5	Liver becomes principal site of hematopoiesis	
5	Immunocompetent cells detected	Liver
6	Progenitor cells committed to granulocyte/monocyte lineage appear	Liver
7	Undifferentiated cells enter the thymus	
8	T lymphocytes appear	Blood/thymus
8–9	B lymphocytes with surface IgM appear	Liver
10–12	T lymphocytes with markers of mature lymphocytes appear	Thymus
12	B lymphocytes with other Ig classes appear	Liver
12–13	Antigen recognition and graft-vs-host reactivity begin	
14	Mature PMNs detectable	Liver/bone marrow
15	Mature PMNs detectable	Blood
20	Bone marrow becomes principal hematopoietic site	

Memory

Memory allows for rapid recognition and isolation of specific pathogens. On the first exposure to a particular antigen, there is a lag time during which the specific immune response is mounted. B cells producing antigen-specific antibodies are essentially "cloned" or replicated after the first exposure; during subsequent antigen exposures, they respond more rapidly and produce much higher antibody titers. This is how long-term immunity to many infectious diseases is achieved.[5]

Diversity

Diversity is the attribute that allows the immune system to identify multitudes of disparate antigenic structures on foreign substances. Diversity also refers to the wide variety of antibodies the body manufactures, allowing it to respond to millions of different antigens.

Collaborative Mechanisms

Innate and adaptive (nonspecific and specific) immune mechanisms are interdependent, working in collaboration to eliminate foreign antigens.[1-4] Monocytes/macrophages participate in the inflammatory process (innate) and also play a significant role in antigen presentation; essentially, macrophages and other cells bind nonspecifically to nonself molecules, permitting them to be recognized by antibodies. Furthermore, the serum complement proteins are utilized as part of both innate and acquired systems, and biologically active molecules called cytokines are produced by cells that also play a role in both types of immunity.[1,2] For example, after nonspecific stimulation caused by a foreign pathogen, macrophages can secrete cytokines, which in turn can control and direct adaptive immune responses.[1] Conversely, T lymphocytes, when presented with a specific antigen, produce other cytokines that enhance the bactericidal ability of macrophages.[1]

DEVELOPMENT OF THE IMMUNE SYSTEM

The cellular components of the immune system develop from hematopoietic stem cells (HSCs) that are first detected in the blood islands in the yolk sac of the fetus during the third week of gestation. During embryogenesis, the site of hematopoiesis moves from the yolk sac to the liver at about the fifth week of gestation, and the liver remains the primary site

FIGURE 2-2 ♦ Genesis of blood cells.

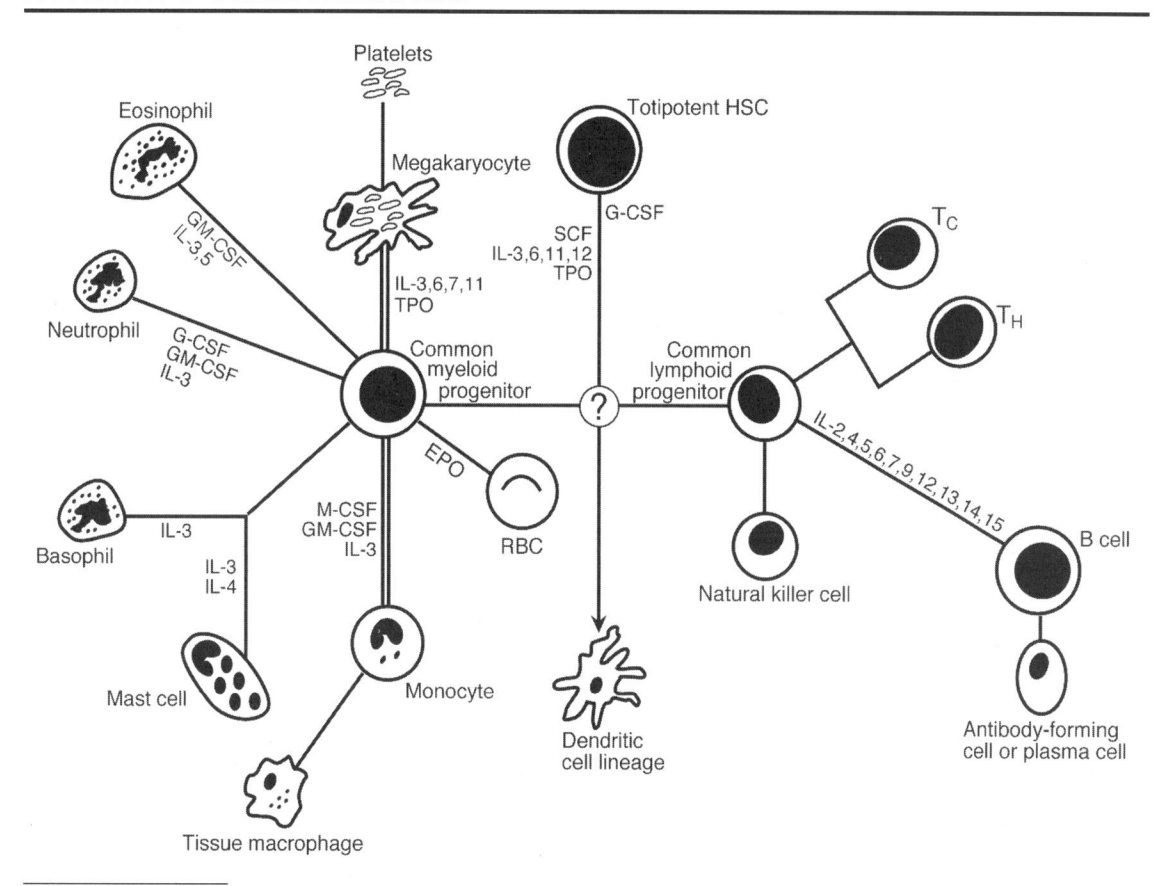

All cells arise from the totipotent hematopoietic stem cell (HSC). HSC is stimulated by growth factors to enter the myeloid or the lymphoid pathway. Growth factors involved in proliferation of various cell lineages are indicated.

Key: GM-CSF = granlulocyte-monocyte colony-stimulating factor, G-CSF = granulocyte colony-stimulating factor, M-CSF = monocyte colony-stimulating factor, IL = interleukin, EPO = erythropoietin, TPO = thrombopoietin, SCF = stem cell factor, T_C = cytoxic T cell, T_H = helper T cell.

between the fifth and twentieth weeks. The spleen also produces erythrocytes and participates in the development and activation of lymphocytes and monocytes during this period. This process ceases by the end of the second trimester, and in the neonate, the spleen does not produce blood cells. By the sixteenth week of gestation, stem cells have "seeded" the thymus, lymph nodes, and bone marrow. Differentiation and activation of immature WBCs take place in the thymus and the lymph nodes. After the twentieth week of intrauterine life, the bone marrow becomes the permanent major site of hematopoiesis.[8–11] Table 2-2 summarizes the timetable of hematopoiesis, highlighting white blood cell development.

Figure 2-2 depicts the genesis and evolution of blood cells. Pluripotent HSCs remain dormant until stimulated by various growth and differentiation factors to enter one of two developmental pathways, giving rise to either a myeloid progenitor (stem) cell or a lymphoid progenitor (stem) cell.[5–7] This next generation of cells is referred to as "primitive," based on the ability to produce cells of several hematopoietic lineages. These primitive progenitor cells are

TABLE 2-3 ◆ Components of the Immune System[3-5,7]

Cellular Mediators	Soluble Mediators
Lymphocytes	
B cells	Antibodies
T cells	Cytokines
Natural killer cells	
Phagocytes	
Monocytes/macrophages	Cytokines, complement, hydrolytic enzymes
Neutrophils	Histamine, lactoferrin, kinins
Eosinophils	
Auxiliary cells	
Basophils	
Mast cells	
Platelets	
Other	
Tissue cells	Cytokines, fibronectin
Dendritic cells	
	Complement

different from HSCs because they are committed to a particular cell lineage and they have a limited capacity for self-renewal.[8]

Myeloid stem cells give rise to erythrocytes, platelets, PMNs, monocytes, eosinophils, mast cells, and basophils. Specialized antigen-presenting cells, such as dendritic cells and Langerhans' cells, also develop from the myeloid lineage. Lymphoid stem cells develop into T cells and B cells.[1,5,6,8,9]

The progression of hematopoiesis is regulated by certain hematopoietic growth factors. Some of these allow the HSCs to remain in a quiescent state. Others trigger progenitor cells to proliferate and commit to a specific differentiation pathway. Still others inhibit hematopoiesis.[1,8] Figure 2-2 also shows the actions of these growth factors.

COMPONENTS OF THE IMMUNE SYSTEM

Components of the immune processes may be categorized as cellular mediators or humoral mediators. Table 2-3 lists the principal cellular and soluble elements of the immune system.

Cellular Components
Granulocytes

Granulocytes may be neutrophils, eosinophils, or basophils. They are identified according to their cellular morphology and cytoplasmic staining characteristics.[1] These cells constitute 50–70 percent of circulating leukocytes.[4] The life span of granulocytes is considerably shorter than that of monocytes, two to three days, compared with months or years.[7] Granulocytes do not display innate specificity for antigens; their role is in the inflammatory response—most specifically, phagocytosis.

Neutrophils. Ninety-five percent of circulating granulocytes are polymorphonuclear leukocytes (PMNs, also called neutrophils).[7] These neutrophils are the most potent killing phagocytes.[11] Precursors of PMNs are initially seen in the yolk sac of the fetus. Mature cells can be detected in the liver and bone marrow at approximately 14 weeks gestation. The concentration of circulating PMNs increases slowly over the next several weeks; by 22–23 weeks gestation, circulating PMNs represent only about 2 percent of the concentration that will be found in the cord blood of term neonates.[11] Neutrophils are produced in the bone marrow from the common progenitor granulocyte-monocyte colony-forming unit, which subsequently gives rise to myeloblasts, promyelocytes, myelocytes, metamyelocytes, bands, and segmented neutrophils. The functional activity of the various developmental stages of PMNs is difficult to assess. However, it appears that full functional potential is displayed only when the cells are mature.[7] After maturing in the bone marrow, PMNs are released into the vascular compartment.

FIGURE 2-3 ◆ Summary of PMN functions.

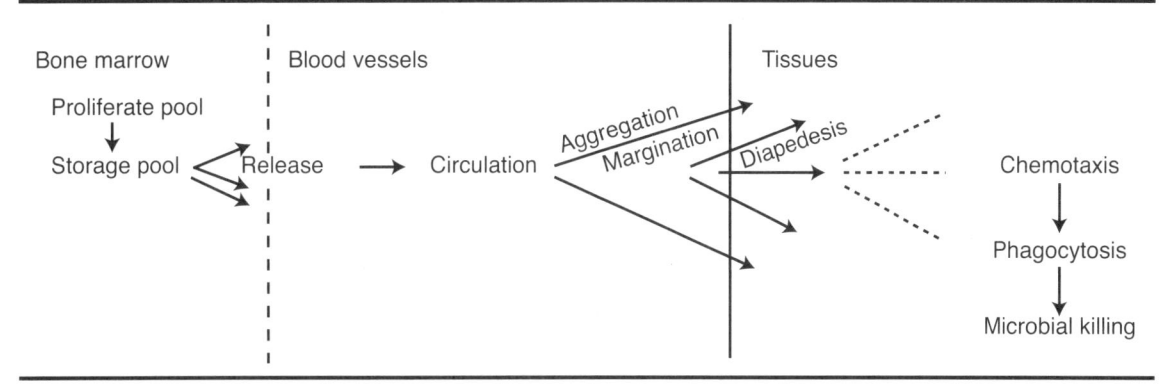

Production and release of PMNs are regulated by cytokines. Under normal conditions, only mature neutrophils and a limited number of bands are released into the circulation. During times of stress, however, the bone marrow can release additional stores of PMNs, and it can increase production. The appearance of a high percentage of bands and/or other immature neutrophils in the circulation indicates the inability of the bone marrow to keep pace with the demand for mature PMNs.[11,12]

PMNs inhabit several body compartments, including the bone marrow proliferative and storage pools, the intravascular circulating and marginated pools, and the tissue pool. Approximately half of the neutrophils in the blood adhere to the vascular epithelium, constituting the marginated pool. Conditions associated with stress, such as infection or epinephrine release, cause demargination of the neutrophils that are adhered to the blood vessel walls, releasing them into the circulating pool. Neutrophilia is common following stressful events such as delivery or circumcision. PMNs remain in circulation for approximately eight hours; tissue neutrophils may survive for an additional two to three days.[11,12]

A series of coordinated steps is involved in the movement of PMNs from the bloodstream to the site of microbial invasion. These steps include adherence (margination), diapedesis, chemotaxis, phagocytosis, and microbial killing (Figure 2-3). Complement, interleukin-8, and platelet-activating factor, molecules that strongly attract PMNs, are responsible for their migration toward sites of injury.[12]

Once at the site of infection, PMNs engulf microorganisms. They accomplish this via receptors that recognize various regions on the antigen. However, PMNs cannot recognize many antigens, including encapsulated bacteria, until those antigens have been opsonized by complement or immunoglobulin (Ig). After phagocytosis, organisms are killed by one of two types of mechanisms: oxygen independent or oxygen dependent. Oxygen-independent mechanisms rely on the action of toxic enzymes, such as lysozyme, proteases, lactoferrin, and defensins, contained within the PMNs. In oxygen-dependent mechanisms, PMNs are activated by cytokines and bacterial cell wall components to undergo a burst of oxygen consumption, producing highly reactive, antibacterial, oxygen free radicals and peroxides. This respiratory burst produces substances that are toxic to ingested bacteria.[11,12]

The PMN storage pools in the bone marrow are much smaller per unit of body weight in neonates than in adults. The basal proliferative rate of progenitor cells is at its maximum level and cannot be increased in times of stress.[2,12] During infection, neonatal PMN stores are rapidly depleted. Neutropenia frequently develops as a result of consumption of

FIGURE 2-4 ♦ Some surface markers of human lymphocytes.

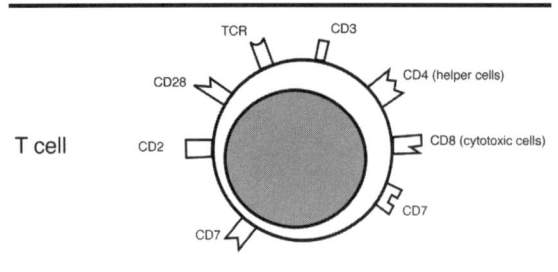

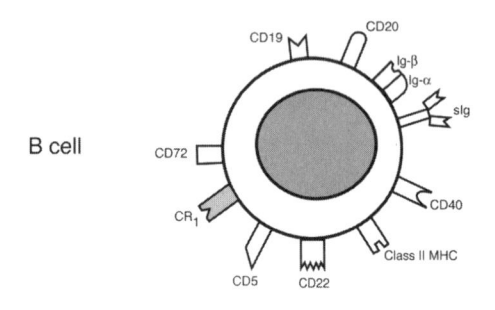

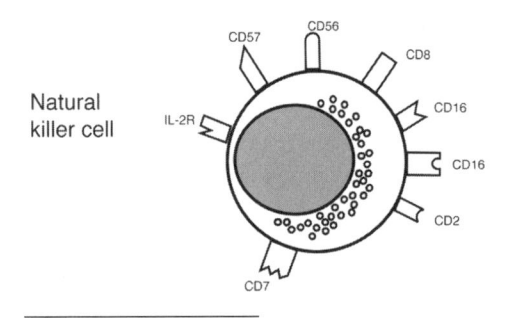

Key: TCR = T-cell antigen receptor, CD = cluster designation, CR_1 = complement receptor for C3b, MHC = major histocompatibility complex, sIg = surface immunoglobulin receptor, IL-2R = IL-2 receptor, Igα and Igβ = α and β chains of immunoglobulin.

these stores and also because of the newborn's limited ability to increase the proliferative rate.[2,12]

Neonatal PMNs also display functional deficiencies. It has been demonstrated that neutrophils from newborns have diminished chemotactic and adhesion capabilities, which are further decreased during infection. Chemotaxis does not appear to attain adult levels until adolescence.[2,13]

The ability of PMNs from healthy newborns to phagocytose and kill pathogens equals that of adults. However, under conditions of stress, as seen in infection and respiratory distress syndrome (RDS), neonatal neutrophils do not display normal phagocytic and microbicidal properties.[2,11,12] There are marked defects in oxygen-dependent killing of organisms such as Group B streptococci and *E. coli* that become clinically significant in stressed neonates.[11] The functional deficiencies of neonatal PMNs contribute significantly to compromised host defense mechanisms and are even more prominent in premature neonates.[2]

Eosinophils. Eosinophils comprise 2–5 percent of circulating leukocytes in healthy adults. They are capable of phagocytosis and destruction of ingested microorganisms, but these are not their principal functions. In response to certain stimuli, eosinophils release cytoplasmic granules, resulting in damage to microbial targets. Eosinophils play a major role in defense against parasites and are also involved in hypersensitivity reactions, including allergy and anaphylaxis.[1,7]

Basophils and mast cells. Circulating basophils exist in small numbers, less than 0.2 percent of leukocytes. Mast cells are found in a variety of tissues, such as skin; connective tissue; and the mucosa of the respiratory, genitourinary, and gastrointestinal tracts. These cells are not phagocytic granulocytes; their primary role is in hypersensitivity reactions. Their granules contain pharmacologically active substances, such as histamine, that mediate the allergic response.[1,7]

Agranulocytes

Agranulocytes, so named because they lack the characteristic granules found in granulocytes, include lymphocytes and monocytes. Both have single, large, nonsegmented nuclei, but are derived from different progenitor cell lines.[8]

INFECTION IN THE NEONATE

Lymphocytes. Lymphocytes initiate the specific immune response. They constitute approximately 20 percent of the leukocyte population in adults. Mature lymphocytes may have long lives and may survive as memory cells for many years.[1,7] There are three types of lymphocytes: T cells, B cells, and natural killer (NK) cells. Cell-mediated immunity is effected by T cells, and the synthesis and secretion of humoral immune factors is initiated by B cells.

Postnatally, all lymphoid cells arise from bone marrow stem cells; they subsequently mature and differentiate in different sites. The thymus is the induction center for T lymphocytes. B lymphocytes evolve from precursor cells in the fetal liver or, postnatally, in the bone marrow. The thymus and bone marrow are the central (or primary) lymphoid organs in which populations of T and B cells acquire the ability to recognize antigens through the development of specific surface receptors.[6,7] The third population of lymphocytes, called natural killer cells, is far less numerous than the other groups of lymphocytes. NK cells are also derived from lymphoid progenitors in the bone marrow, and they have the morphology of large granular lymphocytes. Lymphocytes, as well as other white blood cells, express large numbers of surface molecules, which identify different cell subsets. A nomenclature system has been designed in which differentiation numbers (cluster designations: CD4, CD8) are used to describe specific surface receptors recognized by several different monoclonal antibodies. In addition to these characteristic cluster designation markers, lymphocytes display other unique components on their cell membranes. For instance, B cells are

FIGURE 2-5 ◆ Clonal selection in B lymphocytes.

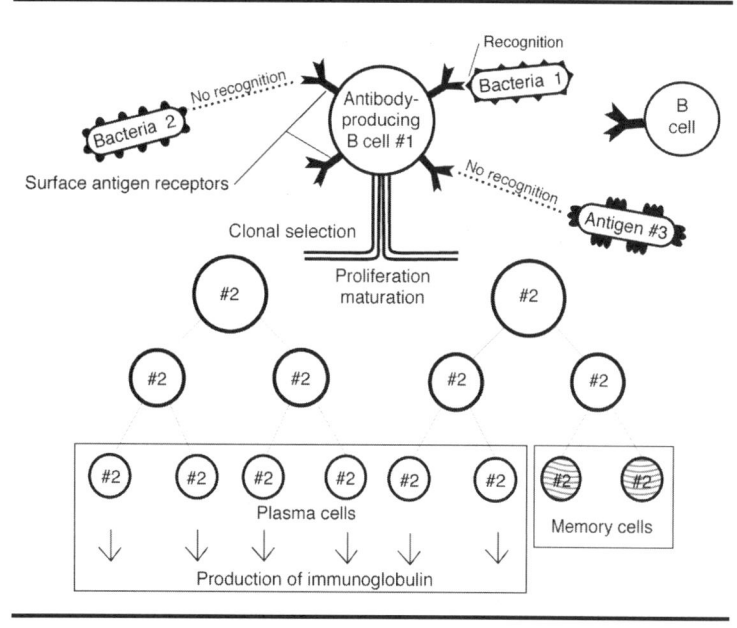

B cell recognizes specific antigen, which will bind to specific surface antigen receptor. B cell is stimulated to proliferate and mature into plasma cells, which produce antibody (immunoglobulin) and memory cells. Memory cells have the same antigen specificity as the original B cell.

defined by the presence of surface immunoglobulins and specific glycoproteins, whereas T cells exhibit the T-cell antigen receptor (TCR).[1,6,7] Figure 2-4 depicts receptors on human lymphocytes.

Each individual T and B lymphocyte is genetically programmed to respond to only one specific antigen, but the immune system in its entirety is able to recognize thousands of antigens. The system develops a large antigen-recognition repertoire over time as the body is exposed to countless numbers of antigens.[1] After an antigen binds to the cells that are able to identify it, these cells are stimulated to multiply quickly. In a few days, a sufficient number of cells has been generated to produce a competent immune response. Thus, the antigen promotes the generation of specific clones of its own antigen-binding cells. This process is called clonal selection and is similar for both T and B

FIGURE 2-6 ◆ Serum immunoglobulin levels (IgG, IgM, IgA) in the fetus and the infant in year 1.

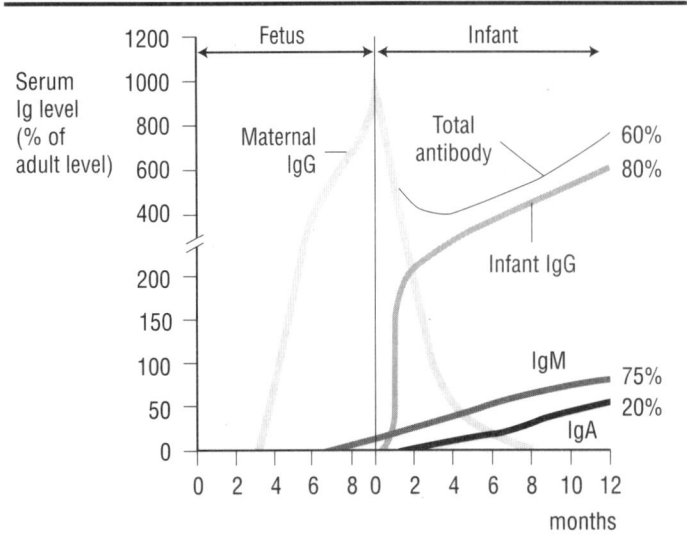

Fetal IgG is maternal in origin. Significant production of antibodies does not occur until after birth. Total serum antibody level in the infant at the end of the first year of life is 60 percent of the adult level.

Adapted from: Turner M. 2001. Antibodies. In *Immunology*, 6th ed., Roitt I, Brostoff J, and Male D, eds. St. Louis: Mosby-Year Book, 75. Reprinted by permission.

lymphocytes.[1,7] Figure 2-5 illustrates clonal selection in B lymphocytes.

B lymphocytes. The development of B lymphocytes takes place in two stages. Undifferentiated HSCs first mature into cells that can be identified as B cells in the fetal liver; this stage occurs without the presence of antigen. Pre–B cells with surface IgM markers are first identified in the fetal liver at 7–8 weeks gestation. These cells develop into immature IgM+ B cells possessing complement receptors and are detected at 8–9 weeks gestation in the liver. B cells exhibiting other surface immunoglobulins are detected by the twelfth week. Beyond 15 weeks gestation, a fetus has circulating B cell levels equivalent to or greater than an adult. The greatest numbers of B lymphocytes are found in the spleen, lymph nodes, and bloodstream of the fetus.[11] Although the fetus acquires the ability to produce immunoglobulin early in gestation, little antibody is normally synthesized *in utero*. The majority of circulating immunoglobulin (IgG) in a term neonate is of maternal origin.

When B lymphocytes recognize a specific antigen, they are stimulated to divide, proliferate, and differentiate into plasma cells. Plasma cells then generate receptor molecules in soluble form (antibodies), which can be secreted in large amounts into the circulation. Because antibodies are almost identical to the original receptor molecule, they are able to bind to the antigen that originally stimulated the B lymphocyte. Some of the newly produced B cells remain after the antigen is killed or neutralized. These memory cells are available for antibody production should the antigen be detected again.[4] Memory cells confer lasting immunity to a specific antigen.

Differences in neonates. Most of the circulating immunoglobulin found in the newborn is of maternal origin; placental transfer, which is limited to IgG isotypes, begins at about 17 weeks gestation. A fetus of 33–34 weeks gestational age has IgG levels approximating those of the mother; and at term, newborn IgG levels are 5–10 percent higher than those of the mother.[14] Premature neonates have lower IgG concentrations than do term infants; very preterm infants may have received little immunoglobulin before delivery. Small-for-gestational-age babies have less passively acquired IgG than their average-for-gestational-age counterparts at any given gestational age. IgG has a half-life of approximately 21 days.[11] Most maternally derived IgG is rapidly catabolized; loss is accelerated in ill infants who require phlebotomy.[11,12] Figure 2-6 displays serum immunoglobulin levels in the fetus and in the infant to one year of age.

FIGURE 2-7 ◆ Presentation of antigen to T lymphocyte.

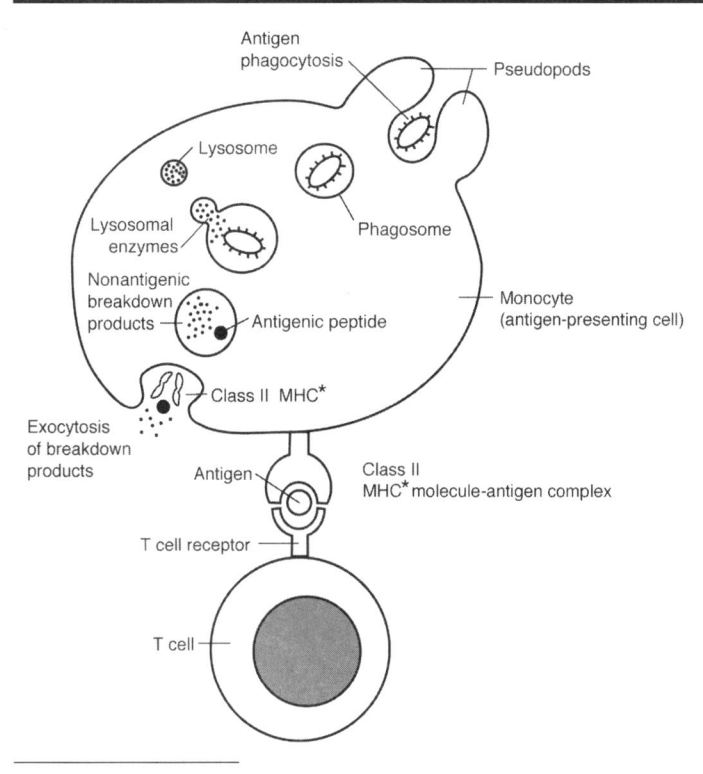

* MHC = major histocompatibility complex.

Antibody production in neonates (both term and preterm) is different from that of older children and adults. Neonatal B lymphocytes preferentially synthesize IgM and IgD, but they do not switch efficiently to production of IgG and IgE. An adult pattern of B-cell differentiation develops during the first year of life. The response of B lymphocytes to certain types of antigen is qualitatively different in newborns as well, apparently in part because of enhanced T-cell suppressor activity. Neonates do not react to certain antigens (bacterial polysaccharides), and their ability to develop immunologic memory is limited.[2,11–13]

T lymphocytes. Early T lymphocytes are produced in the yolk sac and the fetal liver. Undifferentiated cells, lacking the markers of mature T cells, enter the thymus at approximately 7 weeks gestation.[11] T lymphocytes first appear in the blood and among thymic epithelial cells at about the eighth to ninth weeks of gestation.[1,2] Cells bearing specific markers are identified at various times throughout gestation: $CD4^+$ and $CD8^+$ cells in the tenth week, $CD3^+$ in the twelfth week.[11] Antigen recognition and graft-versus-host reactivity are demonstrated by fetal lymphocytes from as early as 12 and 13 weeks gestation, respectively. After 20 weeks gestation, thymocyte precursor cells are derived from the bone marrow and enter the thymus for differentiation and maturation.[2,9] The *percentage* of T lymphocytes in cord blood is lower than that in the peripheral circulation of adults (46 percent versus 72 percent), but the *absolute number* of T cells is equivalent to or may exceed that of the adult because of the higher number of circulating WBCs in the neonate.[11]

T lymphocytes are vital to the development of cell-mediated immune responses. There are several classes of T cells, each with a different role. The first class interacts with B cells, prompting them to multiply, differentiate, and secrete antibody. The second group interacts with monocytes, helping them to destroy intracellular pathogens. Together these two types are called T helper (T_H) cells. These cells express the CD4 marker and primarily help or induce immune responses. Another class of T lymphocytes is able to destroy host cells that have been infected with viruses or other intracellular pathogens. These are referred to as T cytotoxic (T_C) cells. This subset exhibits the CD8 surface marker.[4,6] Activated T lymphocytes secrete cytokines that amplify the host's immune defense system.

FIGURE 2-8 ◆ Summary of the functions of T and B lymphocytes.

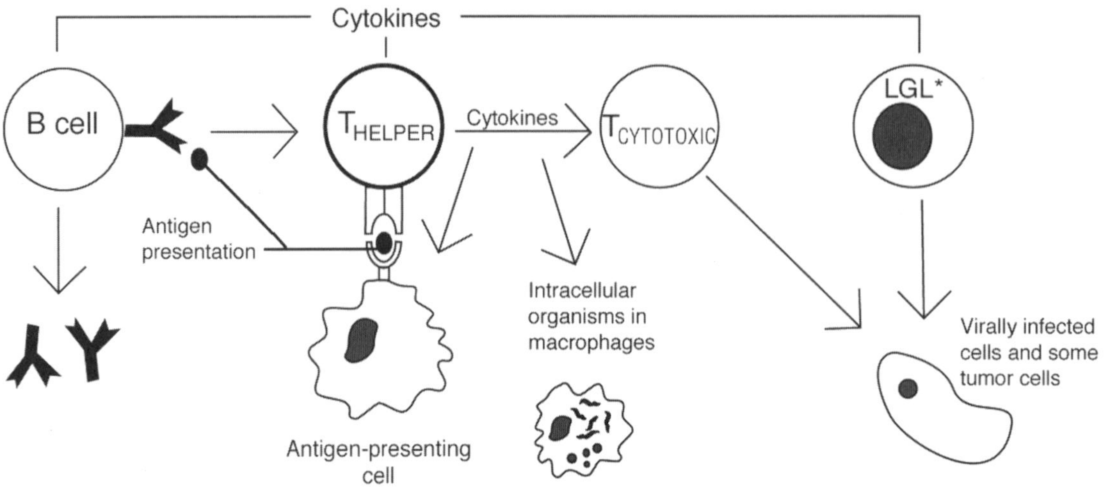

Unlike B cells, T cells are not able to detect free, intact antigen.[15] Using their antigen receptors, T lymphocytes react to antigen fragments that have been processed, bound, and displayed on the surface of antigen-presenting cells (APCs). The T cell receptor (TCR) is related, structurally and functionally, to the surface antibody used by B lymphocytes as their antigen receptor. Figure 2-7 illustrates antigen presentation to a T cell.

The immune response is important in protecting the body from microbial invasion, but the process must be "turned off" after the pathogens are eliminated. If the process is left unchecked, inflammation and the cellular elements it produces can trigger the elaboration of cellular and humoral mediators and vasoactive substances that contribute to the septic shock syndrome. Suppressor cells are T cells that dampen, or terminate, the immune responses of other T and B cells.[7] There is functional evidence for the existence of antigen-specific suppressor T lymphocytes (T_S), but it is not likely that there is a separate T-cell subset that performs this operation. Evidence shows that both CD4+ and CD8+ cells have the ability to suppress immune responses. Suppression may occur via the direct cytotoxicity of the antigen-presenting cells, through suppressive cytokines, or by other mechanisms.[1,7] Figure 2-8 summarizes the functions of T cells and B cells.

Differences in neonates. T cells manifest immunocompetence early in gestation, but their functional capabilities at birth are not always equivalent to those of adult T cells. Several clinical observations support the thesis that neonatal T-cell function is decreased: Infants are predisposed to serious infection with certain viruses (herpes simplex, enterovirus, rubella); delayed hypersensitivity reactions are attenuated; and the acquisition of antigen-specific antibody following infection is delayed.[12,16]

The function of T_H cells in infants is very low, whereas suppressor activity is somewhat greater in infants than in adults. T_H-cell function reaches adult levels by six months of age.[2,12] This suggests that "newborn T cells must undergo age-related maturational changes to be capable of helper functions" (p. 9).[12] Compared with adult T lymphocytes, neonatal cells display a reduced capacity to produce cytokines (interleukin-2 [IL-2], IL-4, interferon-gamma [IFN-γ], and tumor necrosis factor [TNF]) and a decreased ability to stimulate B lymphocytes to produce immunoglobulins. The production of IFN-γ is tenfold lower in infants than in adults, and synthesis of TNF is 50 percent less in neonates than in adults.[2] Because cytokines modulate the immune response, deficiencies in cytokine production have a major impact on the newborn's susceptibility to infection.[16]

The most critical deficiency in cell-mediated immunity in the newborn is the shortage of memory T cells. Neonatal T cells are naïve, lacking prior exposure to foreign antigen, which is the stimulus for clonal expansion of memory T-cell populations. It is this amplified memory cell population that is responsible for the rapid and intense reaction characteristic of the specific immune response.[1] Decreased production of IFN-γ may be a consequence of inexperienced T cells.[11] Diminished activity of IL-12 and IFN-γ are thought to be responsible for decreased cytolytic activity of CD8+ and NK cells in newborns.[12]

Natural killer cells. NK cells are not phagocytic cells, do not possess the antigen-specific receptors of T and B cells, and lack immunologic specificity and memory. However, they share the markers and functions of both macrophages and some T cells.[1,7] Their mechanism of recognition is as yet not fully delineated, but it is thought to involve both activating and inhibitory receptors.[7]

The role of NK cells includes defense against infection by destruction of antibody-coated antigen cells and the killing of certain target cells without previous exposure to an antigen.[1,6] Specifically, NK cells identify and destroy virus-infected host cells and certain types of tumors.[7,17] They are also important in immunoregulation because they produce cytokines such as IFN-γ.[1] The absolute numbers of NK cells are equivalent in neonates and adults. The cytotoxicity of these cells is diminished in the newborn, however, leading to increased risk of infection from viruses and other intracellular pathogens.[12]

Mononuclear phagocyte system. Circulating monocytes and tissue macrophages comprise the mononuclear phagocyte system. Early progenitors of monocytes/macrophages are found in the yolk sac. Committed cells of this lineage are present in the liver by 6 weeks gestation.[9,13] By 30 weeks, monocytes represent 3–7 percent of circulating formed blood cells. After release into the bloodstream, monocytes reach maturity and remain in the circulation for about eight hours, until they migrate into the tissues and differentiate into macrophages.[1,4] Throughout the neonatal period, monocyte counts are high relative to adult values.

Macrophages constitute more than 70 percent of the cells present in the liver before it becomes the major locus of hematopoiesis. When the liver assumes the role of hematopoiesis, the macrophage level declines progressively until, at term, macrophages constitute only 1–2 percent of differentiated blood cells.[11]

Macrophages and macrophage-like cells are dispersed throughout the body, serving different functions in different sites. They are named according to their location: alveolar macrophages, histiocytes, Kupffer cells, mesangial cells, microglial cells, and osteoclasts in the lungs, connective tissue, liver, kidneys, brain, and bone, respectively.[1]

Cells of the mononuclear phagocyte lineage have a wide variety of functions, ranging from microbicidal activity to secretion of immunoregulatory substances. They also play a role in angiogenesis (the formation of blood vessels) and wound healing.[2]

Monocytes usually exist in a resting state, but become activated by a number of stimuli, including the phagocytosis of antigens, cytokines secreted by activated T_H cells, mediators of the inflammatory response, and components of bacterial cell walls. Activated cells become effective in antigen elimination because of their increased (1) phagocyte activity, (2) capacity to kill pathogens, (3) ability to secrete inflammatory mediators, and (4) ability to activate T cells. Finally, only activated monocytes/macrophages secrete cytotoxic proteins, which are directed against virus-infected cells, tumor cells, and intracellular bacteria.[1]

In addition to their involvement in phagocytosis, monocytes/macrophages also function as antigen-presenting cells. Monocytes/macrophages destroy and eliminate most, but not all, of the antigens they ingest. In some cases, the antigen is merely degraded by a processing pathway within the cell and expressed (exocytosis) on the cell surface. This processing and presentation of antigen "are critical to T_H cell activation, a central event in the development of both humoral and cell-mediated immune responses" (p. 44).[1] (For more on antigen presentation to T cells, see "*T lymphocytes*" on page 23, and Figure 2-7.)

Activated monocytes/macrophages secrete a number of soluble mediators, such as complement, cytokines, and hydrolytic enzymes. The secreted cytokines include IL-1 and IL-6, IFN-α, TNF-α, granulocyte-monocyte colony-stimulating factor (GM-CSF), granulocyte colony-stimulating factor (G-CSF), and monocyte colony-stimulating factor (M-CSF). Soluble mediators augment the inflammatory response, stimulate other cells of the immune system, and assist in intracellular destruction of antigen.[1,7]

Differences in neonates. Newborns have circulating levels of monocytes that are similar to those in adults, but the influx of these phagocytes to inflammatory sites is delayed and attenuated compared with adult responses. This is probably the consequence of impaired chemotaxis in newborns. Both phagocytic and antimicrobial activity are equal in newborns and adults. Function of neonatal macrophages appears to be deficient as a result of decreased cytokine production by T lymphocytes.[2]

FIGURE 2-9 ♦ Structure of immunoglobulin.

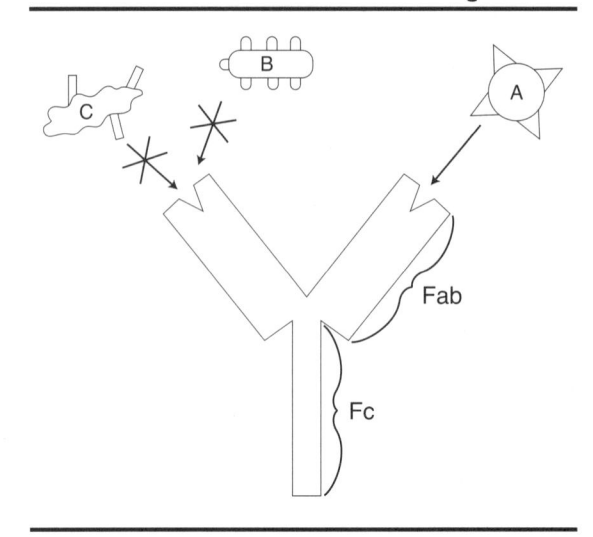

Specific binding sites on Fab portion of Ig bind antigen. Antigen A will be recognized; antigens B and C will not. The Fc region of the Ig will either bind to Fc receptors on host cells or activate the classical complement cascade.

Platelets

In addition to their role in blood clotting, platelets are involved in the immune response. Platelets include granules that contain serotonin and fibrinogen. During thrombogenesis or the formation of antigen-antibody complexes, platelets become activated and degranulate, releasing these substances that promote capillary permeability, activation of complement, and attraction of leukocytes.[4,7]

Dendritic Cells

Dendritic cells get their name from the long extensions of their membranes, which resemble the dendrites of nerve cells.[1] There are several types of dendritic cells. They descend from hematopoietic stem cells, although their precise ontogeny is not yet known.[1,18] Dendritic cells exist in several loci and have different forms and functions, but they share common functional characteristics. Dendritic cells populate most organs, lymphoid tissue, and the thymus and also circulate in the bloodstream.[1] Langerhans' cells (a type of dendritic cell) are present in the skin and mucous membranes.

Most dendritic cells produce antigen. On phagocytosis or endocytosis of antigen in tissues, these dendritic cells migrate to the bloodstream or lymphatic system. They then circulate to lymphoid organs to present the antigen to T lymphocytes.[1,18]

Another type of dendritic cell exists, seemingly of a different origin than the APC dendritic cell. These are located in lymph follicles that contain large numbers of B lymphocytes. These dendritic cells express high levels of membrane receptors for complement and immunoglobulin. Circulating antigen-antibody complexes are bound on these receptors. This binding is thought to facilitate both B-cell activation and development of memory B cells.[1,7]

Soluble Components

Antibodies

Antibodies are immunoglobulins produced by B lymphocytes. There are five classes of immunoglobulins: IgG, IgA, IgM, IgE, and IgD. Class (isotype) switching creates diversity of Ig classes. Immature B cells initially express only surface IgM receptors and no other Ig classes.[19] In the process of isotype switching, cells with surface IgM receptors produce daughter cells expressing another Ig class.[11,12]

Immunoglobulin molecules are composed of two heavy and two light polypeptide chains. The five classes of Igs all share the same basic structure, but differ in the region that binds antigen. The structural variability in this region permits different classes of Ig to react specifically with different antigens (Figure 2-9). The Fab portion of the Ig molecule binds antigen, whereas the Fc portion interacts with other elements of the immune system (phagocytes, complement). When antibody binds antigen on its Fab portion, it links to the Fc receptor on the surface of phagocytic cells. This promotes phagocytosis and intracellular killing of the pathogen. In this way, Ig acts as an opsonin. Phagocytosis is most effective when both complement and Ig are present as opsonins.[11,20]

Functions of immunoglobulins. Immunoglobulins have many diverse functions, but their main role is to bind to invading pathogens so that they can be recognized as foreign by the phagocyte. At times, this is accomplished by direct action: Ig can neutralize bacterial toxins or prevent viral attachment to host cells. However, "the interaction of antibody and antigen is without significance unless secondary 'effector' functions come into play" (p. 74).[20] These effector functions include (1) opsonization, which facilitates phagocytosis by PMNs and monocytes; (2) complement activation, which stimulates the production of substances able to penetrate cell membranes; (3) antibody-dependent cell-mediated cytotoxicity (ADCC), which enables natural killer cells to destroy target cells; and (4) activation of mast cells, eosinophils, and basophils mediating hypersensitivity reactions.[1]

Classes of immunoglobulins. IgG is the most abundant class of immunoglobulin in humans, accounting for 70–75 percent of the antibody activity in serum, and it is the only immunoglobulin that is transplacentally acquired (see Figure 2-6). IgG confers immunity against bacteria (particularly Gram-positive strains), bacterial toxins, and viruses. IgG augments the inflammatory response by activating the classic complement pathway.[1,8,11,13] There are four subclasses of IgG: Bacterial polysaccharides induce primarily IgG2 and, to a lesser degree, IgG4. IgG1 and IgG3 are produced in response to viral antigens.[1,12] Individuals who are deficient in IgG experience recurrent infections unless they receive replacement.

Comprising 10–15 percent of the antibody in serum, IgA is the second most abundant immunoglobulin in serum. Secretory IgA (sIgA) is detectable in large amounts in external

TABLE 2-4 ♦ **Characteristics and Functions of Immunoglobulins**

Name	Activates Classical Complement?	Trans-placentally Acquired?	Found on Mature B-Cell Surface?	Binding to Macrophage Receptors?	Detected in Secretions?	Induction of Mast Cell Degranulation?	Functions
IgG	+ → ++	+	–	+ → ++	–	–	Neutralizes toxins, binds antigens, promotes phagocytosis and clearance of immune complexes, mediates antibody-dependent cellular cytotoxicity
IgA	–	–	–	–	+++	–	Promotes mucosal antigen recognition; prevents antigen from binding to mucosa
IgM	+++	–	+	+	+	–	Binds multi-dimensional antigens, promotes phagocytosis of microorganisms, accessory role as secretory Ig
IgE	–	–	–	–	–	+++	Mediates hypersensitivity reactions
IgD	–	–	+	–	–	–	May participate in activation of B lymphocytes by antigen

Activity key: +++ = high; +/– = minimal; – = none.

Adapted from: Goldsby RA, Kindt TJ, and Osborne BA. 2000. *Kuby Immunology*, 4th ed. New York: WH Freeman, 3–34; and Cole FS. 1998. Infectious and immunologic defense mechanisms. In *Avery's Diseases of the Newborn*, 7th ed., Tausch HW, and Ballard RA, eds. Philadelphia: WB Saunders, 435–534.

secretions and on mucosal surfaces. Serum IgA and sIgA differ structurally. Molecules of sIgA contain a secretory component that renders it resistant to the proteolytic effects of the gastrointestinal tract. IgA provides a vital effector function on mucosal surfaces by preventing attachment of organisms to mucosal cells. In addition to preventing bacterial overgrowth, it may also limit absorption of antigenic dietary proteins.[1,13,20]

IgM accounts for approximately 5–10 percent of the normal adult Ig pool and is the first type of Ig produced in response to an antigen.[1] It is the most efficient immunoglobulin in activation of the classical complement pathway and provides protection against blood-borne organisms, particularly Gram-negative bacteria.[1,13,20]

IgE represents a minute fraction of the immunoglobulin in adult serum: 0.01 percent, or 1/10,000th of the total serum Ig. IgE is synthesized in most lymphoid tissue, but exists in greatest amounts in the lungs and gastrointestinal tract. The appearance of IgE in body fluids generally coincides with the presence of inflammation. These antibodies mediate the hypersensitivity reactions characteristic of allergies and anaphylactic shock. Antigen-specific IgE induces degranulation of mast cells and the release of inflammatory mediators, producing bronchoconstriction, tissue edema, and urticaria.[1,13,20]

IgD, the most recent class to be discovered, is present in very small quantities and represents less than 1 percent of total immunoglobulin in adult serum. Its exact biologic function is unclear, but it is thought to participate in the activation of B cells by an antigen. IgD and IgM are the major membrane-bound Igs exhibited by mature B lymphocytes.[1,13,19,20]

Only IgM and IgG are capable of activating the classical complement pathway and possess the ability to serve as effective opsonins. The other classes of immunoglobulins do not display these functions.[1,19,20] Table 2-4 summarizes the characteristics and functions of immunoglobulins.

Figure 2-10 illustrates the antibody responses after an initial and a subsequent antigenic challenge. IgM is the first antibody produced, appearing early in the primary response to the pathogen; IgG production occurs later and usually requires T- and B-lymphocyte interaction. On secondary exposure to an antigen, antibody is more rapidly synthesized by memory B cells and reaches higher levels. The response persists for a longer period of time and consists predominantly of IgG antibody.[19]

FIGURE 2-10 ◆ Antibody responses (IgM, IgG) after initial and subsequent antigen challenges.

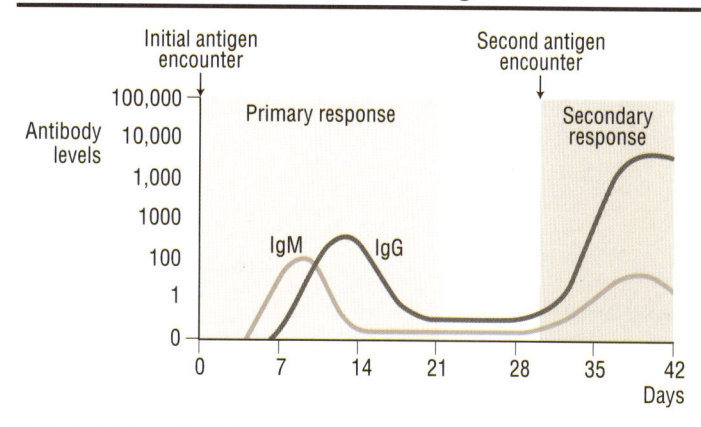

The more rapid and heightened secondary response results from production of memory cells during the initial exposure.

Adapted from: Feldman M, and Marini J. 2001. Cell cooperation in the antibody response. In *Immunology*, 6th ed., Roitt I, Brostoff J, and Male D, eds. St. Louis: Mosby-Year Book, 141. Reprinted by permission.

Complement

The complement system, consisting of more than 30 serum and membrane proteins, is a major component of humoral immunity. The liver synthesizes components of complement as early as the fourth to fifth week of gestation. Complement is not transferred across the placenta. Fetal complement levels are low until the third trimester; the cord blood concentration at term is 60–80 percent of adult levels.[12]

After initial activation, complement components interact with each other in an enzymatic cascade, facilitating antigen clearance and the mounting of an inflammatory response. There are two pathways of complement activation: classic and alternative. Complement activation via the classic pathway is generally triggered by the formation of antigen-antibody complexes or by binding of antibody to antigen on a suitable molecule, such as a bacterial cell. Substances that are foreign to the host, such as endotoxins and the polysaccharide frequently found in

FIGURE 2-11 ♦ Complement cascade.

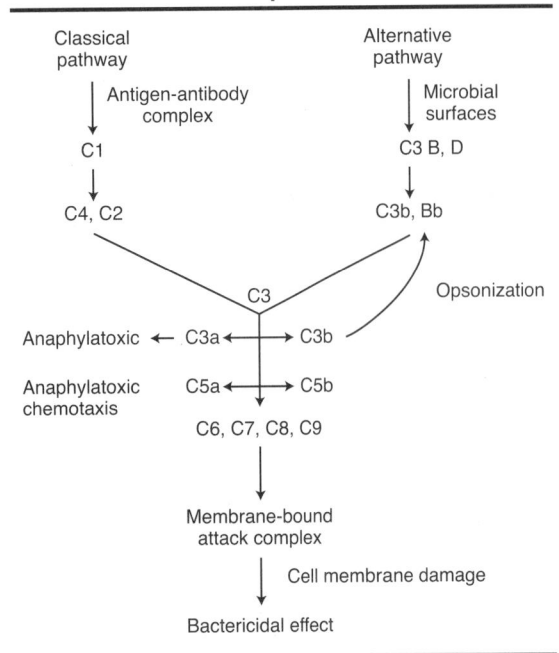

```
    Classical                  Alternative
    pathway                    pathway
       │ Antigen-antibody         │ Microbial
       │ complex                  │ surfaces
       ▼                          ▼
      C1                       C3 B, D
       │                          │
       ▼                          ▼
     C4, C2                    C3b, Bb
          \                   /
           \     C3          /
            \               /  Opsonization
Anaphylatoxic ← C3a ←  → C3b
                        │
Anaphylatoxic   C5a ←  → C5b
chemotaxis              │
                  C6, C7, C8, C9
                        │
                        ▼
                 Membrane-bound
                 attack complex
                        │ Cell membrane damage
                        ▼
                 Bactericidal effect
```

The classical pathway is activated when C1 binds to antigen-antibody complex. The alternative pathway is activated when C3 binds to microbial surfaces. With activation of either pathway, there is generation of soluble factors that augment the immune response.

Differences in neonates. In term neonates and adults, components of the classic complement pathway and their functional activity are comparable. Preterm infants have significantly decreased concentrations of several classic complement components, however.[21,22] Activation of the classic pathway is dependent on the presence of antibody. Because immunoglobulin levels are low after birth, the protection afforded by this pathway is limited. The alternative pathway, and therefore its integrity, assumes a more vital role in triggering the effector functions of the complement cascade.

Levels of the individual components of the alternative complement pathway and the overall activity of the pathway are diminished in both term and preterm infants. Adult serum concentrations of the components of this cascade are not achieved until the end of the first year of life.[11] Lower levels of complement and/or decreased complement activity result in deficiencies of activation products essential in opsonization and chemotaxis.

pathogenic organisms, induce activation of the alternative pathway.[1,5,10] Figure 2-11 illustrates the complement cascade.

Mobilization of either complement pathway generates protein molecules or peptide fragments that produce a number of effects. Complement induces localized vasodilation and increased capillary permeability to plasma molecules, and it attracts cellular elements to the site of infection (chemotaxis). It also opsonizes X antigen to facilitate phagocytosis and intracellular destruction, generates a membrane attack complex (MAC) that lyses a number of bacteria and viruses, and causes the release of inflammatory mediators by mast cells.[1,5,13] Figure 2-12 illustrates the functions of complement.

FIGURE 2-12 ♦ Summary of complement functions.

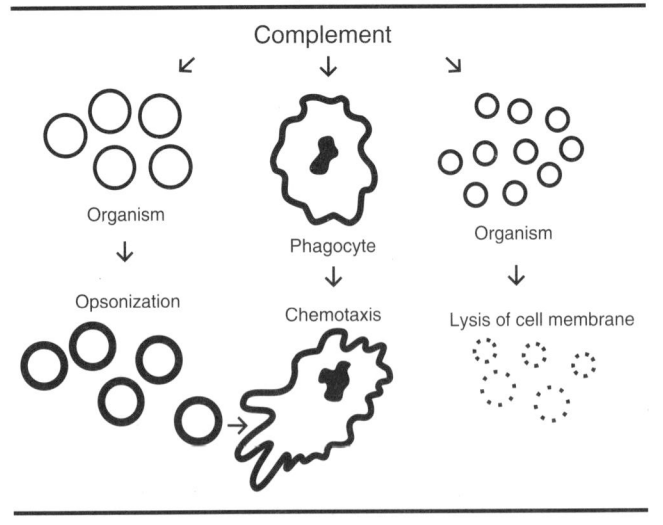

The complement cascade may be activated by either antibody or pathogens. Once activated, complement (1) functions as an opsonin, (2) enhances chemotaxis, and (3) lyses cell membranes on bacteria.

TABLE 2-5 ◆ Sources and Functions of Some Cytokines

Cytokine	Produced By	Site of Action	Major Effects
IL-1α, IL-1β	Macrophages, large granular lymphocyte, B cells	T and B lymphocytes, macrophages, tissue cells, endothelial cells	Activates lymphocytes, stimulates macrophages, enhances leukocyte endothelial adhesion, produces inflammatory response, fever
IL-2	T$_H$ cells	Other T cells, macrophages	Encourages proliferation and differentiation of T cells, activates T$_C$ cells and macrophages
IL-3	T$_H$ cells, stem cells		Promotes growth and differentiation of hematopoietic stem cells
		Mast cells, basophils	Stimulates growth and histamine production
IL-4	T$_H$ cells	B cells	Stimulates growth and differentiation, induces Ig isotype switching
		T cells and thymocytes	Induces proliferation
		Macrophages	Increases phagocytic activity
		Mast cells	Stimulates growth
IL-5	T$_H$ cells	B cells	Promotes growth and differentiation
IL-6	T$_H$ cells, B cells	B cells	Promotes differentiation into plasma cells, stimulates antibody secretion
		Hepatocytes	Stimulates secretion of acute-phase reactants
IL-7	Bone marrow stroll cells	Lymphoid stem cells	Induces differentiation into progenitor B and T cells
		T cells	Promotes secretion of IL-2 and IL-2 receptors
IL-8	Monocytes, fibroblasts, epithelial cells	Neutrophils, basophils, T cells	Enhances chemotaxis, induces adherence to vascular endothelium and extravasation into tissues, stimulates angiogenesis, stimulates superoxide and granule release
IL-10	T$_{H2}$ cells	T$_{H1}$ cells	Suppresses cytokine production
IL-11	Bone marrow stromal cells	Progenitor B cells	Promotes differentiation
		Megakaryocytes	Promotes differentiation
		Hepatocytes	Induces synthesis of acute-phase reactants
IL-13	T$_H$ cells	Macrophages	Inhibits activation and release of pro-inflammatory cytokines
		B cells	Growth and differentiation of B lymphocytes
TNF-α	Macrophages, mast cells, T and B lymphocytes	Macrophages, granulocytes	Activation of granulocytes, macrophages, and cytotoxic cells
		Tissue cells	Promotes WBC-endothelial cell adhesion, produces fever and weight loss, induces production of acute-phase reactants, enhances production of class I MHC* molecules
TNF-β	T and B cells	Tissue cells, leukocytes	Same as TNF-α
IFN-γ	T cells, NK cells, epithelial cells, fibroblasts	Uninfected cells	Inhibits viral replication
		Macrophages	Enhances activity, increases expression of class I and II MHC* molecules
		B cells	Induces isotype switching
		T$_{H2}$ cells	Inhibits proliferation
		Inflammatory cells	Mediates delayed hypersensitivity reaction

(continued on next page)

---

*MHC = major histocompatibility complex.

TABLE 2-5 ◆ Sources and Functions of Some Cytokines (continued)

Cytokine	Produced By	Site of Action	Major Effects
M-CSF	Monocytes, fibroblasts, endothelium		Proliferation of macrophage precursors
G-CSF	Macrophages, fibroblasts	Hematopoietic stem cells	Induces division and proliferation
GM-CSF	T cells, macrophages, endothelium, fibroblasts		Proliferation of granulocyte and macrophage progenitors
Macrophage-inhibiting factor	T cells	Macrophages	Inhibits migration

Adapted from: Roitt I, Brostoff J, and Male D, eds. 2001. *Immunology*, 6th ed. St. Louis: Mosby-Year Book, 441–442. Reprinted by permission.

Cytokines

Cytokine is a generic term for a collection of proteins or peptides that regulate the intensity and duration of the immune response. Cytokines produce a variety of effects on lymphocytes and other components of the immune system, thereby influencing the growth, differentiation, repair, expansion, and activation of cells involved in natural and specific immunity.[1,16,23]

Cytokines bind to specific receptors expressed on the surface of target cells. Once bound to the specific receptor, cytokines stimulate biochemical modifications that alter the expression of genes in the cell and induce, enhance, or inhibit cell function. More than 100 human cytokines have been identified. They are produced by various cells in response to inducing stimuli, and they are classified into different categories. Cytokines can have multiple functions *in vitro*, and several cytokines can have similar functions.[16,23]

Interferons. IFNs are a group of similar proteins produced and excreted by virally infected cells. They are the first line of defense against viruses and are produced early in infection. IFNs serve to warn healthy cells of a potential viral attack, induce a state of antiviral resistance in uninfected host cells, and limit the spread of certain viral infections by inhibiting viral replication.[1] They also augment other immune activities such as enhancing macrophage phagocytic activity and enhancing the actions of NK cells and cytotoxic T cells. Virally infected cells generate some IFNs (IFN-α, IFN-β); another type (IFN-γ) is produced by activated T lymphocytes.[23]

Interleukins. T cells are the major source of the group of cytokines called interleukins, although some macrophages and tissue cells also produce them. Most ILs direct other cells to divide and differentiate, but ILs have a variety of additional functions. There are many different types of ILs (IL-1 through IL-22), and each interacts with cells expressing receptors for its particular type. Table 2-5 lists the functions of some interleukins.

Other cytokines. Colony-stimulating factors direct the division and differentiation of hematopoietic stem cells and the precursors of leukocytes, erythrocytes, and platelets. Some of these cytokines promote further differentiation of cells after they leave the bone marrow. Other cytokines—such as TNF-α, TNF-β, and transforming growth factor (TGF-β)—mediate inflammation and cytotoxic reactions.[15,23] See Table 2-5 for the source, site of action, and role of some major cytokines.

Fibronectins

Fibronectins (Fns) are a class of multifunctional glycoproteins that are found in insoluble

FIGURE 2-13 ♦ Summary of immune response: series of events stimulated by presence of antigen.

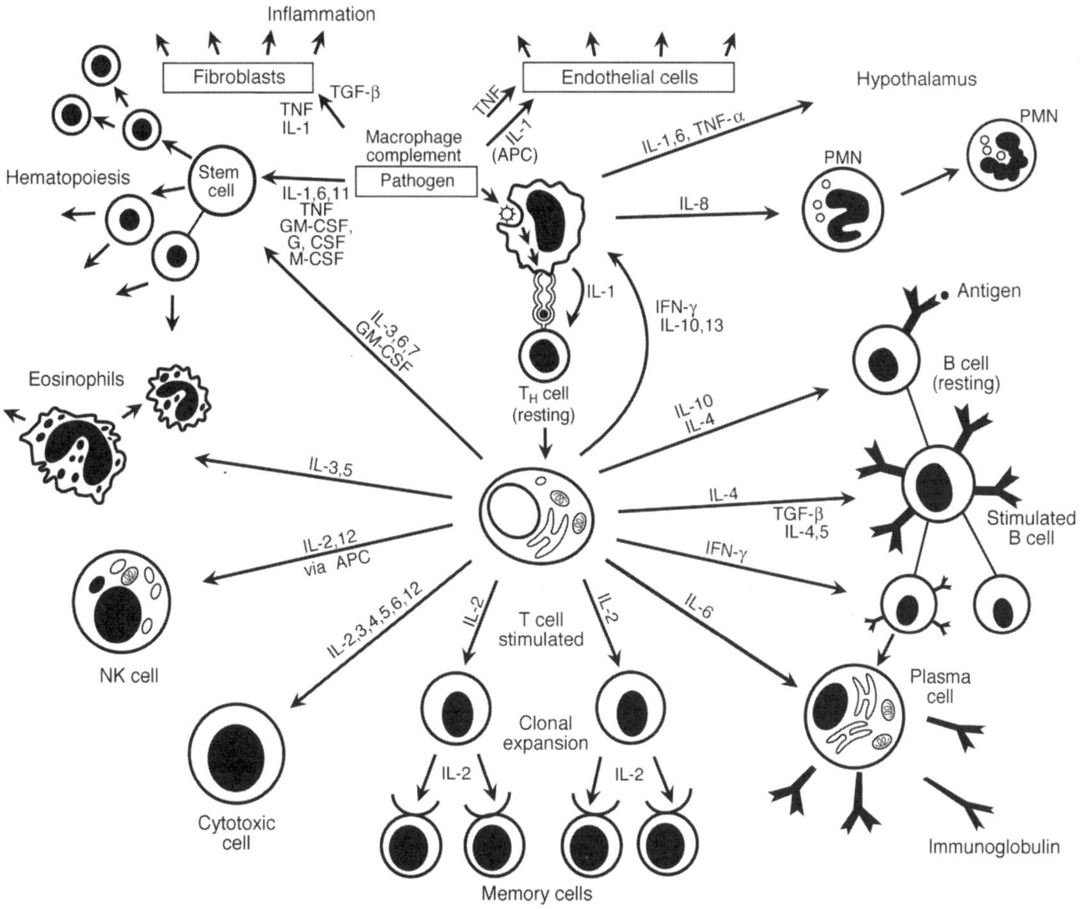

form on most cells and in soluble form in plasma and interstitial fluids. Fibronectins are involved in hemostasis, vascular integrity, and wound healing and in direct cell migration, proliferation, and differentiation during embryogenesis.[11] Fibronectins play a role in the immune response by augmenting the performance of phagocytic cells. They function as chemoattractants; induce the expression of complement receptors; and promote the uptake and clearance of fibrin, platelets, immune complexes, and cellular debris by phagocytic cells. Fibronectins (Fns) are also an opsonic factor for numerous pathogenic organisms, including *S. aureus*, Streptococcus species, and some Gram-negative bacteria.[2,11]

Differences in neonates. Term newborn infants have serum concentrations of fibronectins that are one-third to one-half those found in adults. Levels are directly proportional to gestational age and are also reduced under various pathologic conditions, such as sepsis, malnutrition, asphyxia, and RDS. Although the exact role played by low fibronectin levels in the neonate is unclear, these low levels may contribute to diminished function of phagocytic cells.[2,11]

Other Humoral Factors

Other soluble mediators are involved in the immune response. Some of them are normally present in serum and increase rapidly during infection. One of these is the acute-phase

TABLE 2-6 ♦ Deficiencies in Neonatal Immune Defenses when Compared to Adults

Qualitative and quantitative deficiencies in nonspecific cellular function:
  Limited neutrophil reserves
  Diminished capacity to accelerate neutrophil production
  Decreased neutrophil accumulation at site of infection
  Decreased bactericidal activity of neutrophils during stress/sepsis
  Delayed influx of monocytes to site of inflammation
Decreased activity of serum complement
Reduced ability of B lymphocytes to produce immunoglobulins against bacterial polysaccharide antigen
Antigenically naïve T cells

Adapted from: Male D. 2001. Cell migration and inflammation. In *Immunology*, 6th ed., Roitt I, Brostoff J, and Male D, eds. St. Louis: Mosby-Year Book, 47–64; and Schelonka R, and Infante A. 1998. Neonatal immunology. *Seminars in Perinatology* 22(1): 2–14.

reactant C-reactive protein (CRP). CRP serum concentration increases 100–1,000-fold in response to infection in adults, and an elevated CRP is also a sensitive marker of infection in neonates.[11] CRP binds to the polysaccharide cell wall component of many bacteria and fungi, activating the complement cascade and promoting opsonization, phagocytosis, and clearance of pathogens.[1,4,11]

Histamine and kinins are important chemical mediators of inflammation that are produced by a number of cells in response to tissue injury. After release, histamine binds to receptors on blood vessels, inducing vasodilation and increased permeability. Kinins are usually present in inactive form in plasma. They are activated by tissue injury and, like histamine, promote vasodilation and enhanced blood-vessel permeability.[1]

Lactoferrin is a glycoprotein found in the specific granules of PMNs. It is released by these cells upon phagocytosis of pathogens. Because of its ability to bind iron, lactoferrin deprives bacteria of a vital nutrient. Other functions of lactoferrin appear to include enhancement of chemotaxis, endothelial adhesion, and aggregation of PMNs.[11]

DEVELOPMENTAL IMMUNOLOGY

Developmental immunology investigates the manner in which host defense cells progressively respond to recurrent environmental challenges, promoting health and survival.[10,11] Newborn infants, whether premature or term, have the ability to mount an immune response to environmental challenges (Figure 2-13). However, this response is attenuated as a result of genetic programming and a lack of previous exposure to pathogens, both of which limit the performance of specific immune mechanisms. The immune system of the normal newborn is both immature and inexperienced, putting the neonate at considerable risk for infection. Overall, the deficiencies in the immune system are more marked in premature infants.[2] This is a developmental phenomenon: "The adaptive significance of these alterations for neonatal survival remains obscure" (p. 2).[10] One hypothesis for the delayed responsiveness of the fetal/neonatal immune system is the need to preserve the fetus's status as a graft *in utero*.[13]

Sepsis is a significant cause of mortality and morbidity among newborns despite overall improvements in neonatal care. Microorganisms that pose little or no threat to adults and older children cause serious infections and extensive tissue damage in neonates. Time is required for the components of immunity to develop mature competence. In the case of some factors, adult concentrations or levels of functioning are not achieved until late childhood. The primary factors accounting for the increased susceptibility of the neonate to infection are qualitative and quantitative deficiencies in nonspecific cellular function, decreased activity of serum complement, reduced ability of B lymphocytes to produce immunoglobulins against bacterial polysaccharide antigen, and antigenically naïve

T lymphocytes.[4,12] These factors and their consequences have been outlined in each of the relevant sections. Table 2-6 lists the most clinically significant differences between the immune systems of neonates and adults.

SUMMARY

The immune system of the neonate is immature and inexperienced, but most newborns are able to adapt to their environment. Although the incidence of infection in the newborn is low, the mortality rate approaches 50 percent.[24] In premature infants, the relative risk is higher because of greater deficiencies in their immune response combined with increased risk factors such as invasive procedures and interventions such as the placement of central lines. Research findings continue to enhance our understanding of the developing immune system and, in turn, identify avenues for potential intervention in the prevention and treatment of neonatal infection. Successful treatment of neonates for infection may require adjuvant therapies to enhance the immune response. Some of these therapies are described in Chapters 7 and 8.

REFERENCES

1. Goldsby RA, Kindt TJ, and Osborne BA, eds. 2000. *Kuby Immunology*, 4th ed. New York: WH Freeman, 3–34, 44.
2. Bellanti J, Zeligs B, and Pung Y. 1999. Immunology of the fetus and newborn. In *Neonatology: Pathophysiology and Management of the Newborn*, 5th ed., Avery G, Fletcher M, and MacDonald M, eds. Philadelphia: Lippincott Williams & Wilkins, 1092–1121.
3. Sherwood L. 2001. *Human Physiology: From Cells to Systems*. Pacific Grove, California: Brooks/Cole, 390–432.
4. Male D. 2001. Introduction to the immune system. In *Immunology*, 6th ed., Roitt I, Brostoff J, and Male D, eds. St. Louis: Mosby-Year Book, 1–13.
5. Male D. 2001. Cell migration and inflammation. In *Immunology*, 6th ed., Roitt I, Brostoff J, and Male D, eds. St. Louis: Mosby-Year Book, 47–64.
6. Lawton A, and Cooper M. 1996. Ontogeny of immunity. In *Immunologic Disorders in Infants and Children*, 4th ed., Steihm ER, ed. Philadelphia: WB Saunders, 35–60.
7. Lydyard PM, and Grossi C. 2001. Cells, tissues and organs of the immune system. In *Immunology*, 6th ed., Roitt I, Brostoff J, and Male D, eds. St. Louis: Mosby-Year Book, 15–45.
8. Schibler K. 1998. Developmental biology of the hematopoietic growth factors. In *Fetal and Neonatal Physiology*, 2nd ed., Polin R, and Fox W, eds. Philadelphia: WB Saunders, 1737–1753.
9. Pappas BE. 1999. Primary immunodeficiency disorders in infancy. *Neonatal Network* 18(1): 13–22.
10. Dixon L. 1997. The complete blood count: Physiologic basis and clinical usage. *Journal of Perinatal and Neonatal Nursing* 11(3): 1–18.
11. Kapur R, Yoder CM, and Polin RA. 2002. Developmental immunology. In *Neonatal-Perinatal Medicine: Diseases of the Fetus and Infant*, 7th ed., Fanaroff A, and Martin R, eds. St. Louis: Mosby-Year Book, 676–706.
12. Schelonka R, and Infante A. 1998. Neonatal immunology. *Seminars in Perinatology* 22(1): 2–14.
13. Cole FS. 1998. Infectious and immunologic defense mechanisms. Part 7. In *Avery's Diseases of the Newborn*, 7th ed., Tausch HW, and Ballard RA, eds. Philadelphia: WB Saunders, 435–466.
14. Kohler PF, and Farr RS. 1966. Elevation of cord over maternal IgG immunoglobulin: Evidence for an active placental IgG transport. *Nature* 210(4): 1070–1071.
15. Male D. 2001. T-cell receptors and major histocompatibility molecules. In *Immunology*, 6th ed., Roitt I, Brostoff J, and Male D, eds. St. Louis: Mosby-Year Book, 87–103.
16. Gelfand EW, and Finkel TH. 1996. The T-lymphocyte system. In *Immunologic Disorders in Infants and Children*, 4th ed., Steihm ER, ed. Philadelphia: WB Saunders, 3–34.
17. Male D. 2001. Cell-mediated cytotoxicity. In *Immunology*, 6th ed., Roitt I, Brostoff J, and Male D, eds. St. Louis: Mosby-Year Book, 164–172.
18. Gordon S. 2001. Mononuclear phagocytes in immune defense. In *Immunology*, 6th ed., Roitt I, Brostoff J, and Male D, eds. St. Louis: Mosby-Year Book, 147–162.
19. Feldman M, and Marini J. 2001. Cell cooperation in the antibody response. In *Immunology*, 6th ed., Roitt I, Brostoff J, and Male D, eds. St. Louis: Mosby-Year Book, 131–146.
20. Turner M. 2001. Antibodies. In *Immunology*, 6th ed., Roitt I, Brostoff J, and Male D, eds. St. Louis: Mosby-Year Book, 65–86.
21. Colten HR. 1972. Ontogeny of the human complement system: *In vitro* biosynthesis of individual complement components by fetal tissues. *Journal of Clinical Investigation* 51(4): 725–730.
22. Davis CA, Vallota EH, and Forristal J. 1979. Serum complement levels in infancy: Age related changes. *Pediatric Research* 13(9): 1043–1046.
23. Balkwill F. 2001. Cytokines and cytokine receptors. In *Immunology*, 6th ed., Roitt I, Brostoff J, and Male D, eds. St. Louis: Mosby-Year Book, 119–129.
24. Hall DM, Thureen PJ, and Abzug MJ. 1998. Infectious diseases. In *Assessment and Care of the Well Newborn*, Thureen PJ, et al., eds. Philadelphia: WB Saunders, 301–323.

NOTES

Notes

CHAPTER 3

Intrauterine Infections

DEBBIE FRASER ASKIN, RNC, MN

Transplacental infection with subsequent damage to the fetus was first described in 1941 with the identification of congenital rubella syndrome by Sir Norman Gregg.[1] Since that time, several organisms have been recognized as capable of causing damage to the developing fetus. Traditionally, transplacental infections have been organized using the acronym TORCH—toxoplasmosis, other (among them, syphilis, hepatitis B), rubella, cytomegalovirus (CMV), and herpes (HSV). It is now recognized that this organizational scheme is an oversimplification, with a number of other agents now known to cause intrauterine infections. Some of these agents include Parvovirus, varicella-zoster virus (VZV), enteroviruses, and human immunodeficiency virus (HIV) (Table 3-1). Some authors argue that the TORCH acronym should be abandoned because it is both noninclusive and misleading: Care providers frequently order TORCH serology to diagnose intrauterine infections, yet the test is often ordered inappropriately and as such is nondiagnostic.[2,3] The use of the acronym may also encourage care providers to lump together all causes of intrauterine infection, ignoring the unique features of each organism.[4]

Somewhat tongue in cheek, Klein and Remington report that several new acronyms have been suggested to recognize other fetal pathogens responsible for intrauterine infections. Their proposal was TORCHES CLAP, to include enteroviruses and syphilis, chickenpox, Lyme disease, AIDS, and Parvovirus.[5] Other authors have proposed CHAST LOVER and CHEAP TORCHES.[6,7] In practice, these acronyms may help practitioners remember all of the viruses potentially responsible for intrauterine infections.

GENERAL EFFECTS OF INTRAUTERINE INFECTION

The transplacental passage of viruses during maternal viremia has been clearly documented.[8–10] The effects of such passage on the fetus range from asymptomatic disease to long-term sequelae to fetal death, depending on the timing of the exposure, the type of virus involved, and the viral load. The overall incidence of fetal viral infection is impossible to

TABLE 3-1 ◆ Organisms That Cause Intrauterine Infection

Cytomegalovirus
Enterovirus
Herpes simplex virus
Human immunodeficiency virus (AIDS)
Parvovirus B19
Rubella virus
Toxoplasma gondii (toxoplasmosis)
Treponema pallidum (syphilis)
Varicella-zoster virus

determine for a number of reasons. Maternal infections are often asymptomatic and therefore not recognized. Infants with congenital infection may also be asymptomatic at birth, making it difficult to correlate later deficits to a maternal illness during pregnancy. In the case of some viruses, such as CMV, fetal infection may occur as the result of a reactivation of the virus in the mother, rather than as the result of a primary infection. When maternal serology is available, the results can be difficult to interpret, requiring paired serum testing with samples taken from the mother several weeks apart. Fetal serology is similarly difficult to interpret because the fetal response to infection is often unpredictable before 20 weeks gestation. Finally, it is not always possible to obtain viral cultures, they can be slow to grow, or the infection may result from viruses, such as Parvovirus, that do not readily grow in culture.[10]

Incidence of Intrauterine Infection

Some estimates have been made of the number of intrauterine infections. An infectious cause, documented by culture or serology, is identified in 5–15 percent of fetuses with hydrops, ascites, pleural effusions, or pericardial effusions.[11] The etiology of an additional 22 percent of nonimmune hydrops is unknown, suggesting that infection may play an even larger role than is recognized.[10] In a study of 303 women with abnormal fetal ultrasounds and 154 controls done by Van den Veyver and associates, polymerase chain reaction (PCR) testing of amniotic fluid, fetal blood, and pleural fluid was done. Surprisingly, viral genetic material was found in 39 percent of pregnancies in which ultrasound identified an abnormal fetus. Only 2.6 percent of the control group (routine genetic amniocentesis with no ultrasound abnormalities) demonstrated viral material in the collected samples.[12]

Outcomes of Maternal Infection

Microbial invasion of the maternal bloodstream may have one of four outcomes: no fetal or placental infection, fetal infection without placental infection, placental infection without fetal effect, or infection of both placenta and fetus.[5]

No Fetal or Placental Infection

Many times maternal bacteremia during pregnancy results in neither fetal nor placental infection. Examples include bacterial pneumonia, pyelonephritis, endocarditis, cellulitis, and other pyogenic infections. Some bacterial, viral, and protozoal infections may affect the fetus indirectly through maternal fever, anoxia, circulating toxins, or metabolic derangements. These maternal complications can result in preterm labor, fetal hypoxia or tissue damage, or fetal death.

Fetal Infection without Placental Infection

Congenital infection without placental involvement is theoretically possible. Microorganisms could bypass the placenta by moving across the chorionic villi through pinocytosis or via diapedesis of infected maternal erythrocytes or leukocytes. In most cases of fetal infection, however, some areas of placentitis can be found.[5]

Placental Infection without Fetal Effect

The organisms in the mother's bloodstream may reach the intervillous spaces of the placenta, where they become localized but do not spread.

This has been seen in maternal tuberculosis, syphilis, malaria, CMV, and rubella infection.[5] Fetal defenses may include villus trophoblasts (ectodermal tissue covering the chorionic villi forming the chorion and amnion), placental macrophages, and local production of immune factors such as antibodies and cytokines.

Infection of Both Placenta and Fetus

Microorganisms can be disseminated from the infected placenta to the fetal bloodstream in one of two ways: through infected emboli of necrotic chorionic tissues or by direct extension of placental infection to the fetal membranes, with secondary amniotic fluid infection and aspiration by the fetus.

Placental or fetal infection can result in resorption of the embryo, spontaneous abortion, fetal demise, malformations and/or teratogenesis, intrauterine growth restriction and/or low birth weight, prematurity, chronic postnatal infection, late-onset disease, or neonatal death.

DETECTING INTRAUTERINE INFECTION

Because some women are asymptomatic for disease, relying on maternal history alone will result in failure to identify a number of pregnancies in which congenital infection poses a risk to the fetus. Several screening programs have been suggested or are in place to identify fetuses at risk. The cost-effectiveness of such programs depends on several factors, including the prevalence of the organism and the likelihood of maternal infection during pregnancy, the availability of sensitive and specific screening tests, the probability of fetal infection, the potential effects of the disease on the fetus or neonate, and the availability of appropriate therapeutic alternatives for those fetuses identified as infected. In France, for example, where the prevalence of toxoplasmosis infection is high, a successful screening program is in place to reduce the frequency and severity of infection.[13]

Because of lower prevalence rates of the disease in the U.S. and Canada, however, toxoplasmosis screening is not routine in these countries. Diseases that are part of usual prenatal screening in North America include syphilis, rubella, hepatitis B virus, and, in some areas, HIV.[5]

When screening tests are performed, positive results require follow-up testing. A variety of tests can be carried out on maternal or fetal blood. Careful consideration must be given to the risks associated with obtaining fetal blood samples, and these risks must be weighed against the benefits of prenatal diagnosis of intrauterine infections. In addition to viral cultures and evaluation of fetal or maternal immunoglobulin (IgM and IgG) levels, other hematologic indices may provide insight into fetal infection. The presence of anemia, polycythemia, hemolysis, thrombocytopenia, lymphocytosis, lymphopenia, or neutropenia in the fetus has been associated with fetal viral or parasitic infection.[14]

Electron microscopy is another tool that has been shown to be useful in identifying viral particles in fetal blood or peritoneal fluid even in the presence of normal IgM levels.[10] The availability and cost of this technology may be of issue, however.

Polymerase chain reaction testing has been studied for its usefulness in rapidly detecting viral nucleic acid sequences in infected tissues and body fluids such as blood, peritoneal fluid, and urine. Case reports have indicated the detection of CMV, *Toxoplasma gondii*, rubella, adenovirus, and Parvovirus using PCR.[12,15–17] As PCR becomes more widely available, it may replace many of the current testing methods.

When tissue samples are available, cytology and histologic findings may allow a presumptive diagnosis of infection. For example, there are specific placental changes that characterize certain infections. Cell scrapings from the cervix or from the base of lesions or vesicles may provide the diagnosis of herpes or varicella infections.[5]

TABLE 3-2 ♦ Clinical Manifestations of Toxoplasmosis

Blueberry muffin rash

Hepatosplenomegaly

Hydrops fetalis

Jaundice, anemia, eosinophilia

Lymphadenopathy

Neurologic signs: seizures, bulging fontanel, nystagmus, microcephaly or hydrocephalus, intracerebral calcifications

Ocular findings: chorioretinitis, microphthalmia, cataracts, glaucoma

Pneumonitis

Adapted from: Remington JS, et al. 2001. Toxoplasmosis. In *Infectious Diseases of the Fetus and Newborn Infant*, 5th ed., Remington JS, and Klein JO, eds. Philadelphia: WB Saunders, 205–346; and Isaacs D, and Moxon ER. 1999. *Handbook of Neonatal Infections: A Practical Guide*. London: WB Saunders, 361–374.

Less invasive testing may also provide clues about possible fetal infection. Ultrasound evaluation of the fetus, performed by a skilled operator, combined with a positive screening test strongly suggests fetal infection. Abnormal findings implicating intrauterine infection include fetal growth restriction, oligohydramnios, nonimmune hydrops, ventriculomegaly, echogenic bowel, and structural malformations. However, normal ultrasound findings do not rule out infection.[10]

SPECIFIC ORGANISMS

Toxoplasma Gondii

Toxoplasma gondii is a protozoan parasite commonly found in cats, dogs, pigs, sheep, and cattle, with cats being the definitive host. This parasite has a complex life cycle with three distinct stages: the tachyzoite, present during acute infections; the bradyzoite, present in tissue cysts; and the sporozoite, found in oocysts.[18] Oocysts are formed in the intestine of the cat and shed in its feces. Sporozoites form within the oocysts and are released when the wall of the oocyst is broken down in the host's digestive tract. Transmission to humans is most frequently attributed either to accidental ingestion of feces or material contaminated with feces or to consumption of raw or undercooked meat containing pseudocysts. The third mechanism of transmission is from an infected mother to her fetus.

Prevalence rates of toxoplasmosis vary widely across the world and depend on climate, altitude, and the hygiene and eating habits of the population.[19,20] Approximately 30 percent of the U.S. population is thought to be seropositive for *T. gondii*.[19]

According to Isaacs and Moxon, the incidence of *T. gondii* maternal infection in pregnancy ranges from 2 to 12 per 1,000, whereas the incidence of congenital infection is 1 to 7 per 1,000 births.[1] The National Center for Infectious Diseases places the annual number of cases of congenital toxoplasmosis in the U.S. at between 400 and 4,000.[18] Prevalence rates are difficult to determine because toxoplasmosis is not a reportable disease.

Mothers infected with *T. gondii* during pregnancy may be asymptomatic, although most mothers with an infected baby will recall an episode of mild flulike illness or lymphadenopathy during their pregnancy. When a pregnant woman acquires toxoplasmosis in the first trimester, her fetus has a 15 percent chance of becoming infected, with a greater likelihood of the infection being severe.[21] Infection in the third trimester results in 65 percent of offspring having a subclinical infection, with many of those infants developing chorioretinitis or neurologic sequelae.[22] The highest risk for fetal transmission and development of more severe fetal disease occurs between 10 and 24 weeks gestation.[20]

Eighty to 90 percent of neonates infected *in utero* with *T. gondii* may be asymptomatic at birth, but approximately 50 percent develop progressive chorioretinitis, and 40 percent develop central nervous system (CNS) involvement, such

INFECTION IN THE NEONATE

FIGURE 3-1 ◆ Chorioretinitis. Acute, recurrent, toxoplasmic chorioretinal inflammation adjacent to a healed pigmented lesion.

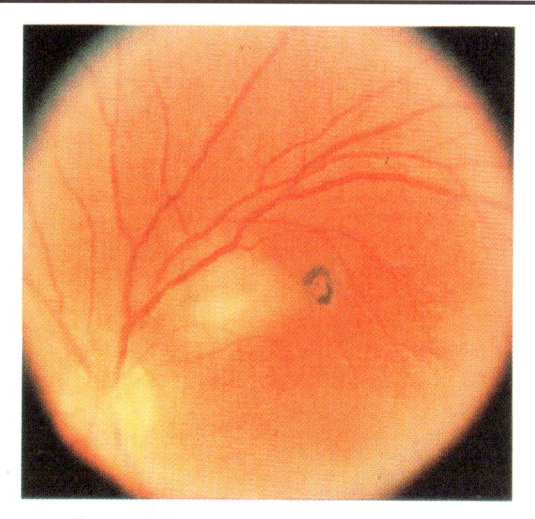

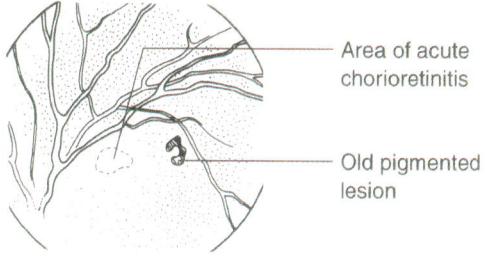

From: Cheng KP, and Biglan AW. 2002. Ophthalmology. In *Atlas of Pediatric Physical Diagnosis*, 4th ed., Zitelli BJ, and Davis HW, eds. St. Louis: Mosby-Year Book, 682. Reprinted by permission.

FIGURE 3-2 ◆ Cerebral calcifications in congenital toxoplasmosis.

CT scan performed at 3 months of age shows cerebral calcifications, both periventricular and diffuse, including involvement of thalamus (thick arrow) and basal ganglia (thin arrow). A shunt catheter (arrowhead) is in the lateral ventricle.

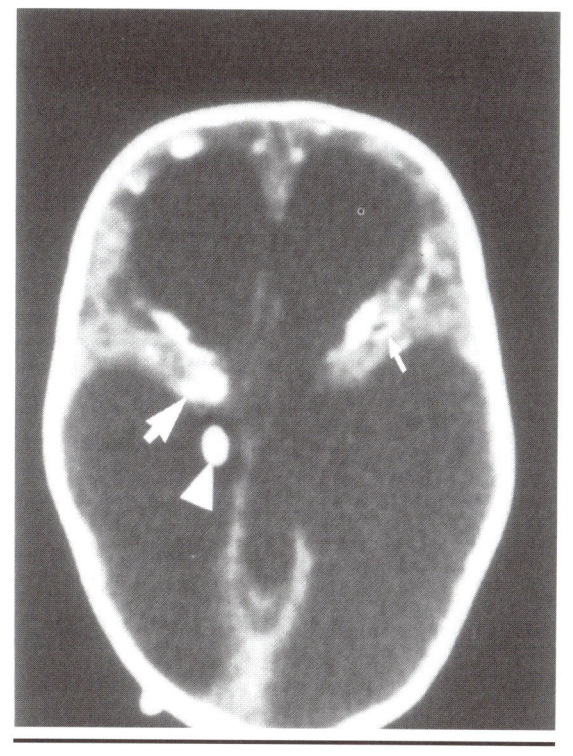

From: Volpe JJ. 1995. *Neurology of the Newborn*, 3rd ed. Philadelphia: WB Saunders, 689. Reprinted by permission.

as hydrocephalus, in the weeks and months following delivery.[20,23] In some cases, chorioretinitis may develop as late as school age or adolescence. Other neonates show severe manifestations at birth. Clinical features ascribed to *T. gondii* infection include four key findings first described by Sabin: hydrocephalus or microcephaly, chorioretinitis (Figure 3-1), seizures or other neurologic manifestations, and cerebral calcifications (Figure 3-2).[24] Subsequently, a variety of other findings has been attributed to infection with this organism. They are summarized in Table 3-2.

Diagnosis of maternal toxoplasmosis infection can be difficult because specific IgM may persist for years and thus does not necessarily reflect recent infection. The conversion of IgG from negative to positive is indicative of infection, but it is unlikely that the IgG level prior to illness would be available. A fourfold or greater increase in serum IgG levels would also be indicative of an acute infection.[1] The presence of a high level of specific IgM combined with a high IgG level indicates a probable recent infection (within the previous three months). A definitive diagnosis of congenital toxoplasmosis can be made by detecting the parasite in amniotic

TABLE 3-3 ♦ Evaluating the Newborn of a Mother Who Acquired Toxoplasmosis during Pregnancy

History and physical examination

Pediatric neurologic evaluation

Pediatric ophthalmologic examination of retinae

Complete blood cell count with differential, platelet count

Liver function tests (bilirubin, γ-glutamyltranspeptidase [GGTP])

Urinalysis, serum creatinine

Serum quantitative immunoglobulins

Serum Sabin-Feldman dye test (IgG), IgM ISAGA, IgA ELISA, IgE ISAGA/ELISA* (Note: With maternal serum, perform the same tests as for infant except substitute IgM ELISA for IgM ISAGA.)

Cerebrospinal fluid cell count, protein, glucose, and T. gondii–specific IgG and IgM antibodies, as well as quantitative IgG to calculate antibody load

Subinoculate into mice or tissue culture 1 ml peripheral blood buffy coat or clot and digest of 100 gm placenta. Consider polymerase chain reaction of buffy coat from approximately 1 ml blood, cell pellet from approximately 1 ml cerebrospinal fluid, and cell pellet from 10–20 ml amniotic fluid.

Brain computed tomography scan with and without contrast medium enhancement

Auditory brain stem response to 20 dB

*When performed in combination in laboratories, these tests have demonstrated a high degree of specificity and sensitivity in establishing the diagnosis of acute infection in the pregnant woman and congenital infection in the fetus and newborn.

From: Remington JS, et al. 2001. Toxoplasmosis. In *Infectious Diseases of the Fetus and Newborn Infant*, 5th ed., Remington JS, and Klein JO, eds. Philadelphia: WB Saunders, 276. Reprinted by permission.

fluid or fetal blood. The Sabin-Feldman dye test is commonly used for this purpose.

The presence of *T. gondii*–specific IgM, IgE, or IgA antibodies in fetal blood is also diagnostic.[25] Before 22 weeks gestation, however, the fetus does not produce IgM and IgA. PCR testing of amniotic fluid can be used to determine fetal infection. This approach is now preferred to testing for immunoglobulins because PCR is faster and more accurate.[26,27]

A detailed sonogram is also helpful in identifying evidence of intrauterine infection.[26] Positive findings include hydrocephalus, microcephaly, intracranial or hepatic calcifications, ascites, hydrops, or placental thickening. Ultrasound findings are present in 30–40 percent of fetuses with congenital *T. gondii* infection.[13]

Diagnosis of neonatal *T. gondii* infection is confirmed by the presence of specific IgM in the cord or neonate's blood. The presence of IgG is likely to reflect maternal antibodies and does not distinguish between an acute and a previous infection. It is also possible to culture the protozoan parasite from the neonate's blood or the placenta. Enzyme-linked immunosorbent assay (ELISA) can detect *T. gondii*–specific IgM, IgA, and IgE and is complemented by immunosorbent agglutination assay (ISAGA) testing. PCR can quickly and accurately identify genetic material from *T. gondii* in the neonate.[20] As PCR becomes more readily available, it will likely replace many of the current diagnostic tests.

Clinically, a cerebral ultrasound is useful to look for ventriculomegaly, and a computerized tomography (CT) scan may be helpful in evaluating for the presence of cerebral calcifications. A pediatric ophthalmologist should perform a complete eye exam, and an examination by a neurologist may be indicated in the presence of CNS findings. Table 3-3 summarizes recommended testing for newborns whose mothers acquired toxoplasmosis during pregnancy.

The diagnosis of toxoplasmosis infection in the first trimester of pregnancy presents several dilemmas for the practitioner. In Europe, spiramycin has been used for a number of years to prevent vertical transmission of toxoplasmosis.[13] In the U.S., this drug is available only by request to the Food and Drug Administration.[20] The use of spiramycin for documented maternal seroconversion in the first trimester of pregnancy is recommended.[20]

Because of the risk of severe disease in the fetus, some clinicians recommend termination of pregnancy for fetuses with first-trimester infections.[20]

Into the second and third trimesters, treatment includes maternal administration of pyrimethamine and sulfadiazine.[28] Maternal treatment remains controversial. A systematic review of the efficacy of treatment concluded that evidence to support treatment during pregnancy was weak.[29] Another study, by Foulon and colleagues, suggests that treatment of acute infection in pregnancy has no impact on maternal-fetal transmission but does reduce the sequelae among infected infants.[30]

Treatment for neonates with congenital toxoplasmosis consists of three or four 21-day courses of pyrimethamine and sulfadiazine alternated with 30- to 45-day courses of spiramycin.* Leucovorin (folinic acid) is needed to counteract the antifolate effects of pyrimethamine.[1] McAuley and colleagues also report good long-term outcomes with a one-year course of pyrimethamine and sulfadiazine.[31] Villena and colleagues extended treatment with pyrimethamine and sulfadiazine to 24 months and found fewer sequelae in the 24-month treatment group than in a group that received only 12 months of treatment. No adverse treatment effects were reported.[32]

The prognosis for untreated congenital toxoplasmosis is poor. In a 1980 study of 24 infants diagnosed with congenital toxoplasmosis, 85 percent developed chorioretinitis, including eight who had unilateral or bilateral functional blindness; and 13 infants had neurologic sequelae, which included hydrocephalus, microcephaly, seizures, and psychomotor dysfunction.[33]

Findings of intracranial calcifications are thought to be particularly ominous according to some authors.[20,34] Dunn and colleagues suggest, however, that most children with intracranial calcifications have normal neurodevelopmental outcomes, with spontaneous resolution of the calcifications. In Dunn and colleagues' review of 603 confirmed maternal toxoplasmosis infections, up to 80 percent of the offspring with congenital toxoplasmosis did have retinal lesions.[35]

The prognosis for those toxoplasmosis-positive infants who receive appropriate treatment is less clear. Preliminary results of a large national prospective study done by a collaborative group based in Chicago indicate that, in 104 children evaluated to date, transient neutropenia is the only adverse drug reaction noted and that all signs of active infection resolved within weeks of initiating treatment.[36] Chorioretinitis did not progress during treatment; however, new lesions did appear in some older children following treatment. Loss of visual acuity remains one of the two most common complications of toxoplasmosis infection.[37] In the Chicago study, 4 of 34 treated infants developed generalized seizures and 8 were identified as having motor or tone impairment.[38,39]

Cytomegalovirus

CMV, an enveloped DNA virus, is a member of the Herpesviridae family. Like other herpesviruses, CMV has the potential for reactivation following a primary infection. Humans are believed to be the only reservoir for CMV.[40] With CMV, infected cells are typically enlarged and contain characteristic intranuclear and cytoplasmic inclusions. CMV infection is sometimes called cytomegalic inclusion disease because of the appearance of these inclusions within infected cells.

CMV infection is common in children, and the percentage of the population with antibodies to CMV increases with increasing age.[40] The prevalence of CMV in the general population varies widely across countries and geographic regions. In some countries in Africa and the South Pacific, the rate of seropositivity approaches 100 percent. In the U.S., seropositivity

---

* Spiramycin (Rovamycine [Rhone-Poulenc Rorer]) is available only as an investigational drug in the United States. It may be obtained from the manufacturer with authorization from the U.S. FDA, Division of Special Pathogens and Immunologic Drug Products; telephone: 301-827-2127; FAX: 301-827-2475.

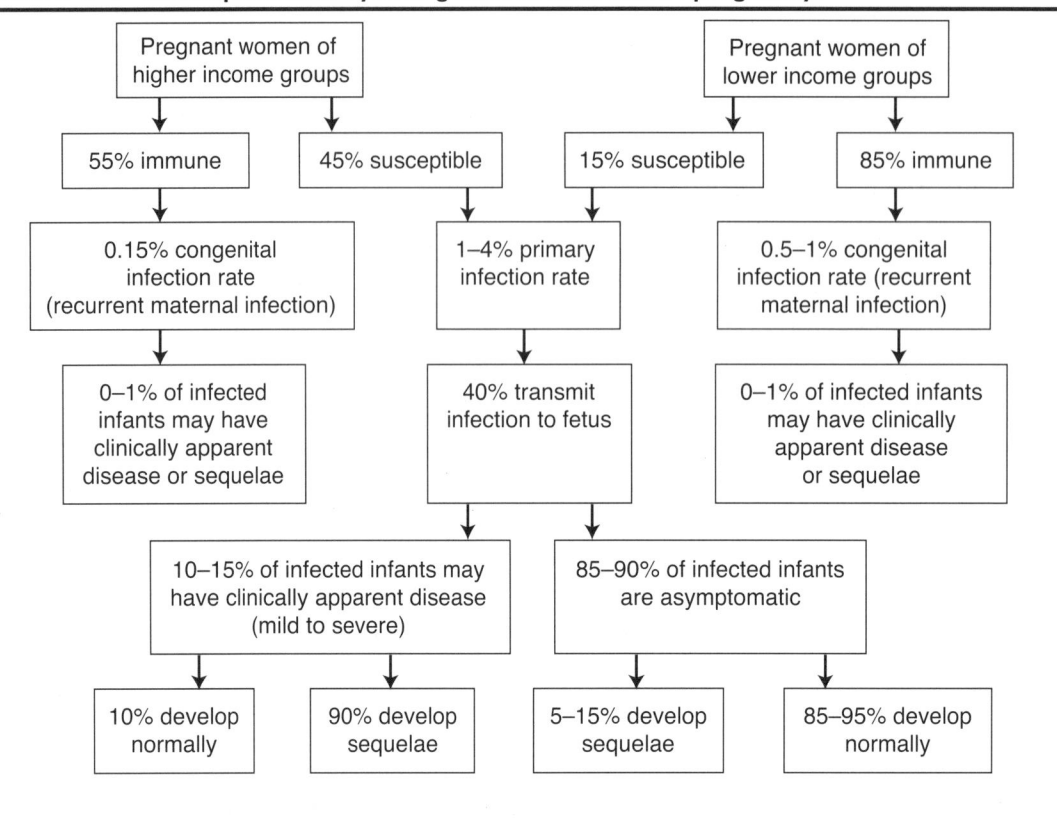

FIGURE 3-3 ◆ Consequences of cytomegalovirus infection in pregnancy.

```
        Pregnant women of                              Pregnant women of
        higher income groups                           lower income groups
         ↓              ↓                              ↓              ↓
    55% immune     45% susceptible              15% susceptible    85% immune
         ↓              ↓                              ↓              ↓
   0.15% congenital   1-4% primary                                0.5-1% congenital
   infection rate    infection rate                               infection rate (recurrent
   (recurrent maternal infection)                                 maternal infection)
         ↓              ↓                                             ↓
   0-1% of infected   40% transmit                                0-1% of infected infants
   infants may have   infection to fetus                          may have clinically
   clinically apparent                                            apparent disease
   disease or sequelae                                            or sequelae
                          ↓
            10-15% of infected infants may        85-90% of infected infants
            have clinically apparent disease      are asymptomatic
            (mild to severe)
              ↓              ↓                       ↓              ↓
         10% develop    90% develop            5-15% develop    85-95% develop
         normally       sequelae               sequelae         normally
```

From: Stagno S. 2001. Cytomegalovirus. In *Infectious Diseases of the Fetus and Newborn Infant,* 5th ed., Remington JS, and Klein JO, eds. Philadelphia: WB Saunders, 397. Reprinted by permission.

rates range from 50 to 85 percent. CMV is the most common congenital infection in developed countries. Primary infection occurs in about 2 percent of middle- to upper-socioeconomic class women of childbearing age per year and in up to 6 percent of women of lower socioeconomic status.[40] Estimates place the incidence of congenital CMV infection in the U.S. at between 0.2 and 2.2 percent of newborns.[40,41] Primary maternal infections carry a greater risk for severe congenital infection than do reactivations of previous infections, but reactivations may also cause fetal disease.[42,43] Boppana and associates found that, of 47 infants with symptomatic congenital CMV, 8 were born to mothers with a confirmed recurrent CMV infection. In 20 of the 47 infants, the type of maternal CMV infection (primary or recurrent) could not be determined.[44] Congenital CMV infection in the offspring of previously immune women appears to be a phenomenon that is unique to CMV. Figure 3-3 outlines the consequences of CMV infection in pregnancy.

CMV has been isolated from cervical secretions, semen, saliva, blood, breast milk, and urine. It can be transmitted through sexual contact or kissing or through contact with infected secretions such as urine. In adults, CMV infection is often asymptomatic. When symptoms are present, they usually take the form of a mononucleosis-like illness with prolonged fever and mild hepatitis.[25] The virus can cross the placenta and infect the fetus. Following delivery, neonates may acquire CMV infection

FIGURE 3-4 ◆ Infant with cytomegalovirus infection.

Note the typical purpuric rash (blueberry muffin) that results from thrombocytopenia.

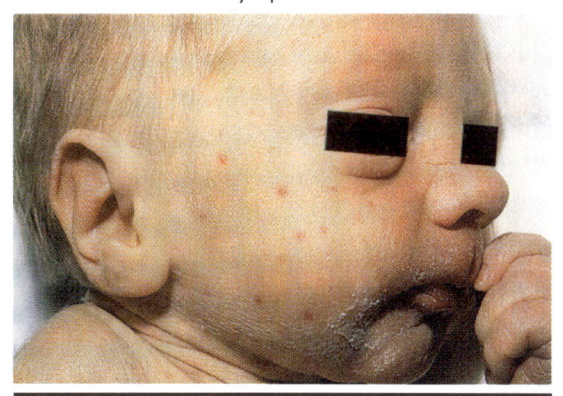

From: Baselga E. 2001. Inflammatory and purpuric eruptions. In *Textbook of Neonatal Dermatology*, Eichenfield LF, Frieden IJ, and Esterly NB, eds. Philadelphia: WB Saunders, 313. Reprinted by permission.

TABLE 3-4 ◆ Clinical Manifestations of Congenital Cytomegalovirus Infection

Chorioretinitis
Deafness
Hepatosplenomegaly
Intrauterine growth restriction
Jaundice
Microcephaly
Periventricular calcifications
Petechiae
Pneumonitis
Prematurity
Purpura (blueberry muffin syndrome)
Seizures
Thrombocytopenia

Adapted from: Isaacs D, and Moxon ER. 1999. *Handbook of Neonatal Infections: A Practical Guide*. London: WB Saunders, 378–388; and Stagno S. 2001. Cytomegalovirus. In *Infectious Diseases of the Fetus and Newborn Infant*, 5th ed., Remington JS, and Klein JO, eds. Philadelphia: WB Saunders, 389–424.

through blood transfusions or by ingesting CMV-positive breast milk.

Unlike viruses that affect developing tissue, CMV can damage organs that have already formed. This means the virus can affect fetal development beyond the first trimester, although earlier infections are usually more severe.[45] Congenital infections are generally (90–95 percent) asymptomatic at birth.[46] But evidence of hearing deficits or learning disabilities may appear in early childhood in as many as 5 to 15 percent of affected infants.[4] Newborn findings of severe CMV disease include the typical purpuric rash that results from thrombocytopenia (Figure 3-4), intrauterine growth restriction, jaundice, hepatosplenomegaly, microcephaly, periventricular calcifications, and chorioretinitis (10–15 percent).[1] Table 3-4 summarizes these and other clinical manifestations. Pneumonitis, appearing at one to four months of age, has been described as a late complication of congenital CMV infection.[47,48] Deafness may be present from birth, usually in infants with other manifestations of the disease, or it may develop as late as five years of age in children who were asymptomatic at birth. Fluctuations in hearing loss in neonates with congenital CMV have been reported and highlight the need for careful ongoing hearing assessment in these children.[49] The incidence of hearing loss in symptomatic congenital CMV infection is reported as being up to 58 percent, and about 6–7.4 percent in those infants who are asymptomatic at birth.[40,46,50]

The diagnosis of CMV is made more difficult because of the ubiquity of the virus, the high prevalence of asymptomatic shedding of virus, and the ability of CMV infection to become reactivated. Recovery of the virus from body fluids or tissues is diagnostic, as is a fourfold rise in CMV antibody titers from paired serum samples collected 4 weeks apart.[25] Culture and PCR testing of amniotic fluid have been shown to have a sensitivity of 80–100 percent when the fluid is tested after 20 weeks gestation.[51] A study by Lazzarotto and colleagues suggests that the detection of 103 genome equivalents of CMV

DNA in amniotic fluid is 100 percent predictive of an infected fetus.[52]

CMV infections should be suspected in the presence of ultrasound abnormalities such as ventriculomegaly, intracranial calcifications, echogenic bowel, microcephaly, hepatosplenomegaly, and signs of hydrops in the fetus.[53] The gold standard for diagnosing congenital CMV infection in neonates is viral culture of the urine in the first week of life.[1] Radio immunoassays and ELISA tests of cord blood or the neonate's blood for CMV-specific IgM may also be used to make the diagnosis of congenital infection. Beyond one to two weeks of life, the potential for postnatal acquisition of CMV infection makes positive cultures less significant in the diagnosis of congenital infection.

Ganciclovir is used to treat the chorioretinitis caused by CMV in adults, but limited data are available about its use in infants and children. The drug has been used to treat congenitally infected infants, but is not routinely recommended because of limited data regarding its efficacy.[25] An evaluation of ganciclovir treatment of symptomatic congenital CMV found that 37 of the 47 infants receiving the drug developed significant hematologic abnormalities, such as thrombocytopenia and neutropenia. The researchers did find, however, that infants receiving treatment evidenced hearing improvement or stabilization at six months of age.[54]

It is estimated that, in general, about 10–20 percent of infants with congenital CMV will have major neurodevelopmental sequelae.[25] These include deafness, visual impairment resulting from chorioretinitis or optic nerve atrophy, mental retardation, and spastic quadriplegia. The mortality rate in symptomatic congenital CMV is about 30 percent; 90 percent of survivors have neurodevelopmental sequelae.[53,55] Microcephaly and intracranial calcifications are associated with significant neurodevelopmental impairment in more than 80 percent of cases.[55] Computerized tomography may be useful in predicting adverse neurodevelopmental outcomes in symptomatic infants. Boppana and colleagues reported data from 56 infants with symptomatic congenital CMV and found that 90 percent of infants with an abnormal CT (n = 39) scan developed at least one neurodevelopmental sequela, compared with 29 percent (n = 17) of infants with a normal scan.[56]

Rubella

Rubella is an RNA member of the Togaviridae, or togavirus, family. Humans are the only source of this infection, and the virus is transmitted by direct or droplet contact with nasopharyngeal secretions. Infected persons are most contagious a few days before and up to seven days after the onset of the rash. Neonates with congenital rubella have been shown to shed virus in their nasopharyngeal secretions and urine for one year or longer.[25] Rubella outbreaks tend to peak in late winter and early spring. Immunity is conferred through natural infection or by vaccine, but reinfections have been reported.[25]

Since the introduction of the rubella vaccine in the late 1960s, the incidence of the disease has decreased by 99 percent in the U.S. Despite the U.S. government's mandate to eliminate indigenous rubella by the year 2000, however, outbreaks still occur among unimmunized young adults at colleges or in work settings.[57] Many of these outbreaks involve immigrants from countries such as Mexico and those in Central America that do not have or only recently introduced a rubella vaccination program.[58] Serologic surveys suggest that about 10 percent of young adults are susceptible to rubella.[25] Between 1997 and 1999, 26 cases of congenital rubella syndrome (CRS) were reported in the U.S., 92 percent in infants of foreign-born mothers.[58]

Adult Infection

Rubella is asymptomatic in 25–50 percent of older children and adults.[58] Prodromal

INFECTION IN THE NEONATE

FIGURE 3-5 ◆ Cataracts in congenital rubella.

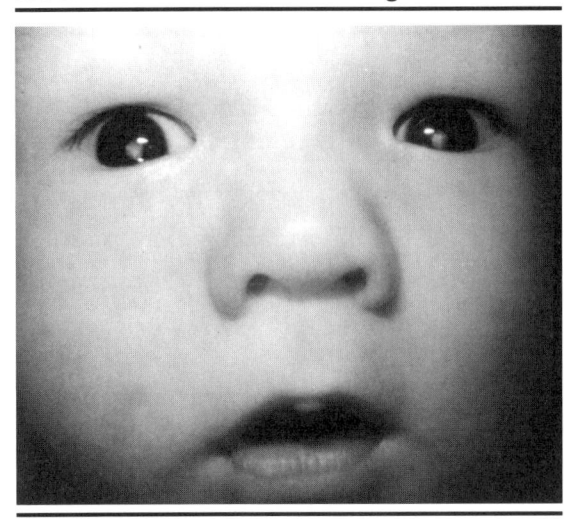

Courtesy of Dr. David A. Clark, Albany Medical Center, Albany, New York. Reprinted by permission.

symptoms, which appear one to five days before the rash develops, include fever, headache, lymphadenopathy, eye discomfort and conjunctivitis, and loss of appetite. Arthralgia and arthritis occur in some adults and adolescent females. Rare complications include thrombocytopenic purpura, encephalitis, neuritis, and orchitis.[58]

In adults, rubella can be diagnosed by isolating virus from nasopharyngeal secretions. Appropriate cell cultures and specific laboratory testing are needed to identify the rubella virus. A fourfold or greater increase in serum antibodies between acute and convalescent titers (or seroconversion) is also diagnostic of infection. Where available, reverse-transcriptase PCR (RT-PCR) assays have been shown to be of use in detecting rubella virus.[59] Diagnosis of congenital rubella is made by isolating virus from throat swabs, blood, urine, or cerebrospinal fluid (CSF).

When a pregnant woman is exposed to rubella, she should be tested as soon as possible to determine her immune status. If no antibody is detected, she should be rescreened in two to three weeks and, if still negative, again at six weeks after exposure to determine if seroconversion has occurred.

In Utero *Transmission*

Rubella can be transmitted *in utero* during the course of maternal primary infection or, theoretically, following maternal immunization for rubella if the immunization is given in the three months preceding pregnancy.[25] The gestational age of the fetus is the primary mediating factor in intrauterine infection. The risk of congenital infection decreases with increasing gestational age; fetal infection is rare beyond the second trimester. If the maternal infection occurs during the first trimester of pregnancy, however, the fetal infection rate is 40–90 percent.[60]

Congenital rubella syndrome encompasses a spectrum that ranges from miscarriage, stillbirth, or birth defects to asymptomatic infection.[58,61] Congenital anomalies associated with CRS include cataracts (Figure 3-5), hearing impairment, and congenital heart disease (most commonly, patent ductus arteriosus or peripheral pulmonic stenosis). Additional findings include chorioretinitis, microphthalmia, purpura, hepatosplenomegaly, jaundice, microcephaly, and radiolucent bone disease (Figure 3-6) (Table 3-5). Developmental delays and mental deficits are common in survivors of CRS.[58] Late-onset manifestations are many and include hearing and language deficits, autism and psychiatric problems, diabetes (20 percent), precocious puberty, thyroid problems (5 percent), visual problems, and hypertension.[60]

The prognosis for CRS depends on the extent of the permanent organ damage that has occurred. Significant permanent damage is found in about 50 percent of infants with maternal infection during the first two months of pregnancy, in 36 percent of those whose mothers were infected at 9–12 weeks gestation, and in 10 percent of those whose mothers were infected at 13–20 weeks.[60,62]

Prevention of congenital rubella is aimed at ensuring that susceptible women are immunized. All postpubertal women without

FIGURE 3-6 ◆ Bone findings in congenital rubella.

Note widespread metaphyseal streaking, best seen in the distal femurs. The radiolucent streaks are vertically arranged, producing the so-called celery stalk appearance.

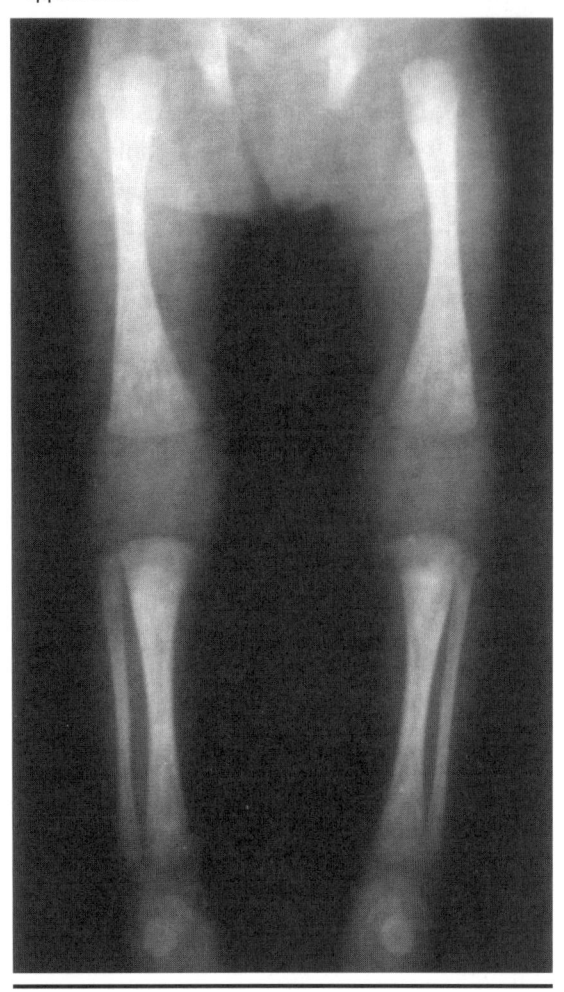

From: Swischuk LE. 1997. *Imaging of the Newborn, Infant, and Young Child*, 4th ed. Philadelphia: Lippincott Williams & Wilkins, 739. Reprinted by permission.

TABLE 3-5 ◆ Clinical Manifestations of Congenital Rubella

Miscarriage
Stillbirth
Anemia
Bone radiolucencies
Cataracts,* chorioretinitis, microphthalmia, glaucoma
Congenital heart defects: patent ductus arteriosus, pulmonary artery stenosis, coarctation of the aorta, pulmonary arterial hypoplasia
Encephalitis
Hepatosplenomegaly*
Intrauterine growth restriction*
Jaundice
Microcephaly
Pneumonitis
Purpura (blueberry muffin syndrome)
Sensorineural hearing loss*
Thrombocytopenia

* Most common

Adapted from: Cooper LZ, and Alford CA. 2001. Rubella. In *Infectious Diseases of the Fetus and Newborn Infant*, 5th ed., Remington JS, and Klein JO, eds. Philadelphia: WB Saunders, 347–388.

evidence of rubella immunity should be immunized unless they are known to be pregnant. Women should be advised not to become pregnant for three months after immunization.[25]

Treponema Pallidum

Treponema pallidum, the Gram-negative spirochete responsible for syphilis, is one of the few bacteria that readily cross the placenta, causing fetal infection. The number of primary and secondary cases of syphilis reported in the U.S. in 2000 was 5,979, down 9.6 percent from the preceding year. The reported rate of congenital syphilis for the year 2000 was 13.4 cases per 100,000 live births.[63]

In adults, syphilis may present in one of several stages: primary, secondary, latent, or tertiary. Primary syphilis presents with genital ulceration (usually a single painless ulcer lasting up to six weeks) and localized lymphadenopathy. Primary syphilis may go unnoticed because of the vague nature of the symptoms. When primary syphilis is untreated, secondary syphilis will follow, sometimes as long as two years after the initial infection. The secondary stage is manifested by a rash, present in 90 percent of cases, usually on the soles and palms.[22] The rash may be macular, papular, pustular, or nonspecific

(Figure 3-7). Other findings include fever, malaise, weight loss, hair loss, mouth or throat lesions, and condylomata in the perineal area.

Following untreated secondary syphilis, patients often enter a period of latency when the disease resolves but viable organisms remain present in the body. Tertiary syphilis is marked by involvement of the cardiovascular or central nervous system.

The mode of transmission of syphilis in adults is sexual. The infant is usually infected *in utero* by transplacental infection, but infection of the amniotic fluid may also occur.[64] The risk to the fetus and neonate varies according to the stage of maternal infection, but it is generally recognized that untreated maternal disease poses a significant risk of stillbirth (12 percent) and of live births with congenital infection (29 percent).[65] Prompt maternal treatment eliminates most fetal infections, but delayed treatment or failure to obtain treatment may result in fetal effects that range from minor anomalies to preterm birth or fetal death. Damage to the fetus depends on when in gestation the infection occurs and the time that elapses before treatment. Silent infection may be present in the neonate at birth, but may not be expressed for up to two years.[25]

FIGURE 3-7 ◆ Secondary syphilis.

Ham-colored palmar macules on palms of hands of adolescent with secondary syphilis.

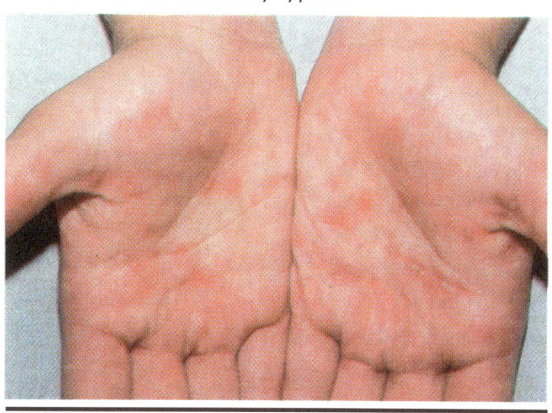

From: Weston WL, and Lane AT. 1991. *Color Textbook of Pediatric Dermatology.* St. Louis: Mosby-Year Book, 51. Reprinted by permission.

Congenital syphilis may result in prematurity, hydrops fetalis, and failure to thrive. Hepatosplenomegaly is common, as is lymphadenopathy. Hematologic findings include anemia, leukopenia, and thrombocytopenia. Characteristic bony lesions occur in the long bones, cranium, and spine and include osteochondritis, osteomyelitis, and periostitis.[64] Other findings include snuffles, mucocutaneous lesions, edema, and rash (Figure 3-8).[25] Some

FIGURE 3-8 ◆ Congenital syphilis rash.

Papulosquamous plaques in two infants with syphilis.

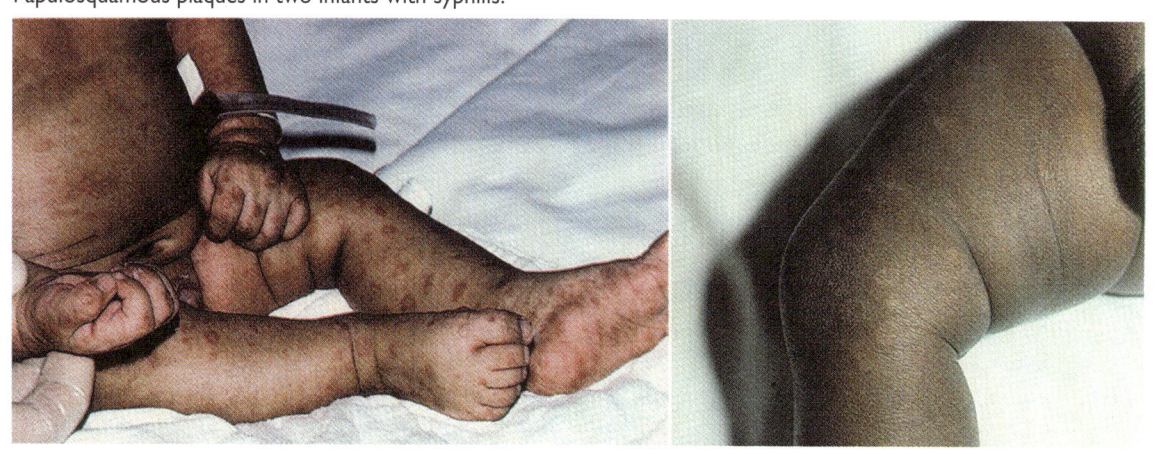

From: Darmstadt GL, and Dinulos JG. 2001. Bacterial infections. In *Textbook of Neonatal Dermatology,* Eichenfield LF, Frieden IJ, and Esterly NB, eds. Philadelphia: WB Saunders, 196. Reprinted by permission.

TABLE 3-6 ◆ Clinical Manifestations of Congenital Syphilis

Early-onset Disease
Anemia, leukopenia, thrombocytopenia
Edema
Failure to thrive
Hepatosplenomegaly
Hydrops fetalis
Lymphadenopathy
Maculopapular rash
Mucocutaneous lesions
Prematurity
Skeletal abnormalities: osteochondritis, osteomyelitis, periostitis
Snuffles

Late-onset Disease
Bowing of shins
Deafness
Frontal bossing
Keratitis
Mulberry molars
Rhagades
Saddle nose

manifestations of congenital syphilis may not appear for many years. These include interstitial keratitis, deafness, bowing of the shins, saddle nose, rhagades, frontal bossing, and mulberry molars. Untreated infants may develop late manifestations (after two years of age) that involve the CNS, bones and joints, teeth, eyes, and skin (Table 3-6).[25]

The diagnosis of *T. pallidum* infection is made by microscopic dark field examination or fluorescent antibody tests of lesions or tissue such as the placenta.[25] False-negative results may occur with these tests, and follow-up serologic testing should be done. Venereal Disease Research Laboratories (VDRL) slides and rapid plasma reagin (RPR) tests can be done quickly, but have higher false-negative results than do specific treponemal tests.[25] All infants born to seropositive mothers should have treponemal and nontreponemal testing of their blood and CSF, as well as long-bone x-rays.

The treatment of choice for syphilis is penicillin G. Neonates should be treated if they have proved or probable disease based on physical findings or serologic testing. Asymptomatic infants born to positive mothers who received adequate treatment for more than four weeks before delivery are at minimal risk of disease and may be monitored or treated with a single dose of penicillin.[25] Figure 3-9 displays an algorithm for treating infants born to a mother with syphilis.

Herpes Simplex

As does CMV, the herpes simplex virus, a DNA virus, belongs to the Herpesviridae family. This family of microorganisms also includes the Epstein-Barr and varicella-zoster viruses. There are two types of herpes simplex viruses: Type 1 is usually associated with oral lesions and type 2, with genital lesions, although increasing numbers of genital infections are caused by type 1 herpes.[25] HSV-1 infection is common in childhood, with about 90 percent of the population seropositive by age 40.[22] HSV-2 infections are less common, with young adults most likely to be infected. Ten to 40 percent of the U.S. population is seropositive for HSV-2.[22] HSV-2 is considered to be a sexually transmitted disease.

The incubation period for HSV infection is about one week following exposure. Transmission is most likely with active ulcerations of the mucous membranes, but asymptomatic viral shedding also occurs. Oral HSV infections present with vesicle development in the pharynx, tongue, oral mucosa, or lips. Fever, malaise, and cervical lymphadenopathy may accompany a severe outbreak. Lesions resolve without treatment in one to two weeks.

In males with genital herpes, vesicular lesions occur on the penile shaft or glans; in females, lesions occur in a variety of areas, including the cervix, vagina, vulva, and perineum. Fever and inguinal lymphedema may accompany primary infections. Lesions may persist for

FIGURE 3-9 ◆ Algorithm for treating an infant born to a mother with syphilis.

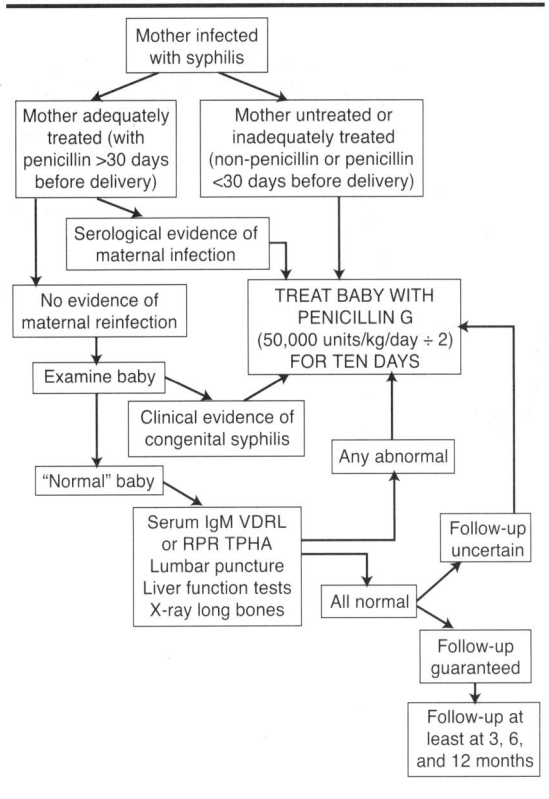

```
                    Mother infected
                    with syphilis
                    /            \
     Mother adequately      Mother untreated or
     treated (with          inadequately treated
     penicillin >30 days    (non-penicillin or penicillin
     before delivery)       <30 days before delivery)
            |                       |
     Serological evidence of
     maternal infection
       /         \
  No evidence of   TREAT BABY WITH
  maternal         PENICILLIN G
  reinfection      (50,000 units/kg/day ÷ 2)
       |           FOR TEN DAYS
  Examine baby
       |       \
       |        Clinical evidence of
       |        congenital syphilis      Any abnormal
       |                                       |
  "Normal" baby                                 |
              \                                 |
               Serum IgM VDRL                   Follow-up
               or RPR TPHA                      uncertain
               Lumbar puncture
               Liver function tests    All normal
               X-ray long bones            |
                                     Follow-up
                                     guaranteed
                                          |
                                    Follow-up at
                                    least at 3, 6,
                                    and 12 months
```

From: Isaacs D, and Moxon ER. 1999. *Handbook of Neonatal Infections: A Practical Guide.* London: WB Saunders, 396. Reprinted by permission.

weeks before crusting over and healing. Recurrent infections are common in both sexes. A prodromal sensation of burning may precede recurrent outbreaks.

Approximately 0.09–0.4 percent of all asymptomatic pregnant women have positive HSV cultures at the time of delivery.[66] The incidence of neonatal herpes simplex infection ranges from 1 per 3,000 to 1 per 20,000 live births.[25] When a mother with a primary infection delivers vaginally, the risk of HSV infection in the neonate is 33–50 percent.[25,66,67] During a reactivated infection, the risk falls to 0–5 percent.[25,68] In more than 75 percent of cases of neonatal HSV infection, the mother has no history or symptoms of infection at the time of delivery.[25] However, serologic testing reveals evidence of the herpes virus.[69]

Most infants contract HSV infection through contact with infected secretions at birth (86 percent of infections). Prolonged rupture of membranes is a risk factor in the presence of active genital lesions. The risk of transmission is decreased if delivery is by cesarean section or if the mother's infection is recurrent rather than primary. Neonatal infections can be severe or fatal. They can be caused by HSV-1 or HSV-2, although HSV-2 is the more common cause of neonatal infection, representing 70–85 percent of cases.[70]

Congenital HSV infections, occurring early in pregnancy, comprise about 4 percent of all neonatal HSV infections.[71] These cases are associated with increased rates of abortion, intrauterine growth restriction, and premature delivery.[72–74] Fetal findings include microcephaly, hydranencephaly, cerebral atrophy, chorioretinitis, microphthalmia, and vesicular skin lesions (Table 3-7).[75] Risk factors associated with intrauterine transmission have not been identified.[67]

Unlike in older children and adults, herpes simplex infections acquired at birth are almost always symptomatic.[55,76,77] HSV infection presents in the first four weeks of life, with two-thirds of cases seen in the first week of life and one-quarter to one-third in the first day of life.[75] Neonatal HSV infection presents in one of three ways (see Table 3-7):

1. **Skin, eye, and mouth (SEM) disease** (40–45 percent of cases). Lesions usually appear in the first ten days after birth, with varying degrees of severity (Figures 3-10 and 3-11). The presenting part is often the site at which skin lesions appear. The presence of a scalp injury provides a portal of entry for the herpes virus.[78] Skin vesicles erupt from an erythematous base, with new lesions forming adjacent to and often coalescing into a larger

TABLE 3-7 ◆ Clinical Manifestations of Congenital Herpes Simplex Infection

Intrauterine Infection (4%)
Chorioretinitis
Hydranencephaly
Keratoconjunctivitis
Microcephaly
Skin vesicles or scarring

SEM Disease
Vesicular lesions involving the skin, eyes, or mucous membranes of the mouth

CNS Disease
Bulging fontanel
Irritability
Lethargy
Poor feeding
Poor tone
Seizures

Disseminated Disease
Bleeding disorders
Elevated liver enzymes
Irritability
Jaundice
Respiratory distress
Seizures
Shock

Adapted from: Kohl S. 1997. Neonatal herpes simplex virus infection. *Clinics in Perinatology* 24(1): 129–150.

FIGURE 3-10 ◆ Neonatal herpes simplex virus.

Cluster of vesicles on the forehead and periocular area.

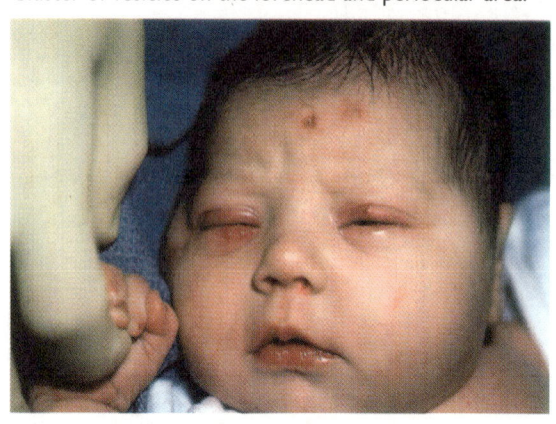

From: Friedlander SF, and Bradley JS. 2001. Viral infections. In *Textbook of Neonatal Dermatology*, Eichenfield LF, Frieden IJ, and Esterly NB, eds. Philadelphia: WB Saunders, 204. Reprinted by permission.

vesicle. For infants with disease limited to the skin, eyes, or mouth, the prognosis is relatively good, with survival approaching 100 percent with treatment. Skin lesions recur over a period of months to years in most infants with vesicles. Neurologic sequelae develop between six months and one year of age in about 5 percent of SEM cases.[79] Without treatment, up to 75 percent of infants who present with SEM disease develop disseminated disease.[71]

2. **CNS disease** (35 percent of cases). For infants with CNS involvement, encephalitis is the only initial manifestation of HSV infection. The signs of CNS disease may be quite nonspecific and typically occur more than a week after birth. Seizures occur as the presenting symptom in 50 percent of infants.[74] Skin lesions are also present in about 50 percent of infants with CNS disease. Herpes should be considered in the differential diagnosis of any infant with suspected sepsis, especially in those who do not respond to antibiotic therapy or who present with unexplained thrombocytopenia, elevated liver function tests, or disseminated intravascular coagulation. Pleocytosis also raises the likelihood of herpes meningitis.[75] With treatment, 85 percent of infants with CNS disease survive, but the morbidity rate is about 65 percent, with sequelae including hydrocephalus, microcephaly, blindness, porencephalic cysts, and developmental delays.[74]

3. **Disseminated disease** (20–25 percent of cases). As the name implies, disseminated disease involves multiple organs, especially the lungs, adrenal glands, and liver.[80] Skin lesions are usually absent in disseminated disease, and initial symptoms may be nonspecific. HSV infection should always be considered in neonates presenting with isolated

FIGURE 3-11 ◆ Neonatal herpes simplex virus.

Multiple vesicles and crusted papules on an erythematous base in the periumbilical area and left flank.

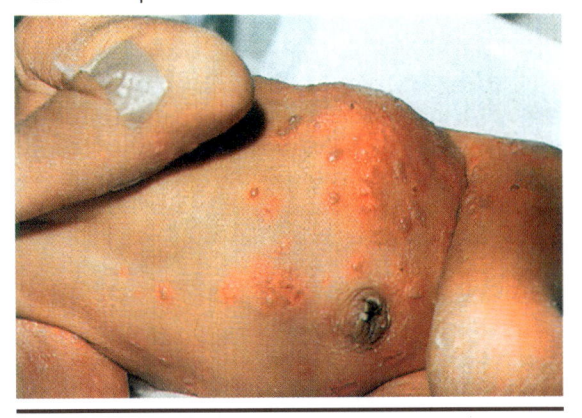

From: Friedlander SF, and Bradley JS. 2001. Viral infections. In *Textbook of Neonatal Dermatology*, Eichenfield LF, Frieden IJ, and Esterly NB, eds. Philadelphia: WB Saunders, 205. Reprinted by permission.

fulminant hepatitis.[70,81] The onset of illness may be as soon as 24 hours after birth, although most infants appear well at delivery.[67] Infants with disseminated disease deteriorate rapidly. Even with treatment, the mortality rate is 50 percent, and 41 percent of survivors have severe neurologic sequelae.[74]

Postnatal acquisition of HSV accounts for about 10 percent of neonatal HSV infection.[71] Herpes virus can be transmitted to the neonate from family members or care providers who have active orolabial lesions. Transmission from an infected neonate to another infant via fomites or the hands of caregivers also occurs.

Herpes infection can be diagnosed by culturing viral material from a lesion. Although culture is the gold standard for diagnosing infection, its efficacy is limited by the duration of viral shedding, which can be several days less than the duration of the lesion itself.[82,83] Staining of material from a lesion can also be done with Giemsa stain (Tzanck smear), although the sensitivity of this test is only 65 percent.[84,85] Many commercial serologic assays cannot distinguish between HSV-1 and HSV-2.[86] These therefore are of limited benefit. Of the available serologic tests, PCR appears to be the most sensitive.[22] It is particularly useful when examining CSF for evidence of HSV meningitis.[25] PCR testing is more sensitive for asymptomatic shedding than are the other approaches.[87] But it is not widely available for testing specimens other than CSF, except on a research basis.[70,88] Enzyme immunoassay methods can be used to detect viral antigens, allowing a presumptive diagnosis to be made pending culture results. In neonates, cultures can be obtained from skin vesicles, eyes, nasopharynx, urine, stool, and CSF. Positive cultures obtained beyond 48 hours of age suggest infection rather than colonization.[25,70]

Herpes simplex should be aggressively treated with the antiviral agent acyclovir. Acyclovir is preferred to other antiviral agents, such as vidarabine, because it has a lower toxicity and is easier to administer. The recommended dose of acyclovir in neonates is 20–30 mg/kg/day.[70,89] Duration of therapy is not well established, but the range is 14 to 21 days. The dose for infants is controversial, however, with some experts recommending higher doses (45–60 mg/kg/day) for critically ill infants.[25] A study by Kimberlin and colleagues supports the use of higher doses of acyclovir to treat CNS and disseminated disease in neonates. These researchers found that survival rates were significantly higher for neonates treated with high-dose acyclovir than with standard dosing, particularly in infants with disseminated disease.[90] Infants with ocular involvement are treated with topical ophthalmic drugs in addition to systemic antiviral agents.

One of the key elements in preventing dissemination of neonatal HSV infection is reducing the interval between clinical presentation and initiation of therapy.[90] This requires that care providers maintain a high index of suspicion with acutely ill neonates. A 1988 study by Whitley and associates found that the average time from disease onset to diagnosis was four to five days.[79] A review by Kimberlin and colleagues published in 2001, suggests that little progress has been made in the past ten years in shortening the interval between onset of HSV symptoms and initiation of antiviral treatment.[91]

Varicella-Zoster Virus

Varicella-zoster virus, a DNA virus from the Herpesviridae family, is the causative agent of chickenpox and shingles. Chickenpox (varicella) is a primary infection, whereas shingles represents a reactivation of the virus, which lies dormant in the dorsal root ganglia. Varicella is primarily a disease of childhood, with less than 5 percent of the 3.5 million cases occurring in adults of childbearing age.[92] The incidence of varicella in pregnancy is estimated to be about 0.7 cases per 1,000 pregnancies.[93]

Varicella is highly infectious, with infection occurring in 90 percent of susceptible contacts.[53] The virus is spread through contact with respiratory droplets, with an incubation period following contact of 14 days. The patient is infectious for 2 days before the rash develops and remains so until the lesions crust over. Despite the relatively low incidence of varicella in adults, adult cases account for 55 percent of the deaths attributed to the disease.[92] Varicella in pregnancy is associated with maternal pneumonia and encephalitis.

Transmission of VZV from mother to fetus occurs via infection of the placenta and subsequent fetal infection. The incidence of congenital varicella syndrome is estimated to be 2 to 3 percent and occurs only with exposure in the first 20 weeks of pregnancy.[94,95] Most reported cases occur as a result of maternal infection between 8 and 20 weeks gestation.[96]

Congenital varicella syndrome is characterized by skin findings that include scarring (Figure 3-12). Limb hypoplasia, CNS damage, chorioretinitis, and microcephaly have also been reported (Table 3-8).[74,94,97–99] There does not appear to be an increased incidence of spontaneous abortion or premature delivery associated with varicella infection.[93]

Neonatal varicella occurs in newborns of mothers who develop a varicella infection in the five days before or two days after delivery.[100] For these infants, the risk of mortality is quite high because they do not receive any maternal antibody.

Maternal infection is diagnosed clinically. If laboratory confirmation is needed, VZV-specific antibody can be detected in serum using ELISA testing, fluorescent antimembrane antibody, or latex agglutination. Fetal infection may be suspected if ultrasound evaluation reveals

FIGURE 3-12 ◆ Congenital varicella syndrome.

Segmental and stellate-shaped deep scars on the right ear, head, shoulder, and arm that appear to follow a dermatome.

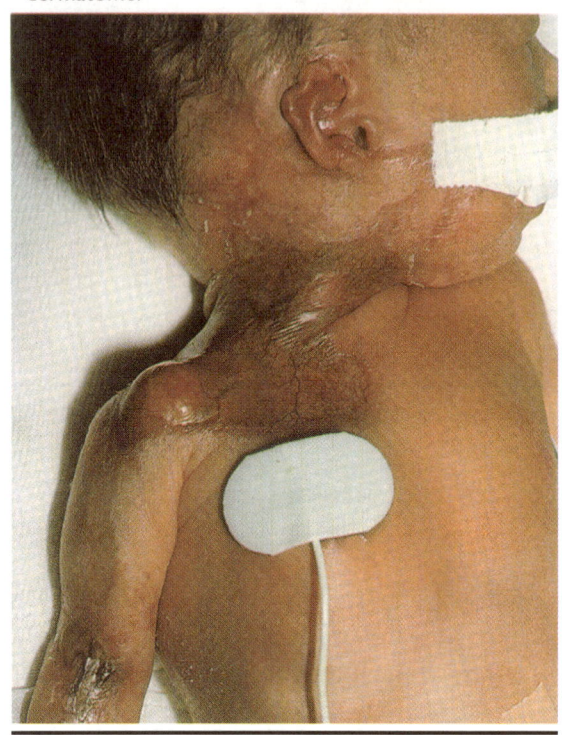

From: Friedlander SF, and Bradley JS. 2001. Viral infections. In *Textbook of Neonatal Dermatology,* Eichenfield LF, Frieden IJ, and Esterly NB, eds. Philadelphia: WB Saunders, 206. Reprinted by permission.

TABLE 3-8 ◆ Clinical Manifestations of Congenital Varicella-Zoster Infection

Chromosomal abnormalities

Cortical atrophy, mental retardation

Limb hypoplasia

Low birth weight

Microcephaly

Ocular abnormalities: microphthalmia, chorioretinitis, cataracts

Prematurity

Punctate lesions of lungs, liver, adrenals, esophagus, thymus, kidneys, spleen

Skin scars

Adapted from: Gershon A. 2001. Chickenpox, measles and mumps. In *Infectious Diseases of the Fetus and Newborn Infant*, 5th ed., Remington JS, and Klein JO, eds. Philadelphia: WB Saunders, 683–732.

characteristic findings including hydrops, echogenic foci in the bowel or liver, intrauterine growth restriction, limb or cardiac malformations, or microcephaly.[101] Detection of VZV antibodies or DNA in fetal blood or amniotic fluid can confirm fetal infection, but cannot predict the sequelae.[96]

Treatment with acyclovir has been shown to be of benefit in reducing the duration of infection and number of lesions, as well as associated symptoms in the mother if treatment is instituted within 24 hours of the onset of the exanthem.[102] Intravenous acyclovir can be used in pregnancy to treat maternal pneumonia.[103] This treatment does not, however, appear to protect the fetus from congenital infection.[104] The neonate whose mother has varicella within the window of five days before delivery or two days following it should be given varicella-zoster immune globulin (VZIG) after delivery. Neonates who develop varicella in the first two weeks of life are treated with IV acyclovir.[106] See Chapter 5 for a thorough discussion of postnatally acquired varicella infection.

Human Parvovirus B19

Human Parvovirus (HPV) B19, a DNA virus, was first identified in the mid-1970s. It is responsible for a common childhood illness known as erythema infectiosum, also called fifth disease or "slap-cheek" disease. Parvovirus B19 can be transmitted through respiratory droplets or by hand-to-mouth contact. Outbreaks can occur at any time, but are more common in late winter through early summer. Fifty percent of individuals are HPV B19 seropositive by the time they reach 15 years of age, with the rate increasing to 90 percent in the elderly. The annual seroconversion rate in women of childbearing age is reported to be 1.5 percent.[25]

In children and adults, infection occurs seven to ten days after exposure, with the most common symptoms being sore throat, low-grade fever, and rash (a reticular, lacelike rash on the trunk and an intensely red facial rash resembling a slapped cheek).[53] In adults, especially women, arthralgia and arthritis occur commonly.[25] Fifteen to 25 percent of those infected display no symptoms.[106] HPV B19 affects the hematologic system, causing a drop in production of reticulocytes that results in red-cell hypoplasia or aplasia.

In pregnancy, HPV B19 is transmitted vertically in 25–30 percent of maternal infections.[107] It is associated with spontaneous abortions, stillbirths, and severe nonimmune hydrops, and the incidence of fetal loss following Parvovirus infection is estimated to be 3 to 9 percent.[108] The incidence of hydrops fetalis is 3 to 10 percent.[109,110] In 60 percent of the cases of hydrops fetalis, the hydrops resolves spontaneously or with appropriate management.[109]

Hydrops fetalis develops as a result of aplastic anemia, which follows the virally induced interruption of reticulocyte production.[111,112] Because human Parvovirus infection mimics congenital rubella infection, it should be part of the differential diagnosis of congenital infection.

Table 3-9 summarizes the clinical manifestations of HPV B19 infection.

Diagnosis of maternal Parvovirus infection is made difficult by the long-term presence of anti-Parvovirus IgM. After known exposure, serum IgM and IgG levels can be followed to determine infection. Virus particles may also be detected using electron microscopy.[111] PCR testing is the most sensitive technique for diagnosing HPV infection.[22]

If seroconversion occurs or if the virus is detected in maternal serum, weekly fetal ultrasounds should be done to detect the development of hydrops. In the case of HPV infection, the severity of maternal clinical disease does not necessarily correspond with fetal outcome. Smoleniec and colleagues found that no woman in their study with clinically symptomatic disease experienced a fetal loss, whereas the loss rate for women with asymptomatic seroconversion was 44 percent.[113]

Fetal diagnosis of Parvovirus infection can be made by isolating viral particles from fetal or placental tissue.[112] Several studies have shown PCR to be highly sensitive in identifying virus in fetal serum, amniotic fluid, or placental tissue.[16,114]

Treatment for both mother and baby is determined by the symptoms displayed. Hydrops may require intrauterine transfusions to correct the anemia; however, spontaneous resolution of hydrops following resumption of red-cell production has also been reported.[115] High-dose intravenous immunoglobulin has been used to treat immunocompromised children with HPV B19 infection and has been suggested by some as an alternative to intrauterine transfusion.[117] Further investigation of this treatment is needed.

Experimental data in animals have demonstrated that the Parvoviruses have the potential to cause birth defects.[117] Data in humans are less clear; however, the association between intrauterine Parvovirus infection and defects, particularly in the CNS, has been suggested.[107,118,119] Other studies have reported no long-term sequelae in neonates with congenital Parvovirus infection.[109,120,121]

TABLE 3-9 ◆ Clinical Manifestations of Congenital Human Parvovirus B19 Infection

Spontaneous abortion
Stillbirth
Nonimmune hydrops fetalis
Aplastic anemia

Adapted from: Torok TJ. 2001. Human Parvovirus B19. In *Infectious Diseases of the Fetus and Newborn Infant*, 5th ed., Remington JS, and Klein JO, eds. Philadelphia: WB Saunders, 779–811.

Other Viruses

Other viral agents have been suspected of causing intrauterine infection. For two in particular, the evidence is quite strong. HIV and Enterovirus have both been implicated as a cause of intrauterine infection. These viruses are also known to cause significant infections in the postnatal period and are discussed in detail in Chapter 5.

SUMMARY

Intrauterine infections are a cause of significant morbidity and mortality in the fetus and newborn, often resulting in lifelong effects. As diagnostic tests improve and further research is conducted, increasing numbers of viruses are being implicated along with *T. pallidum* and *T. gondii* as capable of causing intrauterine infection. Several authors have pointed out the need to abandon the TORCH acronym in favor of something more encompassing. Those providing care for pregnant women must remain vigilant to the often subtle signs and symptoms of the microorganisms responsible for intrauterine infection. Likewise, those caring for newborn infants need to maintain a heightened awareness of the potential for intrauterine infections when an infant is born with stigma such as intrauterine growth restriction or unexplained dermatologic or neurologic findings.

This chapter has examined the general effects of maternal infection and the implications for the fetus. In addition, the more common agents known to cause intrauterine infection in the human fetus were examined. For further discussion of postnatally acquired infections, the reader is directed to Chapters 4 and 5.

REFERENCES

1. Isaacs D, and Moxon ER. 1999. *Handbook of Neonatal Infections: A Practical Guide.* London: WB Saunders.
2. Cullen A, et al. 1998. Current use of TORCH screen in the diagnosis of congenital infection. *Journal of Infection* 36(2): 185–188.
3. Leland D, et al. 1983. The use of TORCH titers. *Pediatrics* 72(1): 41–43.
4. Stamos JK, and Rowley AH. 1994. Timely diagnosis of congenital infections. *Pediatric Clinics of North America* 41(5): 1017–1033.
5. Klein JO, and Remington JS. 2001. Current concepts of infections of the fetus and newborn. In *Infectious Diseases of the Fetus and Newborn Infant*, 5th ed., Remington JS, and Klein JO, eds. Philadelphia: WB Saunders, 1–24.
6. Ronel DN, Klein JO, and Ware KG. 1995. New acronym needed for congenital infections (letter). *Pediatric Infectious Disease Journal* 14(10): 921.
7. Ford-Jones EL, and Kellner JD. 1995. "CHEAP TORCHES": An acronym for congenital and perinatal infections (letter). *The Pediatric Infectious Disease Journal* 14(7): 638–640.
8. Karesh JW, Kapur S, and MacDonald M. 1983. Herpes simplex virus and congenital malformations. *Southern Medical Journal* 76(12): 1561–1563.
9. Khuroo MS, Kamili S, and Jameel S. 1995. Vertical transmission of hepatitis E virus. *Lancet* 345(8956): 1025–1026.
10. Weiner CP. 1997. The elusive search for fetal infection: Changing the gold standards. *Obstetrics and Gynecology Clinics of North America* 24(1): 19–32.
11. Boyd PA, and Keeling JW. 1992. Fetal hydrops. *Journal of Medical Genetics* 29(2): 91–97.
12. Van den Veyver IB, et al. 1998. Detection of intrauterine viral infection using the polymerase chain reaction. *Molecular Genetics and Metabolism* 63(2): 85–95.
13. Alger LS. 1997. Toxoplasmosis and Parvovirus B19. *Infectious Disease Clinics of North America* 11(1): 55–75.
14. Thilaganathan B, et al. 1994. Fetal immunological and haematological changes in intrauterine infection. *British Journal of Obstetrics and Gynaecology* 101(5): 418–421.
15. Rozenberg F, and Lebon P. 1991. Amplification and characterization of herpesvirus DNA in cerebrospinal fluid from patients with acute encephalitis. *Journal of Clinical Microbiology* 29(11): 2412–2417.
16. Torok TJ, et al. 1992. Prenatal diagnosis of intrauterine infection with Parvovirus B19 by the polymerase chain reaction technique. *Clinical Infectious Diseases* 14(1): 149–155.
17. Bosma TJ, et al. 1995. Use of PCR for prenatal and postnatal diagnosis of congenital rubella. *Journal of Clinical Microbiology* 33(11): 2881–2887.
18. Lopez A, et al. 2000. Preventing congenital toxoplasmosis. *MMWR* 49(RR-02): 57–75.
19. Grant A. 1996. Varicella infection and toxoplasmosis in pregnancy. *Journal of Perinatal and Neonatal Nursing* 10(2): 17–29.
20. Remington JS, et al. 2001. Toxoplasmosis. In *Infectious Diseases of the Fetus and Newborn Infant*, 5th ed., Remington JS, and Klein JO, eds. Philadelphia: WB Saunders, 205–346.
21. Lynfield R, and Guerina NG. 1997. Toxoplasmosis. *Pediatrics in Review* 18(3): 75–84.
22. Isada CM, et al. 1999. *Infectious Diseases Handbook.* Hudson, Ohio: Lexi-Comp.
23. Martin S. 2001. Congenital toxoplasmosis. *Neonatal Network* 20(4): 23–30.
24. Sabin AB. 1942. Toxoplasmosis: Recently recognized disease of human beings. Part V: Clinical manifestations of toxoplasmosis in man. *Advances in Pediatrics* 1: 1–56.
25. American Academy of Pediatrics. 2000. *Red Book: Report of the Committee on Infectious Diseases*, 25th ed., Pickering L, ed. Elk Grove Village, Illinois: American Academy of Pediatrics, 227–230, 547–560, 310–319, 496–501, 424–426.
26. Beazley DM, and Egerman RS. 1998. Toxoplasmosis. *Seminars in Perinatology* 22(4): 332–338.
27. Litwin CM, and Hill HR. 1997. Serologic and DNA-based testing for congenital and perinatal infections. *Pediatric Infectious Disease Journal* 16(12): 1166–1175.
28. Gilbert GL. 1996. Congenital fetal infections. *Seminars in Neonatology* 1(2): 91–105.
29. Wallon M, et al. 1999. Congenital toxoplasmosis: Systematic review of evidence of efficacy of treatment in pregnancy. *British Medical Journal* 318(7197): 1511–1514.
30. Foulon W, et al. 1999. Treatment of toxoplasmosis during pregnancy: Impact on fetal transmission and children's sequelae at one year of age: A multicenter study. *American Journal of Obstetrics and Gynecology* 180(2 part 1): 410–415.
31. McAuley J, et al. 1994. Early and longitudinal evaluations of treated infants and children and untreated historical patients with congenital toxoplasmosis: The Chicago Collaborative Treatment Trial. *Clinical Infectious Diseases* 18(1): 38–72.
32. Villena I, et al. 1999. Pyrimethamine-sulfadoxine treatment of congenital toxoplasmosis: Follow-up of 78 cases between 1990 and 1997. *Scandinavian Journal of Infectious Diseases* 30(3): 295–300.
33. Wilson CB, et al. 1980. Development of adverse sequelae in children born with subclinical congenital Toxoplasmosis infection. *Pediatrics* 66(5): 767–774.
34. Virkola K, et al. 1997. Radiological signs in newborns exposed to primary toxoplasma infection *in utero*. *Pediatric Radiology* 27(2): 133–138.
35. Dunn D, et al. 1999. Mother-to-child transmission of toxoplasmosis: Risk estimates for clinical counseling. *Lancet* 353(9167): 1829–1833.
36. McLeod R, et al. 1992. Levels of pyrimethamine in cerebrospinal and ventricular fluids from infants treated for congenital toxoplasmosis. *Antimicrobial Agents and Chemotherapy* 36(5): 1040–1048.
37. Mets MB, et al. 1996. Eye manifestations of congenital toxoplasmosis. *American Journal of Ophthalmology* 122(3): 309–324.
38. Roizen N, et al. 1992. Developmental and neurologic function in treated congenital toxoplasmosis. *Pediatric Research* 31: 353A.
39. Swisher CN, Boyer K, and McLeod R. 1994. Congenital toxoplasmosis. *Seminars in Pediatric Neurology* 1(1): 4–25.
40. Stagno S. 2001. Cytomegalovirus. In *Infectious Diseases of the Fetus and Newborn Infant*, 5th ed., Remington JS, and Klein JO, eds. Philadelphia: WB Saunders, 389–424.
41. Nelson C, and Demmler G. 1997. Cytomegalovirus infection in the pregnant mother, fetus and newborn infant. *Clinics in Perinatology* 24(1): 151–160.

42. Fowler KB, et al. 1992. The outcome of congenital cytomegalovirus infection in relation to maternal antibody status. *New England Journal of Medicine* 326(10): 663–667.

43. Stagno S, et al. 1982. Congenital cytomegalovirus infection: The relative importance of primary and recurrent maternal infection. *New England Journal of Medicine* 306(16): 945–949.

44. Boppana SB, et al. 1999. Symptomatic congenital cytomegalovirus infection in infants born to mothers with preexisting immunity to cytomegalovirus. *Pediatrics* 104(1 Part 1): 55–60.

45. Boppana SB, et al. 1993. Virus-specific antibody responses in mothers and their newborn infants with asymptomatic congenital cytomegalovirus infections. *Journal of Infectious Diseases* 167(1): 72–77.

46. Preece PM, Pearl KN, and Pecham CS. 1984. Congenital cytomegalovirus infection. *Archives of Disease in Childhood* 59(12): 1120–1126.

47. Preece PM, et al. 1986. Congenital cytomegalovirus infection: Predisposing maternal factors. *Journal of Epidemiology and Community Health* 40(3): 205–209.

48. Alford CA, et al. 1990. Congenital and perinatal cytomegalovirus infections. *Reviews of Infectious Diseases* 12(S7): S745–S753.

49. Fowler KB, et al. 1997. Progressive and fluctuating sensorineural hearing loss in children with asymptomatic congenital cytomegalovirus infection. *Journal of Pediatrics* 130(4): 624–630.

50. Kumar ML, et al. 1984. Congenital and postnatally acquired cytomegalovirus infections: Long-term follow-up. *Journal of Pediatrics* 104(5): 674–679.

51. Donner C, et al. 1993. Prenatal diagnosis of 52 pregnancies at risk for congenital cytomegalovirus infection. *Obstetrics and Gynecology* 82(4 part 1): 481–486.

52. Lazzarotto T, et al. 2000. Prenatal indicators of congenital cytomegalovirus infection. *Journal of Pediatrics* 137(1): 90–95.

53. Kuhlmann RS, and Autry AM. 2001. An approach to nonbacterial infections in pregnancy. *Clinics in Family Practice* 3(2): 1–17.

54. Whitley RJ, et al. 1997. Ganciclovir treatment of symptomatic congenital cytomegalovirus infection: Results of a phase II study. *Journal of Infectious Diseases* 175(5): 1080–1086.

55. Whitley RJ, and Kimberlin DW. 1997. Treatment of viral infections during pregnancy and the neonatal period. *Clinics in Perinatology* 24(1): 267–283.

56. Boppana SB, et al. 1997. Neuroradiographic findings in the newborn period and long-term outcome in children with symptomatic congenital cytomegalovirus infection. *Pediatrics* 99(3): 409–414.

57. Reef S, et al. 2002. The changing epidemiology of rubella in the 1990s: On the verge of elimination and new challenges for control and prevention. *JAMA* 287(4): 464–472.

58. Centers for Disease Control and Prevention. 2001. Control and prevention of rubella: Evaluation and management of suspected outbreaks, rubella in pregnant women, and surveillance for congenital rubella syndrome. *MMWR* 50(RR-12): 1–23.

59. Tanemura M, et al. 1996. Diagnosis of fetal rubella infection with reverse transcription and nested polymerase chain reaction: A study of 34 cases diagnosed in fetuses. *American Journal of Obstetrics and Gynecology* 174(2): 578–582.

60. Cooper LZ, and Alford CA. 2001. Rubella. In *Infectious Diseases of the Fetus and Newborn Infant*, 5th ed., Remington JS, and Klein JO, eds. Philadelphia: WB Saunders, 347–388.

61. Reef SE, et al. 2000. Preparing for elimination of congenital rubella syndrome: Summary of the workshop on CRS elimination in the United States. *Clinical Infectious Diseases* 31(1): 85–95.

62. Peckham GS. 1972. Clinical and laboratory study of children exposed *in utero* to maternal rubella. *Archives of Disease in Childhood* 47(254): 571–577.

63. Centers for Disease Control and Prevention. 2001. National overview of sexually transmitted diseases, 2000. Available at www.cdc.gov/std/stats/2000NatOverview.htm.

64. Ingall D, and Sanchez PJ. 2001. Syphilis. In *Infectious Diseases of the Fetus and Newborn Infant*, 5th ed., Remington JS, and Klein JO, eds. Philadelphia: WB Saunders, 643–681.

65. Sheffield JS, et al. 1999. Congenital syphilis: The influence of maternal stage of syphilis on vertical transmission. *American Journal of Obstetrics and Gynecology* 180: 85A.

66. Brown ZA, et al. 1991. Neonatal herpes simplex virus infection in relation to asymptomatic maternal infection at the time of labor. *New England Journal of Medicine* 324(18): 1247–1252.

67. Arvin AM, and Whitley RJ. 2001. Herpes simplex virus infections. In *Infectious Diseases of the Fetus and Newborn Infant*, 5th ed., Remington JS, and Klein JO, eds. Philadelphia: WB Saunders, 425–446.

68. Prober CG, et al. 1987. Low risk of herpes simplex virus infections in neonates exposed to the virus at the time of vaginal delivery to mothers with recurrent genital herpes simplex virus infections. *New England Journal of Medicine* 316(5): 240–244.

69. Ashley RL, and Wald A. 1999. Genital herpes: Review of the epidemic and potential use of type-specific serology. *Clinical Microbiology Reviews* 12(1): 1–8.

70. Fingeroth J. 2000. Herpesvirus infection of the liver. *Infectious Disease Clinics of North America* 14(3): 689–719.

71. Jones CL. 1996. Herpes simplex virus infection in the neonate: Clinical presentation and management. *Neonatal Network* 15(8): 11–15.

72. Brown ZA, et al. 1985. Genital herpes in pregnancy: Risk factors associated with recurrences and asymptomatic viral shedding. *American Journal of Obstetrics and Gynecology* 153(1): 24–30.

73. Hutto C, et al. 1987. Intrauterine herpes simplex virus infections. *Journal of Pediatrics* 110(1): 97–101.

74. Scott L, Hollier L, and Dias K. 1997. Perinatal herpesvirus infections: Herpes simplex, varicella and cytomegalovirus. *Infectious Disease Clinics of North America* 11(1): 27–53.

75. Kohl S. 1997. Neonatal herpes simplex virus infection. *Clinics in Perinatology* 24(1): 129–150.

76. Jacobs RF. 1998. Neonatal herpes simplex virus infections. *Seminars in Perinatology* 22(1): 64–71.

77. Corey L. 2000. Herpes simplex virus. In *Principles and Practice of Infectious Diseases*, 5th ed., Mandell GL, Bennett JE, and Dolin R, eds. Philadelphia: Churchill Livingstone, 1564–1572.

78. Parvey LS, and Chien LT. 1980. Neonatal herpes simplex virus infection introduced by fetal-monitor scalp electrodes. *Pediatrics* 65(6): 1150–1153.

79. Whitley RJ, et al. 1988. Changing presentation of herpes simplex virus infection in neonates. *Journal of Infectious Diseases* 158(1): 109–116.

80. Arvin AM, and Prober CG. 1990. Herpes simplex virus infections. *Pediatric Infectious Disease Journal* 9(10): 765–767.

81. Greenes DS, et al. 1995. Neonatal herpes simplex virus infection presenting as fulminant liver failure. *The Pediatric Infectious Disease Journal* 14(3): 242–244.

82. Kroon S. 1994. Management strategies in herpes: Limiting the continued spread of genital herpes. Worthing, United Kingdom: PPS Europe Ltd., 17–22.

83. Straus SE, et al. 1989. Effect of oral acyclovir treatment on symptomatic and asymptomatic virus shedding in recurrent genital herpes. *Sexually Transmitted Diseases* 16(2): 107–113.

84. Hensleigh PA. 1994. Undocumented history of maternal genital herpes followed by neonatal herpes meningitis. *Journal of Perinatology* 14(2): 216–218.

85. Nahass GT, et al. 1992. Comparison of Tzanck smear, viral culture, and DNA diagnostic methods in detection of herpes simplex and varicella-zoster infection. *JAMA* 268(18): 2541–2544.

86. Ashley R, et al. 1991. Inability of enzyme immunoassays to discriminate between infections with herpes simplex virus types 1 and 2. *Annals of Internal Medicine* 115(7): 520–526.

87. Cone RW, et al. 1994. Frequent detection of genital herpes simplex virus DNA by polymerase chain reaction among pregnant women. *JAMA* 272(10): 792–796.

88. Diamond C, et al. 1999. Viremia in neonatal herpes simplex virus infections. *Pediatric Infectious Disease Journal* 18(6): 487–489.

89. Zenk K, Sills JH, and Koeppel RM. 2003. *Neonatal Medications & Nutrition: A Comprehensive Guide*, 3rd ed. Santa Rosa, California: NICU INK, 4.

90. Kimberlin DW, et al. 2001. Safety and efficacy of high-dose acyclovir in the management of neonatal herpes simplex virus infections. *Pediatrics* 108(2): 230–238.

91. Kimberlin D, et al. 2001a. Natural history of neonatal herpes simplex virus infections in the acyclovir era. *Pediatrics* 108(2): 223–229.

92. Centers for Disease Control and Prevention. 1997. Varicella-related deaths among adults—United States, 1997. *MMWR* 46(19): 409–412.

93. Balducci J, et al. 1992. Pregnancy outcome following first-trimester varicella infection. *Obstetrics and Gynecology* 79(1): 5–6.

94. Jones KL, Johnson KA, and Chambers CD. 1994. Offspring of women infected with varicella during pregnancy: A prospective study. *Teratology* 49(1): 29–32.

95. Pastuszak AL, et al. 1994. Outcome after maternal varicella infection in the first 20 weeks of pregnancy. *New England Journal of Medicine* 330(13): 901–905.

96. McCarter-Spaulding DE. 2001. Varicella infection in pregnancy. *Journal of Obstetric, Gynecologic, and Neonatal Nursing* 30(6): 667–673.

97. DaSilva O, Hammerberg O, and Chance GW. 1990. Fetal varicella syndrome. *Pediatric Infectious Disease Journal* 9(11): 854–855.

98. Andreou A, et al. 1995. Fetal varicella syndrome with manifestations limited to the eye. *American Journal of Perinatology* 12(5): 347–348.

99. Gershon A. 2001. Chickenpox, measles and mumps. In *Infectious Diseases of the Fetus and Newborn Infant*, 5th ed., Remington JS, and Klein JO, eds. Philadelphia: WB Saunders, 683–732.

100. Miller E, Cradock-Watson JE, and Ridehalgh MK. 1989. Outcome in newborn babies given anti-varicella-zoster immunoglobulin after perinatal maternal infection with varicella-zoster virus. *Lancet* 2(8659): 371–373.

101. Pretorius DH, et al. 1992. Sonographic evaluation of pregnancies with maternal varicella infection. *Journal of Ultrasound Medicine* 11(9): 459–463.

102. Wallace MR, et al. 1992. Treatment of adult varicella with oral acyclovir: A randomized, placebo-controlled trial. *Annals of Internal Medicine* 117(5): 358–363.

103. Nathwani D, et al. 1998. Varicella infections in pregnancy and the newborn. A review prepared for the UK Advisory Group on Chickenpox on behalf of the British Society for the Study of Infection. *Journal of Infection* 36(supplement 1): S59–S71.

104. Smego RA, and Asperilla MO. 1991. Use of acyclovir for varicella pneumonia during pregnancy. *Obstetrics and Gynecology* 78(6): 1112–1116.

105. Williams H, et al. 1987. Acyclovir in the treatment of neonatal varicella. *Journal of Infection* 15(1): 65–67.

106. Chorba T, et al. 1986. The role of Parvovirus B19 in aplastic crisis and erythema infectiosum (fifth disease). *Journal of Infectious Diseases* 154(3): 383–393.

107. Public Health Laboratory Service Working Party on Fifth Disease. 1990. Prospective study of human Parvovirus (B19) infection in pregnancy. *British Medical Journal* 300(6733): 1166–1170.

108. Centers for Disease Control and Prevention. 1989. Current trends risks associated with human Parvovirus B-19 infection. *MMWR* 38(6): 81–88, 93–97.

109. Gilbert GL. 2000. Parvovirus B19 infection and its significance in pregnancy. *Communicable Diseases Intelligence* 24(supplement): S69–S71.

110. Yaegashi N, et al. 1994. The frequency of human Parvovirus B19 infection in nonimmune hydrops. *Journal of Perinatal Medicine* 22(2): 159–163.

111. Naides SJ, and Weiner CP. 1989. Antenatal diagnosis and palliative treatment of non-immune hydrops fetalis secondary to fetal Parvovirus B-19 infection. *Prenatal Diagnosis* 9(2): 105–114.

112. Rodis JF, et al. 1988. Human Parvovirus infection in pregnancy. *Obstetrics and Gynecology* 72(5): 733–738.

113. Smoleniec JS, et al. 1994. Subclinical transplacental Parvovirus B19 infection: An increased fetal risk? *Lancet* 343(8905): 1100–1101.

114. Kovacs BW, et al. 1992. Prenatal diagnosis of human Parvovirus B19 in nonimmune hydrops fetalis by polymerase chain reaction. *American Journal of Obstetrics and Gynecology* 167(2): 461–466.

115. Rodis JF, et al. 1990. Management and outcomes of pregnancies complicated by human B19 Parvovirus infection: A prospective study. *American Journal of Obstetrics and Gynecology* 163(4 part 1): 1168–1171.

116. Selbing A, et al. 1995. Parvovirus B19 infection during pregnancy treated with high-dose intravenous gammaglobulin. *Lancet* 345(8950): 660–661.

117. Torok TJ. 2001. Human Parvovirus B19. In *Infectious Diseases of the Fetus and Newborn Infant*, 5th ed., Remington JS, and Klein JO, eds. Philadelphia: WB Saunders, 779–811.

118. Morey AL, et al. 1992. Clinical and histopathological features of Parvovirus B19 infection in the human fetus. *British Journal of Obstetrics and Gynaecology* 99(7): 566–574.

119. Rogers BB, Mark Y, and Oyer CE. 1993. Diagnosis and incidence of fetal parvovirus infection in an autopsy series. Part I: Histology. *Pediatric Pathology* 13(3): 371–379.

120. Miller E, et al. 1998. Immediate and long-term outcome of human Parvovirus B19 infection in pregnancy. *British Journal of Obstetrics and Gynaecology* 105(2): 174–178.

121. Sheikh AU, Ernest JM, and O'Shea M. 1992. Long-term outcome in fetal hydrops from Parvovirus B19 infection. *American Journal of Obstetrics and Gynecology* 167(2): 337–341.

NOTES

Notes

CHAPTER 4

Bacterial Infections

Debbie Fraser Askin, RNC, MN

The reported occurrence of bacterial infection in neonates varies widely and is dependent on the definitions used in reporting. In newborn infants the incidence range is 1 to 8 cases per 1,000 live births in the U.S.[1] Among premature and low birth weight infants, the incidence increases markedly. The cost of neonatal infections is large, in terms of morbidity and mortality, increased length of hospital stay, and costs for long-term care needs that may result from complications of infection.

Neonates become infected in one of four ways:

1. **Transplacental infection.** Very few bacteria are capable of crossing the placental barrier and causing infection in the fetus. The exceptions are *Listeria monocytogenes* and *Treponema pallidum*. As explained in Chapter 3, the movement of viral infections across the placenta is well documented.
2. **Ascending infections.** Ascending infections cause amnionitis, and thus infection of the fetus. This route of infection becomes particularly important with prolonged rupture of amniotic membranes. Organisms transmitted by this route include Group B Streptococcus (GBS).
3. **Birth-canal-acquired infections.** During vaginal deliveries, infants may become colonized with organisms found in the mother's lower genital tract. GBS, *Escherichia coli*, and *Neisseria gonorrhoeae* (gonorrhea) may be acquired via this route.
4. **Nosocomial infections.** A variety of organisms may be transmitted to newborn infants as a result of poor handwashing, the use of contaminated equipment, or the feeding of colonized breast milk. Nosocomial infections are particularly common in the NICU.

HISTORICAL PATTERNS OF BACTERIAL INFECTION

Just as humans are constantly changing and evolving, so too are bacteria. Over the past century, the patterns of neonatal infection have changed, with different organisms predominating. In the 1930s and 1940s, *Streptococcus pyogenes* was responsible for a number of outbreaks of infection in nurseries.[2] The 1950s saw the identification of GBS as a neonatal pathogen.

TABLE 4-1 ◆ Risk Factors for Neonatal Infection

Maternal	Intrapartum	Neonatal
Poverty	Maternal fever	Congenital anomalies of the integument
Impaired nutrition	Prolonged rupture of membranes	Asplenia
Lack of prenatal care	Chorioamnionitis	Galactosemia
Use of illicit substances	Prolonged labor	Prematurity
Urinary tract infection	Birth asphyxia	Low birth weight
	Meconium aspiration	Male sex
		Multiple gestation
		Prolonged hospital stay
		Failure to thrive

During this period, methicillin-resistant *Staphylococcus aureus* (MRSA) was noted to be an important nursery pathogen, with several reports of nursery outbreaks.[3] In the 1960s and 1970s, GBS and *E. coli* were the organisms most commonly responsible for neonatal infections.[4] That pattern continues today.[5,6]

In the 1980s, increased survival rates among very low birth weight infants and the growing use of invasive technology provided an opportunity for *Staphylococcus epidermidis* infections to assume increasing importance. By 1990, methicillin-resistant *S. aureus* had been identified in the neonatal population. In the 1990s and into the twenty-first century, GBS continues to play a major role in newborn infection. With growing antepartum and intrapartum prophylaxis for GBS, there is concern about the potential for increased antibiotic resistance as well as the ongoing threat of Gram-negative sepsis.

RISK FACTORS FOR BACTERIAL SEPSIS

Maternal risk factors for the development of sepsis in the neonate include premature onset of labor or premature rupture of membranes and maternal infection. Although there are many etiologies of preterm labor, infection should always be considered when labor begins before 36 weeks gestation. For example, the Centers for Disease Control and Prevention (CDC) report that the attack rate for GBS sepsis increases from the 1–2 percent range in term pregnancies to 15.2 percent in pregnancies in which the onset of labor begins before 37 weeks.[7] In another study, Watts and colleagues identified amniotic fluid cultures that were positive for bacterial growth in 19 percent of women experiencing preterm labor.[8] Table 4-1 identifies additional maternal and intrapartum risk factors.

The single most important neonatal risk factor for sepsis is low birth weight.[1] Yancey and colleagues demonstrated a progressive increase in the risk of sepsis with decreasing gestational age.[9] Other neonatal risk factors are outlined in Table 4-1.

EARLY-ONSET VERSUS LATE-ONSET BACTERIAL INFECTIONS

Bacterial infections in the neonate are typically divided into two categories—early onset and late onset—based on time of presentation. Early-onset infections are those that present within the first 48 hours of life; they are usually acquired from the birth canal. A history of prematurity, premature rupture of membranes, chorioamnionitis, or maternal fever is common. Organisms responsible for early-onset infection include GBS, *E. coli*, *Haemophilus influenzae*, and *L. monocytogenes*. Early-onset infections present as fulminant, multisystem illnesses, with a mortality rate of 5–50 percent.[10]

TABLE 4-2 ◆ Bacterial Agents That Cause Neonatal Infections

Gram-Positive Cocci	Gram-Negative Cocci	Spirochete
Staphylococcus	Neisseria	*Treponema pallidum* (discussed in Chapter 3)
S. aureus	*N. gonorrhoeae*	
S. epidermidis	*N. meningitidis*	**Mycobacterium**
Streptococcus	**Gram-Negative Rods**	*M. tuberculosis*
Group A Streptococcus (*S. pyogenes*)	*Haemophilus influenzae*	**Chlamydia**
	Bacteroides fragili	*C. trachomatis*
Group B Streptococcus (GBS)	Pseudomonas	**Mycoplasma**
Group D Streptococcus	Enteric bacteria	*M. hominis*
S. viridans	*Escherichia coli*	*Ureaplasma urealyticum*
S. pneumoniae	Citrobacter	
Enterococcus (E. faecalis)	Klebsiella	
Gram-Positive Rods	Proteus	
Listeria monocytogenes	Salmonella	
Clostridium	Serratia	
C. botulinum	Shigella	
C. difficile		
C. perfringens		
C. tetani		

Late-onset infections may present as early as five days of age, but typically show themselves after one week of age and may be acquired from the birth canal or from the environment. The mortality rate with late-onset infections is 2 to 6 percent.[10] Infants who develop nosocomial infections are usually those with risk factors such as prematurity or congenital anomalies of the skin or mucous membranes or those requiring invasive procedures. Bacteria responsible for late-onset infections include *S. epidermidis* and *S. aureus*; Group A Streptococcus; and enteric bacteria including *E. coli*, Klebsiella, Pseudomonas, and Proteus. Table 4-2 categorizes the bacterial agents that cause neonatal infections.

SPECIFIC BACTERIAL AGENTS

Streptococcus

The Streptococcus genus consists of a group of Gram-positive organisms that arrange themselves in pairs or chains. Most are facultative anaerobes. Streptococci can be divided into three groups according to their pattern of hemolysis of red blood cells: organisms with complete hemolysis—β-Streptococcus; those with partial hemolysis—α-Streptococcus; and those with no hemolytic characteristics—nonhemolytic Streptococcus.

Group A (α-Hemolytic) Streptococcus (S. Pyogenes)

Commonly known as the cause of bacterial pharyngitis and flesh-eating disease, Group A Streptococcus was the most common cause of lethal maternal and perinatal infections in the late nineteenth and early twentieth centuries.[11] Once again, in the 1990s, this Gram-positive organism became an important pathogen in neonates. Streptococcus A disease in the newborn ranges from chronic omphalitis to fulminant sepsis and meningitis. Group A Streptococcus has also been linked to numerous infectious outbreaks in hospital nurseries.[12,13]

Group A Streptococcus is covered in an outer capsule made of hyaluronic acid identical to that found in connective tissue. This protects the organism against phagocytosis. The organism also produces a number of proteins, exotoxins, and enzymes that enhance its virulence.

TABLE 4-3 ◆ Risk Factors for Early-Onset GBS

Prolonged rupture of membranes (>18 hours)
Prematurity
Maternal fever (>38°C [100.4°F])
Chorioamnionitis
Maternal GBS bacteriuria
Previous infant with GBS sepsis
Maternal age <21
African American

Group A Streptococcus commonly colonizes the oropharynx and is spread directly by respiratory droplets.

Group B (β-Hemolytic) Streptococcus (S. Agalactiae)

The most common cause of neonatal sepsis and meningitis in the U.S., Group B (β-hemolytic) Streptococcus is a Gram-positive facultative anaerobe that grows in short chains on a blood agar plate surrounded by a narrow zone of hemolysis.[1,7] Two forms of neonatal GBS disease have been identified: early onset (occurring in the first seven days of life) and late onset (occurring after seven days of age). Perinatal transmission of GBS occurs as a result of aspiration of infected material, either from the amniotic fluid or during passage through the birth canal.[14]

The human reservoir for Group B Streptococcus is most likely the lower gastrointestinal tract, although GBS has been isolated from various body sites, including the throat, skin, cervix, vagina, and rectum, as well as from urine, stool, and blood. GBS is not typically associated with infection in healthy adults, but has been reported to cause skin or soft tissue infection, genitourinary infection, bacteremia, and pneumonia.[15]

In pregnant women, GBS causes urinary tract infections, amnionitis, endometritis, and wound infections.[7] Maternal colonization has been shown to increase the risk of premature labor and premature rupture of membranes and has been implicated as a cause of stillbirths.

Approximately 15–20 percent of pregnant women are colonized with GBS at delivery.[16] The rate of positive cultures is influenced by the site that cells are taken from to be cultured as well as the type of medium used to grow the culture. The number of positive cultures is increased by up to 27 percent when a combined anovaginal swab technique, rather than a vaginal swab alone, is used for testing.[7] Colonization rates are higher in women who are sexually active, are under 21, use an intrauterine contraceptive device, are of African-American descent, or are of lower parity.[7,16-18] The risk of neonatal GBS infection increases in cases where there is heavy colonization of the maternal genital tract or delivery of a previous infant with GBS disease.[7,19,20] Other factors that increase the likelihood of neonatal infection include prematurity, prolonged rupture of membranes, intrapartum fever,[21] and maternal GBS bacteriuria.[22,23]

Of infants born to untreated GBS-positive women, 40–79 percent will become colonized with GBS, with about 1 percent becoming ill with GBS sepsis.[16] Early-onset disease accounts for 70–80 percent of the cases of GBS sepsis.[7,16] It occurs at a rate of 1.8 per 1,000 live births.[7] About 75 percent of the cases of early-onset disease are associated with maternal risk factors (Table 4-3), leaving fully one-quarter of early-onset cases with no risk factors.[16] A comprehensive discussion of risk factors for early-onset GBS can be found in a report by Benitz and colleagues.[24]

Early-onset infection usually presents in the first 24 hours of life (85 percent of cases).[14] Premature infants are more likely to present early, with term infants occasionally presenting as late as day 6 of life. Between 35 and 55 percent of early-onset GBS takes the form of pneumonia, one-third of infants have septicemia without a specific focus, and 5–10 percent present with meningitis.[14]

Regardless of the focus of infection, neonates with early-onset GBS usually present with respiratory signs, including apnea, tachypnea, cyanosis, and grunting respirations. Up to 25 percent of GBS-infected infants also present with hypotension.[14] Additional signs include lethargy, poor tone, feeding intolerance, unstable temperature, pallor, and tachycardia. Chest x-ray findings in GBS infection are indistinguishable from those of transient tachypnea of the newborn or respiratory distress syndrome (Figure 4-1). One-third of infants with congenital pneumonia will have infiltrates on x-ray.[14]

The mortality rate for early-onset GBS sepsis declined from 55 percent in 1977[25] to about 4–6 percent by the mid-1990s,[26] reflecting enhancements in neonatal care. Factors predictive of a fatal outcome include the presence of shock, apnea, neutropenia, a low five-minute Apgar score, and pleural effusions.[18,27,28]

Late-onset infection is more likely to occur in term infants between seven days and 12 weeks of life and is associated with a mortality rate of 2–6 percent.[18,27] Clusters of late-onset disease among premature infants in the NICU have also been reported.[29,30] About 50 percent of late-onset GBS presents as meningitis, 40 percent as generalized septicemia, and 10 percent of infants have osteomyelitis or septic arthritis. It is speculated that most cases of late-onset GBS result from colonization of the nasopharynx at birth, with later invasion of the bloodstream. Nosocomial transmission of GBS has been reported, although infection via this route is rare.[16]

Signs and symptoms of late-onset infection include fever, poor feeding, poor tone, lethargy or irritability, and tachypnea. More severe signs and symptoms, associated with a poor outcome, include seizures, shock, neutropenia, elevated colony-stimulating factor (CSF) protein levels (>300 mg/dl), and coma.[14]

Meningitis occurs in 5–10 percent of GBS infections.[31] This is the most frequent manifestation of late-onset disease.[32] Early reports regarding the morbidity and mortality of GBS meningitis indicated a fatality rate of 26 percent.[33,34] From 25 to 50 percent of the survivors had significant neurologic sequelae.[34,35] No recent data are available to indicate whether changes in care have altered these figures.[14]

FIGURE 4-1 ♦ Chest x-ray showing Group B β-hemolytic Streptococcus pneumonia.

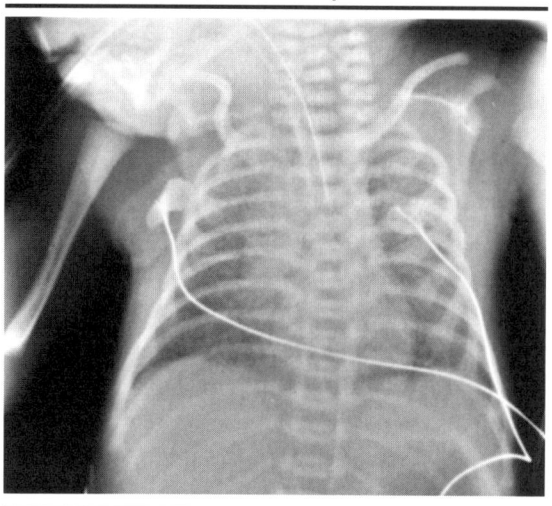

From: Trotter C, and Carey BE. 2000. Radiology basics: Overview and concepts. *Neonatal Network* 19(2): 36. Reprinted by permission.

The prevention of GBS disease has been the focus of much attention in the past two decades. Several studies have demonstrated the efficacy of intrapartum chemoprophylaxis for GBS.[36,37] Based on these findings, in 1992, the American Academy of Pediatrics (AAP) presented recommendations for the screening (and treatment) of pregnant women for GBS. These guidelines recommended anogenital cultures of all pregnant women between 26 and 28 weeks of gestation, with subsequent intrapartum chemoprophylaxis of culture-positive women.[38] Guidelines issued by the Centers for Disease Control and Prevention in 1996 offered two strategies for prevention of GBS disease, the first based on screening cultures done at 35–37 weeks gestation along with consideration of risk factors, the second involving consideration of risk factors with no screening cultures.[7]

In the first approach to prevention of GBS disease, intrapartum antibiotic prophylaxis (IAP) was recommended for all women with prenatal risk factors that include a previous GBS-positive baby, GBS bacteriuria, or labor at <37 weeks. Women with no prenatal risk factors had screening cultures done between 35 and 37 weeks gestation. Those with positive results and intrapartum risk factors such as a fever or prolonged rupture of membranes were treated in labor. Those with positive cultures and no intrapartum risk factors could opt for treatment. Women with negative cultures were not treated. In the risk factor–based approach, women with prenatal or intrapartum risk factors received IAP without screening cultures being done.

Studies have estimated that compliance with these guidelines would reduce the incidence of early-onset GBS disease by approximately 86 percent for the combination risk factor–plus–culture approach and 69 percent for the risk factor–only approach.[39–42] Edwards and Baker suggest that the culture-based approach would result in 20–25 percent of pregnant women receiving antibiotics during labor, with a resulting reduction in GBS sepsis of 85–90 percent.[14] Truong and associates report that following implementation of the CDC guidelines, the incidence of GBS sepsis in their review dropped from 1.7 cases per 1,000 live births to 0.3 cases.[43] Schrag and colleagues estimated a decline in cases from 1.7 per 1,000 to 0.6 per 1,000 live births.[26] For a comprehensive analysis of the literature on antimicrobial prevention of GBS sepsis, see the work done by Benitz and colleagues and by Schimmel and associates.[44,45]

Despite the potential benefits of following the CDC recommendations, studies examining the implementation of these guidelines have found that compliance rates are lower than desired.[42,46] One study by Chandran and colleagues found that, in centers combining risk factors and the use of cultures, compliance with intrapartum administration of chemoprophylaxis ranged from 75 to 84 percent and that 22 percent of laboring women received unindicated antibiotics. Only 65 percent of women with risk factors received antepartum cultures, and only 9 percent of those cultures were done using combined anovaginal screening. In the risk factor–based approach (no cultures done), indicated antibiotics were administered to 76 percent of women, and 15 percent of women received antibiotics where none were indicated.[47]

Recent data directly comparing the culture and risk factor approach compared to risk factor management alone for 5,144 births demonstrated that culture screening was over 50 percent more effective than a risk-based strategy in preventing early-onset GBS disease in neonates.[48] These data prompted reconsideration of prior guidelines.

In 2002, the CDC released new guidelines, now recommending that all pregnant women be screened at 35 to 37 weeks gestation for GBS colonization and that identified carriers be given intravenous penicillin as soon as possible after hospital admission through delivery.[49]

The new recommendations also contain the following changes:

- A neonate born to a woman suspected of having chorioamnionitis should have a full diagnostic evaluation and receive empiric broad-spectrum therapy (e.g., ampicillin and gentamicin) pending culture results, regardless of the infant's clinical condition at birth or gestational age.
- When a neonate has clinical signs of sepsis, a full diagnostic evaluation should include a lumbar puncture, if feasible. If the lumbar puncture has been deferred and the therapy is continued more than 48 hours because of suspected infection, cerebrospinal fluid should be obtained for routine studies and culture.
- In addition to penicillin or ampicillin, IAP with cefazolin at least four hours before

FIGURE 4-2 ♦ Indications for intrapartum antibiotic prophylaxis to prevent perinatal GBS disease under a universal prenatal screening strategy based on combined vaginal and rectal cultures collected at 35–37 weeks gestation from all pregnant women.

Vaginal and rectal GBS screening cultures at 35–37 weeks gestation for ALL pregnant women (unless patient had GBS bacteriuria during the current pregnancy or a previous infant with invasive GBS disease)

Intrapartum prophylaxis indicated
- Previous infant with invasive GBS disease
- GBS bacteriuria during current pregnancy
- Positive GBS screening culture during current pregnancy (unless a planned cesarean delivery, in the absence of labor or amniotic membrane rupture, is performed)
- Unknown GBS status (culture not done, incomplete, or results unknown) and any of the following:
  - Delivery at <37 weeks gestation*
  - Amniotic membrane rupture ≥18 hours
  - Intrapartum temperature ≥100.4°F (≥38.0°C)†

Intrapartum prophylaxis not indicated
- Previous pregnancy with a positive GBS screening culture (unless a culture was also positive during the current pregnancy)
- Planned cesarean delivery performed in the absence of labor or membrane rupture (regardless of maternal GBS culture status)
- Negative vaginal and rectal GBS screening culture in late gestation during the current pregnancy, regardless of intrapartum risk factors

---

* If onset of labor or rupture of amniotic membranes occurs at <37 weeks gestation and there is a significant risk for preterm delivery (as assessed by the clinician), a suggested algorithm for GBS prophylaxis management is given in source noted below, page 12.

† If amnionitis is suspected, broad-spectrum antibiotic therapy that includes an agent known to be active against GBS should replace GBS prophylaxis.

From: Centers for Disease Control and Prevention. 2002. Prevention of perinatal Group B streptococcal disease. Revised guidelines from CDC. *MMWR* 51(RR-11): 8.

---

delivery is considered adequate because cefazolin achieves bactericidal concentrations against GBS in amniotic fluid three hours after an IAP dose.

- Hospital discharge as early as 24 hours after birth may be reasonable when the infant is born after 4 or more hours of maternal IAP, is 38 weeks gestational age or more, appears healthy, and meets all discharge criteria, including care by an individual able to comply fully with instructions for home observation.

Figure 4-2 outlines an algorithm for intrapartum antibiotic prophylaxis, and Figure 4-3 provides a sample algorithm for managing a newborn whose mother received IAP.

Group D Streptococcus

Group D Streptococcus has an occurrence pattern similar to that of GBS and is associated with complicated deliveries.[11] In the past, Group D Streptococcus included Enterococcus (*E. faecalis*), which are now recognized as a separate taxonomic group. Despite the separation, these two groups are often considered together. Streptococcus D causes both early- and late-onset infection. Infants with early-onset infection usually have known risk factors such as prolonged rupture of membranes, maternal fever, or premature labor.[50] In Dobson and Baker's review of 56 cases of neonates with Group D Streptococcus born in a single hospital between 1977 and 1986, neonates with early-onset sepsis tended to be older (36.5 weeks gestational age) than those with late-onset disease.[50] Late-onset disease may present as meningitis, pneumonia, scalp abscesses, or catheter-related sepsis.

FIGURE 4-3 ◆ Sample algorithm for management of a newborn whose mother received intrapartum antimicrobial agents for prevention of early-onset Group B streptococcal disease* or suspected chorioamnionitis.

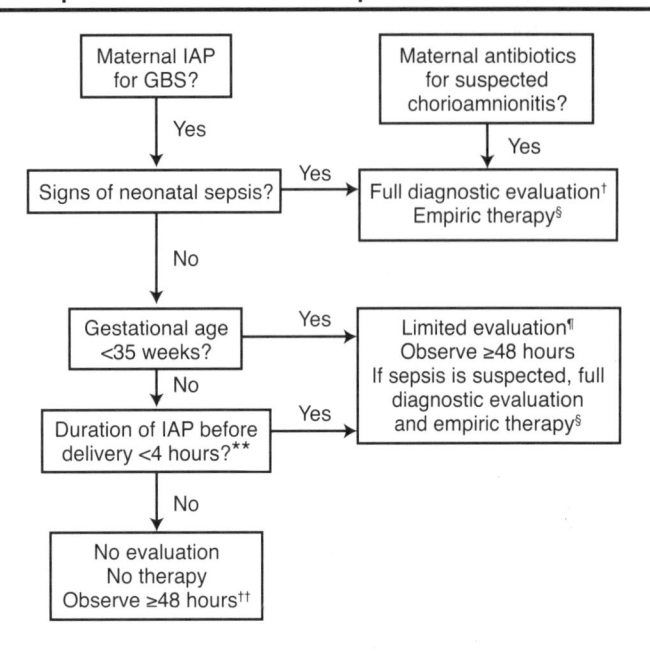

```
┌─────────────────┐         ┌──────────────────────┐
│ Maternal IAP    │         │ Maternal antibiotics │
│ for GBS?        │         │ for suspected        │
└────────┬────────┘         │ chorioamnionitis?    │
         │ Yes              └──────────┬───────────┘
         ▼                             │ Yes
┌─────────────────┐    Yes   ┌─────────▼────────────┐
│ Signs of        ├─────────►│ Full diagnostic      │
│ neonatal sepsis?│          │ evaluation†          │
└────────┬────────┘          │ Empiric therapy§     │
         │ No                └──────────────────────┘
         ▼
┌─────────────────┐    Yes   ┌──────────────────────┐
│ Gestational age ├─────────►│ Limited evaluation¶  │
│ <35 weeks?      │          │ Observe ≥48 hours    │
└────────┬────────┘          │ If sepsis is         │
         │ No                │ suspected, full      │
         ▼                   │ diagnostic evaluation│
┌─────────────────┐    Yes   │ and empiric therapy§ │
│ Duration of IAP ├─────────►│                      │
│ before delivery │          └──────────────────────┘
│ <4 hours?**     │
└────────┬────────┘
         │ No
         ▼
┌─────────────────┐
│ No evaluation   │
│ No therapy      │
│ Observe ≥48     │
│ hours††         │
└─────────────────┘
```

Note: This algorithm is not an exclusive course of management. Variations that incorporate individual circumstances or institutional preferences may be appropriate.

* If no maternal intrapartum prophylaxis for GBS was administered despite an indication being present, data are insufficient on which to recommend a single management strategy.

† Includes complete blood cell count and differential, blood culture, and chest radiograph if respiratory abnormalities are present. When signs of sepsis are present, a lumbar puncture, if feasible, should be performed.

§ Duration of therapy varies depending on results of blood culture, cerebrospinal fluid findings, if obtained, and the clinical course of the infant. If laboratory results and clinical course do not indicate bacterial infection, duration may be as short as 48 hours.

¶ CBC with differential and blood culture.

** Applies only to penicillin, ampicillin, or cefazolin and assumes recommended dosing regimens.

†† A healthy-appearing infant who was ≥38 weeks gestation at delivery and whose mother received ≥4 hours of intrapartum prophylaxis before delivery may be discharged home after 24 hours if other discharge criteria have been met and a person able to comply fully with instructions for home observation will be present. If any one of these conditions is not met, the infant should be observed in the hospital for at least 48 hours and until criteria for discharge are achieved.

From: Centers for Disease Control and Prevention. 2002. Prevention of perinatal Group B streptococcal disease. Revised guidelines from CDC. *MMWR* 51(RR-11): 13.

Streptococcus Viridans

Streptococcus viridans is a group of α-hemolytic organisms that form part of the normal flora of the mouth in infants and children. Sepsis caused by *S. viridans* is usually early onset, with the average age of presentation being 3.5 days.[11] Although its symptoms are similar to those of GBS, *S. viridans* tends to cause less leukopenia and respiratory distress than GBS. Sepsis caused by *S. viridans* has a reported fatality rate of 8.8 percent.[10]

Streptococcus Pneumoniae

Early-onset infection with *Streptococcus pneumoniae* (also referred to as pneumococcus) is acquired by ascending infection from the maternal genital tract. Although pneumococcus infection is uncommon, its features are similar to those of GBS. The infection is usually fulminant, with a poor outcome. Risk factors are similar to those for GBS. Pneumococcus meningitis may occur as part of an early-onset infection or may present at two to four weeks of age. The incidence of neonatal pneumococcal meningitis in the U.S. is 3 per 100,000 infants.[16]

Staphylococcus

The word *staphylococcus* comes from the Greek term for "a bunch of grapes," reflecting the shape of Staphylococcus colonies, which grow in grapelike clusters on culture plates. These organisms are nonmotile, facultative anaerobes. Of 32 known Staphylococcus species, 16 are found colonizing human skin and mucous membranes. Infections caused by staphylococcal bacteria can be divided into those caused by coagulase-positive organisms (i.e., *S. aureus*) and

FIGURE 4-4 ◆ Scalded skin syndrome secondary to staphylococcal infection.

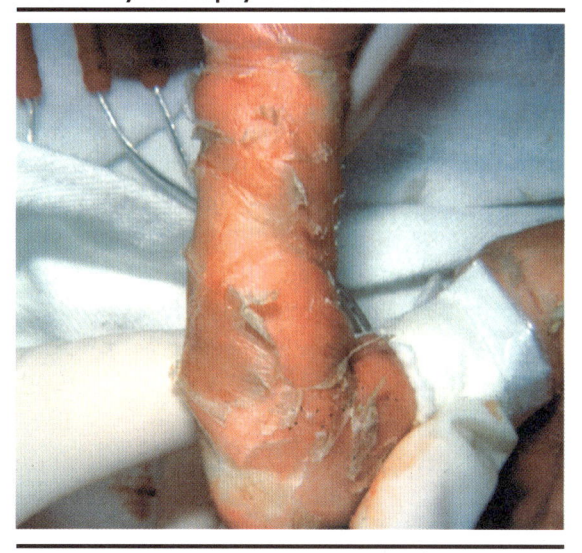

Courtesy of Dr. David A. Clark, Albany Medical Center, Albany, New York.

FIGURE 4-5 ◆ Multiple vesicles and bullae of staphylococcal pustulosis.

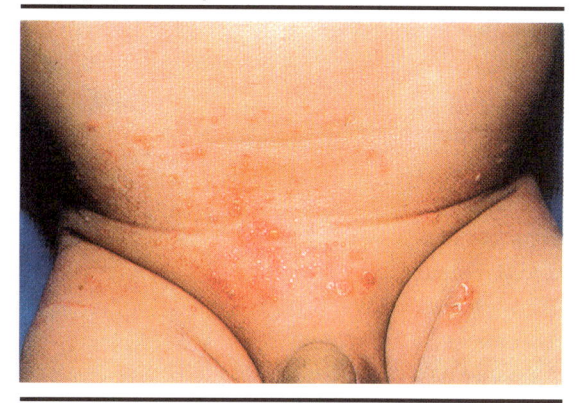

From: Darmstadt GL, and Dinulos JG. 2001. Bacterial infections. In *Textbook of Neonatal Dermatology*, Eichenfield LF, Frieden IJ, and Esterly NB, eds. Philadelphia: WB Saunders, 180. Reprinted by permission.

those caused by coagulase-negative bacteria (predominantly *S. epidermidis*).

Staphylococcus Aureus

Staphylococcus aureus colonizes the skin, umbilicus, and nares in 40–90 percent of neonates in the full-term nursery by five days of age.[51] Despite this high colonization rate, the incidence of *S. aureus* infection is relatively low. This organism, however, is responsible for periodic epidemic outbreaks within the nursery population in many countries of the world.[51] The major source of colonization by *S. aureus* is the hands of medical and nursing personnel.

S. aureus, which grows in golden colonies on agar plates, is the only Staphylococcus species that produces the enzyme coagulase (see Chapter 1). The surface of *S. aureus* bacteria is coated with a substance, protein A, that binds to some IgG molecules, preventing antibody-mediated immune clearance.[52] In addition, *S. aureus* produces toxins and enzymes that enhance the organism's virulence.

In the nursery outbreaks of the 1950s, *S. aureus* caused a wide range of illnesses, including mastitis, omphalitis, osteomyelitis, septic arthritis, and sepsis. A different strain of *S. aureus*, known as phage group II, emerged in the 1970s. This organism produces an exotoxin that is responsible for much of the tissue damage that occurs in scalded skin syndrome and bullous impetigo (Figures 4-4 and 4-5).

Since the mid-1980s, methicillin-resistant *S. aureus* has become a difficult infection control issue in NICUs. The development of resistance has occurred as a result of a genetic modification of the bacteria's cell wall that renders it immune to the action of β-lactam antibiotics. MRSA appears to have a particular affinity for bones and joints; together, nonresistant *S. aureus* and MRSA are responsible for the majority of neonatal osteomyelitis and septic arthritis.[53,54] Cohorting of infected babies and increased attention to staff handwashing are important strategies in preventing the spread of MRSA in the NICU.[55]

S. aureus can be carried on the hands of or in the nasopharynx of health care workers. Overcrowding in the nursery has been shown to be a factor in the organism's spread to infants.[56] Up

TABLE 4-4 ♦ Coagulase-Negative Staphylococcal Normal Flora

S. auricularis
S. capitis
S. cohnii
S. epidermidis
S. haemolyticus
S. hominis
S. lugdunensis
S. saccharolyticus
S. saprophyticus
S. schleiferi
S. simulans
S. warnerii
S. xylosus

to 15 percent of healthy adults are persistent carriers of *S. aureus* in their nasopharynx.[52] Good handwashing remains the single most important means of preventing the spread of this organism.[16]

Conjunctivitis is one of the most common manifestations of *S. aureus* infection, presenting with purulent eye discharge. Breaks in the skin, such as those resulting from intravenous catheters or scalp electrodes, present an opportunity for the development of *S. aureus* abscesses. *S. aureus* causes a wide range of systemic manifestations. Infection may be localized to the lungs, bones, kidneys, or heart or may present without a focus. Generalized sepsis may follow a local infection. Pneumonia as a result of *S. aureus* is associated with the development of pneumatoceles.

Coagulase-Negative Staphylococci

Coagulase-negative staphylococci (CoNS) include 31 species, the most common pathogenic species being *S. epidermidis*. Other species known to cause disease in humans include *S. saprophyticus, S. haemolyticus, S. hominis, S. warnerii, S. simulans, S. lugdunensis, and S. schleiferi*.[51] CoNS make up much of the normal flora of the skin and are generally nonpathogenic. Table 4-4 lists the coagulase-negative staphylococcal species found as part of the human normal flora.

Originally thought to be a skin contaminant in positive blood cultures rather than a true pathogen, CoNS are now recognized as a significant cause of late-onset infection in low birth weight infants. Several surveillance reports suggest that CoNS account for 48 to 58 percent of positive blood cultures in the NICU.[1,57–59] Raimundo and colleagues isolated 55 coagulase-negative staphylococci over two separate 12-month periods (26 in 1993 and 29 in 1996) from the blood of neonates in an NICU in Melbourne, Australia. The most common species in their unit were *S. epidermidis, S. haemolyticus,* and *S. warnerii*. Most such isolates were resistant to penicillin and to either or both methicillin and gentamicin.[60]

CoNS infections have been highly correlated with the following clinical risk factors: decreased gestational age; birth weight <1,000 gm; presence of indwelling foreign material, such as central or other intravascular lines, ventriculoperitoneal (VP) shunts, chest tubes, urinary catheters, and vascular graft material; and neonatal receipt of intravenous fat emulsion infusions.[61,62]

Several characteristics of coagulase-negative staphylococci contribute to their virulence in immunocompromised hosts. Some species, such as *S. epidermidis*, produce an extracellular slime that facilitates adherence to polyvinyl chloride (PVC) tubing and helps to prevent phagocytosis. This slime also inhibits the antimicrobial action of vancomycin. Once attached to a device such as a catheter, the organisms multiply and form multiple layers attached by intercellular adhesions known as biofilms, therefore making it difficult to eradicate the bacteria without removal of the infected material.[51] Some strains of CoNS produce a polysaccharide capsule that protects the bacteria from the body's immune system. Still others produce exoproteins and toxins that play a role in pathogenesis.

Host deficiencies account for the increased risk of CoNS experienced by very low birth weight (VLBW) infants. The single most important factor in controlling staphylococcal infections is an intact neutrophil phagocytic response.[63] All neonates, but particularly premature ones, lack the ability to release additional neutrophils in response to a bacterial invasion. Neutrophils in neonates also show a diminished chemotactic response compared to those in older children and adults[64] as well as a diminished capacity for adherence and phagocytosis.[51]

Often insidious, CoNS infections typically present with nonspecific signs, including temperature instability, apnea and bradycardia episodes, lethargy, increased oxygen requirements, feeding intolerance, and thrombocytopenia. Fallat and colleagues reviewed the cases of 65 central venous catheter infections and found that fever and pulmonary dysfunction were the most common presenting signs.[65] Laboratory findings often include an abnormal white blood cell count, unexplained metabolic acidosis, and hyperglycemia.[66]

CoNS sepsis has been associated with necrotizing enterocolitis, although causation has not been shown. Pneumonia, meningitis, and endocarditis are rare complications of CoNS infection.[59] Endocarditis is almost always associated with a structurally abnormal heart.

Because CoNS are not very virulent organisms, the mortality rate from a CoNS infection is not high (less than 5 percent).[67] However, a CoNS infection does result in morbidity in the form of prolonged hospitalization[57] or ventilator support[68] and often in the need to remove central lines or other foreign objects such as VP shunts. Persistent sepsis despite antibiotic therapy is associated with an increased risk of end-organ damage and death.[69]

S. epidermidis is frequently resistant to penicillin and gentamicin. Because of this resistance to multiple antibiotics, including methicillin, treatment with vancomycin is needed; this increases the possibility of toxicity, as well as increasing the risk of the development of vancomycin-resistant enterococci.[70] Distinguishing an ill infant from one with a contaminated blood culture is not always easy; the result can be treatment for false-positive cultures, further contributing to the development of drug resistance.[62]

Prophylactic administration of vancomycin has been shown to reduce the incidence of CoNS sepsis in low birthweight infants.[65,71] However, prophylactic use of vancomycin is associated with an increased risk of Gram-negative sepsis[72] and Candida infection.[73] Concerns remain regarding the potential for the development of vancomycin-resistant bacterial strains with the ongoing use of prophylactic vancomycin to prevent sepsis or to treat suspected sepsis in culture-negative infants.[57,71]

The need to remove central venous catheters (CVCs) in infants with CoNS bears careful consideration. In some infants, especially those of VLBW, removal of the central line may be the only way to rid the blood of bacteria. The need to rapidly eliminate the infection is weighed against the need for central venous access for ongoing antibiotic and nutritional support in this vulnerable population. Studies have shown that the duration of CoNS infections is reduced when the central line is removed. In a study by Karlowicz and coworkers, however, the CVC was successfully retained in 46 percent of infants with CoNS sepsis, but only if the bacteria in the blood were present for fewer than four days.[74] Benjamin and colleagues recommend that infants with one blood culture positive for CoNS be managed medically, but that infants with three positive cultures should have the CVC removed.[69]

In an era of increasing drug resistance, strategies for the prevention of CoNS sepsis are an important consideration in the NICU. Strict handwashing protocols and meticulous attention to surgical technique are critical in preventing contamination of indwelling lines and catheters.[75] Kilbride and colleagues demonstrated a significant decrease in the incidence of CoNS sepsis in six NICUs that adopted a protocol that included instruction in handwashing and line management and improvements in the accuracy of diagnosis.[76] National guidelines for the prevention and management of CoNS have been developed.[77,78]

Listeria

Listeria, a Gram-positive rod, can be acquired from animals or contaminated food. Listeriosis is reported to occur in the U.S. at a rate of 7.4 cases per million persons, with 30–50 percent of those cases occurring in pregnant women or their offspring.[11] The incidence of neonatal infection is reported to be 12.7 per 100,000 live births.[52] Epidemics of listeriosis have been reported, usually associated with contaminated food. Pregnant women, neonates, and immunocompromised patients are particularly vulnerable to these epidemics. It is postulated that specific defects in the immune system allow Listeria to grow unchecked in these populations.[1]

In neonates, listeriosis may present as either early- or late-onset disease. Early-onset disease may be acquired transplacentally or from the birth canal. In the case of transplacental acquisition, fetal death or spontaneous abortion may occur, or the infant may present at birth with a constellation of symptoms, including hepatosplenomegaly; apnea; seizures; abnormal tone; vomiting; mucous stools; and, rarely, the classic skin findings consisting of white or pink granulomatous papules on the face, on the trunk, and in the mouth.[11,16] Serious morbidity is common in the early-onset group.[79] Listeria infection is associated with the presence of meconium in the amniotic fluid and should be suspected in cases of preterm delivery with meconium staining.[16]

Late-onset listeriosis presents as meningitis, usually in the second week of life, but symptoms may occur as late as week 5. *L. monocytogenes* is responsible for up to 10 percent of neonatal meningitis cases in the United Kingdom and the U.S.[80] This type of listeriosis may be acquired from nasal colonization at birth or from the environment. Unlike GBS meningitis, the prognosis of late-onset *L. monocytogenes* meningitis is good with few sequelae.[11]

Gram-Negative Bacilli

Since the 1970s, widespread colonization of neonates with enteric bacilli has been reported. Of concern is the rapidity with which antibiotic resistance is developing among these organisms.[81] In addition to β-lactamase resistance, there are now reports of outbreaks of infection with organisms resistant to aminoglycosides and third-generation cephalosporins.[82]

Controversy exists as to whether or not increased use of intrapartum antibiotic therapy has resulted in a proportional increase in early-onset neonatal sepsis caused by Gram-negative organisms. Baltimore and colleagues examined all cases of non-GBS sepsis in 19 hospitals in Connecticut between 1996 and 1999 and found no increase in the annual rate of Gram-negative sepsis.[83] Chen and colleagues had similar results in their retrospective review conducted between 1990 and 1996 at a tertiary hospital in Boston.[84] Sinha and associates demonstrated a decrease in non-GBS infections between 1990 and 1998 in their study population.[85]

Nambiar and Singh studied 640 cases of sepsis in a tertiary children's hospital between 1996 and 2001 and found an increasing predominance of Gram-negative rods as a cause of sepsis in the NICU.[86] Stoll and colleagues studied 5,447 neonates as part of a large multicenter surveillance program conducted between 1998 and 2000. They compared them to

7,606 infants born between 1991 and 1993 and found an increase in the rate of *E. coli* sepsis (3.2 to 6.8 per 1,000 live births), accompanied by a rise in the number of ampicillin-resistant *E. coli* infections.[87]

Enteric bacilli form the bulk of the normal flora of the intestine, with *E. coli* comprising the bulk of human fecal flora. Enteric bacilli are sometimes found in small numbers as part of the normal flora of the genital and upper respiratory tracts. Enteric bacteria do not generally cause disease—unless they enter tissue where they are not part of the normal flora. The most frequent site of Gram-negative infection is the urinary tract, followed by other sites in the abdominal cavity; however, the lung, bone, or meninges may also become infected. Gram-negative sepsis often accompanies necrotizing enterocolitis and urinary tract infections.

Escherichia Coli

Escherichia coli, a member of the coliform family, is the most common cause of Gram-negative sepsis in neonates and is second only to GBS as a cause of sepsis and meningitis in neonates.[11] The stated incidence of *E. coli* sepsis is 1 to 2 cases per 1,000 births; however, there have been suggestions that this rate may be declining.[1]

In healthy neonates, *E. coli* from the maternal genital tract colonizes the lower intestinal tract within the first few days of life. Nosocomial acquisition takes place via person-to-person transmission or from environmental reservoirs.[88] There are many strains of *E. coli*, some of which are pathogenic and others that are less likely to cause disease. The more toxic strains of *E. coli* are indistinguishable from normal coliform flora through the usual bacteriologic methods. Special serotyping must be done to identify these strains.[89] The strains of *E. coli* that are most pathogenic are those that have the K1 polysaccharide capsule, a defense mechanism that prevents a mother exposed to this strain from developing antibodies that would normally confer some immunity to the fetus. The K1 strain of *E. coli* is uniquely associated with neonatal meningitis.[10]

As a pathogen, *E. coli* is a recognized cause of maternal infections such as chorioamnionitis as well as a number of local infections in neonates, including omphalitis, diarrheal illness, pneumonia, peritonitis, urinary tract infections, and meningitis. Unhanand and colleagues report that *E. coli* was responsible for 57 percent of the Gram-negative meningitis in term infants and 61 percent of that in preterm infants in their 20-year review of cases of sepsis in their institution.[90] *E. coli* is responsible for almost all (90–93 percent) of community-acquired urinary tract infections in infants less than three months of age.[91] Predisposing factors in neonatal *E. coli* infections include maternal infection, low birth weight, prolonged rupture of membranes, and septic or traumatic delivery. Clinical signs of *E. coli* sepsis are relatively nonspecific and include fever, temperature instability, apnea, cyanosis, jaundice, hepatomegaly, lethargy or irritability, vomiting, abdominal distention, and diarrhea. Meningitis may be present along with sepsis without specific central nervous system signs.[88] Initial treatment for suspected *E. coli* sepsis consists of ampicillin and an aminoglycoside. Alternatively, ampicillin and a cephalosporin (such as cefotaxime) active against most Gram-negative bacilli can be used; however, concern about the emergence of cephalosporin-resistant Gram-negative strains precludes the routine use of broad-spectrum cephalosporins unless Gram-negative bacterial meningitis is strongly suspected.[88]

Klebsiella

In the neonatal population, Klebsiella is second only to *E. coli* as a cause of Gram-negative meningitis in the U.S.[80] Klebsiella is present in the respiratory tract and feces of about 5 percent of normal adults.[52] The most common source of Klebsiella colonization in neonates is the hands of health care providers, but this organism has also been found in breast milk and in the reservoirs of nursery equipment.[92] Klebsiella is responsible for some cases of bacterial pneumonia, particularly in intubated neonates. In a review of 825 cases of late-onset sepsis in an NICU, Klebsiella was responsible for 8 percent of these infections.[93] This is similar to surveillance work done by Stoll and colleagues as part of the National Institute of Child Health and Human Development Neonatal Research Network. They found that in 3,856 neonates who had a blood-culture proven late-onset sepsis, Klebsiella was responsible for 52 infections, or 4 percent.[57]

Proteus

Although much less common than *E. coli* or Klebsiella, several Proteus species, including *P. mirabilis*, *P. vulgaris*, and *P. morganii*, may become neonatal nosocomial pathogens if they leave the intestinal tract. These organisms may cause urinary tract infections, pneumonia, or bacteremia. The rapid motility of these species may contribute to their ability to enter the urinary tract.

Salmonella

Salmonella infection is estimated to occur at a rate of 75 cases per 100,000 infants in the first month of life.[89] Nontyphoidal Salmonella organisms may be carried asymptomatically, but are also known to cause gastroenteritis, sepsis, and local infections, including meningitis and osteomyelitis.[88]

Salmonella outbreaks in the nursery cause diarrhea. Infected neonates present with abrupt onset of loose, green, mucusy stools. Bloody diarrhea and fever are also common. The organism is readily spread via the fecal-oral route as a result of poor handwashing or contact with contaminated nursery equipment. It may occasionally be acquired from the mother at birth. In the case of a nursery outbreak, the index case is often traced to a mother.[89] When Salmonella is introduced to the nursery, the risk of an infant becoming infected is reported to be as high as 20–27 percent. A variety of factors contributes to the virulence of this organism in neonates. Stomach acidity is an important barrier to Salmonella; therefore, the hypochlorhydria and rapid gastric emptying times experienced by neonates may explain the high rate of acquisition.[89] Once in the nursery, Salmonella can be difficult to eradicate, with epidemics lasting as long as 30 months reported in the literature.[94]

Antibiotic treatment of Salmonella infection has been shown to prolong fecal excretion of the organism.[95–97] Despite the risk of prolonging the carrier state, antibiotic treatment of premature infants with Salmonella infection is recommended.[89]

Shigella

Shigella infections are usually limited to the gastrointestinal tract and are a common cause of outbreaks of gastrointestinal infections in daycare settings. The organism is transmitted via the fecal-oral route. More than half the cases of Shigella diarrhea in neonates occur within the first three days of life, suggesting that the organism was transmitted from the mother at birth.[89]

Abdominal pain, low-grade fever, and watery diarrhea signal the onset of a Shigella infection. Severity of symptoms in neonates ranges from mild diarrhea to severe colitis. Sepsis, occurring when gut organisms have access to the bloodstream because of damaged intestinal mucosa, occurs in 12 percent of Shigella cases.[89] In neonates, chronic diarrhea may develop following a Shigella infection.

Antibiotic treatment is dictated by local sensitivity patterns. Multiple-resistant strains complicate the choice of therapies; however, a third-generation cephalosporin is a good choice while awaiting antibiotic sensitivity tests.[89]

Citrobacter and Serratia

Citrobacter and Serratia form part of the normal flora of the intestine, but are less numerous than *E coli*. Citrobacter can cause urinary tract infections as well as bacteremia and has been associated with epidemic outbreaks of sepsis and meningitis.[10] A species of Citrobacter, *C. diversus* (*C. koseri*), has been found to cause brain abscesses.[98] Citrobacter is usually resistant to ampicillin and variably sensitive to aminoglycosides.[10]

Serratia is an opportunistic pathogen that causes infection in immunocompromised patients such as neonates or the elderly. It may cause pneumonia, bacteremia, or endocarditis. *S. marcescens* is resistant to a number of antibiotics, including penicillin and aminoglycosides, and requires treatment with a third-generation cephalosporin.[52]

Pseudomonas

Pseudomonas is a frequent contaminant in the NICU environment. Sinks, respiratory equipment, and even soap containers may serve as reservoirs for this organism. Isolate typing suggests, however, that most infections result from maternal colonization or cross-contamination from other babies rather than from these reservoirs.

P. aeruginosa is resistant to a number of antimicrobials. Following exposure to broad-spectrum antibiotics, small or sick neonates may develop a Pseudomonas infection because of the elimination of commensal organisms that serve to keep the growth of Pseudomonas in check. Infections also follow tissue damage, such as necrotic damage resulting from IV burns or catheter complications or the introduction of intravenous or urinary catheters.

Haemophilus Influenzae

Haemophilus influenzae (Hib) forms part of the normal flora of the upper respiratory tract. Transmission is thought to be person to person, by direct contact, through inhalation of droplets of respiratory tract secretions containing the organism, or, in the neonate, by intrapartum aspiration of amniotic fluid or genital tract secretions containing the organism.[88] In neonates, *H. influenzae* causes septic arthritis, osteomyelitis, sepsis, meningitis, and pneumonia.

Most *H. influenzae* infections occur *in utero* or in the immediate postpartum period. The mortality rate for this organism has been reported to be as high as 55 percent overall—and as high as 90 percent in infants <30 weeks gestation.[1] Treatment for suspected Hib meningitis is cefotaxime or ceftriaxone. Ampicillin alone should not be used as initial therapy because 10–40 percent of Hib isolates are ampicillin resistant.[88]

Anaerobic Bacteria

For many years, difficulty in culturing and growing anaerobic bacteria limited our understanding of their role in disease. A brief general discussion of anaerobic bacteria can be found in Chapter 1. The exact frequency of anaerobic sepsis in neonates is unknown. A literature review of anaerobic sepsis in neonates done by Brook in 1990 identified 179 cases with a 26 percent mortality rate.[99] In these 179 cases, two organisms, Bacteroides and Clostridium, were the most common pathogens. Both organisms are part of normal human flora and have been found to colonize the maternal genital tract.[10]

Bacteroides

Acquired from the maternal birth canal, Bacteroides has been identified as a cause of neonatal sepsis and meningitis. The presence of Bacteroides in the maternal vagina has been implicated in premature rupture of membranes and premature delivery in several studies.[100,101]

Clostridium

Clostridia are Gram-positive spore-forming bacilli. Most diseases associated with clostridia result from the exotoxins produced by these bacteria.

Clostridium Botulinum

The *Clostridium botulinum* species of Clostridium causes botulism, usually as a result of contamination of canned or preserved foods with Clostridium spores. In infants, honey used in mixing home-prepared formula is a common vehicle for infant botulism, although the number of cases reported each year in the U.S. is relatively low at 71.[88]

Clostridium Perfringens

Clostridium perfringens is a common cause of food poisoning, but is not often seen in neonatal patients. When present in neonates, *C. perfringens* has been associated with omphalitis, cellulitis, necrotizing fasciitis, sepsis, and meningitis.[10] Presenting signs are similar to those of other bacterial infections.

Clostridium Difficile

Clostridium difficile is associated with the development of pseudomembranous colitis following antibiotic therapy. Diarrhea usually begins four to nine days into a course of antibiotics and stops after the antibiotic is discontinued.[89] Some authors have suggested a relationship between *C. difficile* and necrotizing enterocolitis, but this remains controversial.[102,103] This organism is resistant to many antimicrobials.

Clostridium Tetani

Neonatal tetanus, caused by *Clostridium tetani*, is the most important cause of infant mortality in developing countries, causing more than 800,000 deaths per year worldwide.[16] Most of these deaths are attributable to ritual practices of cord care resulting in contamination of the umbilical stump with Clostridium spores. In the U.S., only three cases of neonatal tetanus have been reported since 1984.[104]

Neonatal tetanus presents at between 3 and 14 days of age with muscle rigidity involving mainly muscles of the jaw, face, abdomen, and spine, with death resulting from respiratory failure.

Neisseria

Several Neisseria species are indigenous to humans, including *N. meningitidis*, a well-known cause of meningitis in neonates. *N. gonorrhoeae* also has a long-standing history of causing illness in neonates.

Neisseria Gonorrhoeae

The most frequently reported sexually transmitted disease in the U.S., gonorrhea has experienced a resurgence in recent years. In 2000, the number of reported new adult cases of gonorrhea was 358,995.[105] However, it is estimated that only half of all new cases are reported. Gonococcal infections are more common in the late summer, in African-Americans, and in those 15 to 19 years of age.[106]

Transmission of Gonococcus to the neonate occurs during passage through the birth canal of an infected mother. It is estimated that 30–35 percent of infants born vaginally to infected mothers will develop ophthalmic gonococcal infection.[106] Cases of eye and oropharynx infections have also been reported following cesarean section when the membranes ruptured prior to delivery.[107,108]

Gonococcal ophthalmia neonatorum presents two to five days after birth as an acute, purulent conjunctivitis. Partial suppression of the infection with eye prophylaxis occasionally results in a later presentation. In cases of prolonged rupture of membranes, presentation may occur soon after birth. Prompt antibiotic treatment has reduced the risk of permanent eye damage, which was the hallmark of the disease in the preantibiotic era. Systemic gonococcal disease is rare in the neonate; septic arthritis is the most common manifestation, and only a few case reports of gonococcal meningitis have been reported in the literature.[106]

Spirochetes

The spirochete genus consists of five species: Treponema, Borrelia, Spirochaeta, Leptospira, and Cristispira, with Treponema being of interest in the neonatal population. *T. pallidum* is one of the few bacteria that readily cross the placenta to cause intrauterine infection, in this case, syphilis. Syphilis is discussed with the congenital infections in Chapter 3.

Mycoplasma

The family Mycoplasmataceae comprises a unique group of microorganisms that have the distinction of being the smallest free-living organisms. They comprise two genera: Mycoplasma and Urealyticum. Mycoplasmata are unique in that they lack a rigid cell wall, a property that is responsible for a number of their characteristics, including resistance to β-lactam antibiotics and the need for a parasitic or saprophytic existence.[109] In humans, mycoplasmata most commonly colonize mucous membranes, particularly the respiratory and genital tracts.

Mycoplasma Hominis

One of 12 species of Mycoplasma, *M. hominis* colonizes the female genital tract in about 21–53 percent of healthy women.[109] Rates of colonization are higher in women of lower socioeconomic status. The role of *M. hominis* in neonatal disease is unclear. This organism has been cultured from the CSF in some babies with posthemorrhagic hydrocephalus, but the significance of this finding is unclear.[110] There have also been case reports of the isolation of *M. hominis* from pericardial effusions and scalp abscesses.[111]

Ureaplasma Urealyticum (T-Mycoplasma)

Ureaplasma urealyticum was first identified in the 1950s.[112,113] It is now known to colonize the genital tract in about 40–80 percent of sexually active women.[109] Neonatal colonization has been found in 45–58 percent of infants whose mothers were cervical-culture positive.[114,115]

The presence of *U. urealyticum* has been linked to chorioamnionitis and premature delivery.[116] In the neonate, it is associated with pneumonia, persistent pulmonary hypertension, chronic lung disease, and central nervous system disease.[111] Although the relationship between this organism and neonatal pneumonia has been established, the link to chronic lung disease remains inconclusive.[109] Gilbert reports that *U. urealyticum* has been isolated from babies with congenital pneumonia and early bronchopulmonary dysplasia.[117] Wang and colleagues found that low birth weight infants colonized with *U. urealyticum* had double the risk of developing chronic lung disease than did noncolonized infants.[118] Other studies support the role of *U. urealyticum* as a cause of neonatal pneumonia and chronic lung disease.[119–122] The pathogenicity of *U. urealyticum* appears to be largely restricted to low birth weight infants, perhaps because of the paucity of maternal antibodies transferred to these infants before their birth.[109] Cases of meningitis have also been attributed to infection with *U. urealyticum*. Investigators in Birmingham, Alabama, reported that *U. urealyticum* was one of the most commonly isolated microorganisms in the CSF of neonates suspected of sepsis.[110,123] Several investigators have reported finding *U. urealyticum* in the CSF of premature infants with intraventricular hemorrhage.[110,124] Other investigators have found no mycoplasmata in the CSF of neonates.[121,125]

Mycobacterium

Mycobacteria are long, slender, weakly Gram-positive organisms that are nonmotile and non–spore forming. Unique properties of this organism's cell wall make it more resistant than many bacteria to light, pH changes, and human antibodies, therefore rendering it more resistant to the body's defense systems.[126]

Mycobacterium Tuberculosis

The incidence of tuberculosis (TB) is on the rise in North America.[127] The infection is found primarily among those of lower socioeconomic status, those with human immunodeficiency virus (HIV) infection, and immigrants from countries where TB is endemic. Outbreaks in Native American communities are also common. Of particular concern is the emergence of antibiotic-resistant strains, which have been found in some people with HIV.

Congenitally acquired tuberculosis is rare, but it can occur as a result of infection of the placenta, inhalation of infected amniotic fluid, or ingestion of infected amniotic fluid. When TB is spread to the fetus through the bloodstream, the result may be a primary focus of the disease in the liver or the lung. Multiple lesions may also occur throughout the body. Ingestion or inhalation of infected amniotic fluid can result in otitis media, pneumonia, hepatosplenomegaly, or disseminated disease. The mortality rate for congenital TB approaches 50 percent, largely because of delays in making the diagnosis.[126]

Neonatal tuberculosis can be acquired by inhalation or ingestion of infected droplets or by direct contamination of wounds or mucous membranes.[126] Airborne infection is the most common route. The time frame for onset of disease varies when infection occurs in the newborn period.

Signs of TB in the neonate relate to the site and size of the lesion. The symptoms of larger lesions or those close to vital organs may be more evident than those of smaller lesions. Occasionally present at birth, signs and symptoms are more likely to present by the second or third week of life. Signs include hepatosplenomegaly, respiratory distress, fever, lymphadenopathy, ear discharge, irritability or lethargy, and abdominal distention.[126]

Isoniazid (INH) is the mainstay of treatment for neonatal tuberculosis; however, none of the antituberculosis drugs has been well studied in the preterm or term neonate.[126] Neonates receiving INH should have their liver function monitored on a regular basis, and those who are breastfed should receive pyridoxine supplements while on INH.

Chlamydia

Chlamydia trachomatis is a small Gram-negative bacterium that was responsible for a reported 702,093 chlamydial infections in the U.S. in 2000.[128] Transmission of Chlamydia is sexual, and neonatal infections occur as a result either of ascending infection or of contamination in the birth canal. Chlamydial infection of the newborn typically presents as either conjunctivitis (20–50 percent of exposed infants) or pneumonia (10–20 percent of exposed infants). Neonates born to women with chlamydial infection have a 60–70 percent chance of acquiring the infection.[129]

Chlamydial conjunctivitis usually presents within 5–14 days of delivery with a watery discharge that later becomes purulent. The conjunctivitis is usually self-limiting; however, cases of conjunctival scarring have been reported.[130] Chlamydial pneumonia has a gradual onset, between 2 and 12 weeks of age, beginning with rhinorrhea and progressing to tachypnea and coughing. It is speculated that pneumonia may occur as a result of movement of the organism from the conjunctiva into the lower respiratory tract; however, conjunctivitis is not a prerequisite to pneumonia.[129] Chlamydia can also directly infect the respiratory tract at delivery. Chlamydia pneumonia is rarely fatal; in fact, in most infants it is relatively benign. However, abnormalities in pulmonary functioning may persist for years following chlamydial pneumonia.[130]

Chlamydia can be identified with scrapings of the conjunctiva or by using a special culture medium for nasopharyngeal secretions. Eye prophylaxis with erythromycin can be used to prevent conjunctivitis, but it will not prevent the development of pneumonia. Infants born vaginally to Chlamydia-positive women should be treated with systemic erythromycin.

SUMMARY

Clearly, the risk of bacterial infection in the newborn is significant, particularly for the premature and low birth weight segment of the neonatal population. Although prevalence patterns of bacterial infection have changed over the years, organisms such as GBS and *E. coli* remain primary as causes of neonatal infections.

Current attention focuses on the emergence of antibiotic-resistant strains of common organisms, as well as on new and emerging pathogens. Through all of this, the need for vigilant assessment with a high index of suspicion for signs of sepsis remains paramount. Equally important are measures aimed at the prevention of infection: handwashing, adequate space and staff, and cohorting of infants with certain types of infection.

References

1. Guerina NG. 1998. Bacterial and fungal infections. In *Manual of Neonatal Care*, 4th ed., Cloherty JP, and Stark AR, eds. Philadelphia: Lippincott Williams & Wilkins, 271–300.
2. Nyhan WL, and Fousek MD. 1958. Septicemia of the newborn. *Pediatrics* 22(2): 268–278.
3. Freij BJ, and McCracken GH. 1994. Acute infections. In *Neonatology: Pathophysiology and Management of the Newborn*, Avery GB, Fletcher MA, and MacDonald MG, eds. Philadelphia: Lippincott Williams & Wilkins, 1082–1116.
4. Freedman RM, et al. 1981. A half century of neonatal sepsis at Yale: 1928 to 1978. *American Journal of Diseases of Children* 135(2): 140–144.
5. Gladstone IM, et al. 1990. A ten-year review of neonatal sepsis and comparison with the previous fifty-year experience. *Pediatric Infectious Disease Journal* 9(11): 819–825.
6. Stoll BJ, et al. 1996. Early-onset sepsis in very low birthweight neonates: A report from the National Institute of Child Health and Human Development Neonatal Research Network. *Journal of Pediatrics* 129(1): 72–80.
7. Centers for Disease Control and Prevention. 1996. Prevention of perinatal Group B streptococcal disease: A public health perspective. *MMWR* 45(RR-7): 1–24.
8. Watts D, et al. 1992. The association of occult amniotic fluid infection with gestational age and neonatal outcome among women in premature labor. *Obstetrics & Gynecology* 79(3): 351–357.
9. Yancey MK, et al. 1996. Risk factors for neonatal sepsis. *Obstetrics & Gynecology* 87(2): 188–194.
10. Klein JO. 2001. Bacterial sepsis and meningitis. In *Infectious Diseases of the Fetus and Newborn Infant*, 5th ed., Remington JS, and Klein JO, eds. Philadelphia: WB Saunders, 943–998.
11. Cole FS. 1998. Bacterial infections of the newborn. In *Avery's Diseases of the Newborn*, Taeusch HW, and Ballard R, eds. Philadelphia: WB Saunders, 490–512.
12. Campbell JR, et al. 1996. An outbreak of M serotype 1 Group A Streptococcus in a neonatal intensive care unit. *Journal of Pediatrics* 129(3): 396–402.
13. Geil CC, Castle WK, and Mortimer EA Jr. 1970. Group A streptococcal infections in newborn nurseries. *Pediatrics* 46(6): 849–854.
14. Edwards MS, and Baker CJ. 2001. Group B streptococcal infections. In *Infectious Diseases of the Fetus and Newborn Infant*, 5th ed., Remington JS, and Klein JO, eds. Philadelphia: WB Saunders, 1091–1156.
15. Farley MM, et al. 1993. A population-based assessment of invasive disease due to Group B Streptococcus in nonpregnant adults. *New England Journal of Medicine* 328(25): 1807–1811.
16. Isaacs D, and Moxon ER. 1999. *Handbook of Neonatal Infections: A Practical Guide*. London: WB Saunders.
17. Hickman ME, et al. 1999. Changing epidemiology of Group B streptococcal (GBS) colonization. *Pediatrics* 104(2): 203–209.
18. Schuchat A, et al. 1990. Population-based risk factors for neonatal Group B streptococcal disease: Results of a cohort study in metropolitan Atlanta. *Journal of Infectious Diseases* 162(3): 672–677.
19. Carstensen H, et al. 1988. Early-onset neonatal Group B streptococcal septicaemia in siblings. *Journal of Infection* 17(3): 201–204.
20. Faxelius G, et al. 1988. Neonatal septicemia due to Group B streptococci—Perinatal risk factors and outcome of subsequent pregnancies. *Journal of Perinatal Medicine* 16(5-6): 423–430.
21. Boyer KM, and Gotoff SP. 1985. Strategies for chemoprophylaxis of GBS early-onset infections. *Antibiotics and Chemotherapy* 35: 267–280.
22. Moller M, et al. 1984. Rupture of fetal membranes and premature delivery associated with Group B streptococci in urine of pregnant women. *Lancet* 2(8394): 69–70.
23. Wood EG, and Dillon HC Jr. 1981. A prospective study of Group B streptococcal bacteriuria in pregnancy. *American Journal of Obstetrics and Gynecology* 140(5): 515–520.
24. Benitz WE, Gould JB, and Druzin ML. 1999. Risk factors for early-onset Group B streptococcal sepsis: Estimation of odds ratio by critical literature review. *Pediatrics* 103(6): e77.
25. Anthony BF, and Okada DM. 1977. The emergence of Group B streptococci in infection of the newborn infant. *Annual Review of Medicine* 28: 355–369.
26. Schrag SJ, et al. 2000. Group B streptococcal disease in the era of intrapartum antibiotic prophylaxis. *New England Journal of Medicine* 342(1): 15–20.
27. Weisman LE, et al. 1992. Early-onset Group B streptococcal sepsis: A current assessment. *Journal of Pediatrics* 121(3): 428–433.
28. Payne NR, et al. 1988. Correlation of clinical and pathologic findings in early onset neonatal Group B streptococcal infection with disease severity and prediction of outcome. *Pediatric Infectious Disease Journal* 7(12): 836–847.
29. Noya FJ, et al. 1987. Unusual occurrence of an epidemic of Type Ib/c Group B streptococcal sepsis in a neonatal intensive care unit. *Journal of Infectious Diseases* 155(6): 1135–1144.
30. Weems JJ Jr, Jarvis WR, and Colman G. 1986. A cluster of late onset Group B streptococcal infections in low birth weight premature infants: No evidence for horizontal transmission. *Pediatric Infectious Disease* 5(6): 715–717.
31. Sanchez PJ. 2002. Perinatal infections and brain injury: Current treatment options. *Clinics in Perinatology* 29(4): 799–826.
32. Siegel JD. 1998. Prophylaxis for neonatal Group B streptococcus infections. *Seminars in Perinatology* 22(1): 33–49.
33. Chin KC, and Fitzhardinge PM. 1985. Sequelae of early-onset Group B streptococcal neonatal meningitis. *Journal of Pediatrics* 106(5): 819–822.
34. Edwards MS, et al. 1985. Long-term sequelae of Group B streptococcal meningitis in infants. *Journal of Pediatrics* 106(5): 717–722.
35. Wald ER, et al. 1986. Long-term outcome of Group B streptococcal meningitis. *Pediatrics* 77(2): 217–221.
36. Allen UD, Navas L, and King SM. 1993. Effectiveness of intrapartum penicillin prophylaxis in preventing early-onset Group B streptococcal infection: Results of a meta-analysis. *Canadian Medical Association Journal* 149(11): 1659–1665.
37. Boyer KM, and Gotoff SP. 1986. Prevention of early-onset Group B streptococcal disease with selective intrapartum chemoprophylaxis. *New England Journal of Medicine* 314(26): 1665–1669.
38. American Academy of Pediatrics, Committee on Infectious Diseases and Committee on Fetus and Newborn. 1992. Guidelines for pre-

vention of Group B streptococcal (GBS) infection by chemoprophylaxis. *Pediatrics* 90(5): 775–778.

39. Centers for Disease Control and Prevention. 1997. Decreasing incidence of perinatal Group B streptococcal disease—United States, 1993–1995. *MMWR* 46(21): 473–477.

40. Cheon-Lee E, and Amstey MS. 1998. Compliance with the Centers for Disease Control and Prevention antenatal culture protocol for preventing Group B streptococcal neonatal sepsis. *American Journal of Obstetrics and Gynecology* 179(1): 77–79.

41. Glantz JC, and Kedley KE. 1998. Concepts and controversies in the management of Group B Streptococcus during pregnancy. *Birth* 25(1): 45–53.

42. Lieu TA, et al. 1998. Neonatal Group B streptococcal infection in a managed care population. *Obstetrics & Gynecology* 92(1): 21–27.

43. Truong V, Yancey MK, and Lentz SL. 2000. Reduction of early-onset Group B streptococcal sepsis with universal screening and intrapartum antimicrobial therapy for preterm and colonized term parturients. *Obstetrics & Gynecology* 94(4 part 2): S8.

44. Benitz WE, Gould JB, and Druzin ML. 1999. Antimicrobial prevention of early-onset group B streptococcal sepsis: Estimates of risk reduction based on a critical literature review. *Pediatrics* 103(6): e78.

45. Schimmel MS, Samueloff A, and Eidelman AI. 1998. Prevention of neonatal Group B streptococcal infections. *Clinics in Perinatology* 25(3): 687–697.

46. Whitney CG, et al. 1997. Prevention practices for perinatal Group B streptococcal disease: A multi-state surveillance analysis. Neonatal Group B Streptococcal Disease Study Group. *Obstetrics & Gynecology* 89(1): 28–32.

47. Chandran L, et al. 2001. Compliance with Group B streptococcal disease prevention guidelines. *MCN: American Journal of Maternal Child Nursing* 26(6): 313–319.

48. Schrag SJ, et al. 2002. A population-based comparison of strategies to prevent early-onset Group B streptococcal disease in neonates. *New England Journal of Medicine* 347(4): 233–239.

49. Centers for Disease Control and Prevention. 2002. Prevention of perinatal Group B streptococcal disease: Revised guidelines from the CDC. *MMWR* 51(RR-11): 1–22.

50. Dobson SRM, and Baker CJ. 1990. Enterococcal sepsis in neonates: Features by age at onset and occurrence of focal infection. *Pediatrics* 85(2): 165–171.

51. Shinefield HR, and St. Geme JW. 2001. Staphylococcal infections. In *Infectious Diseases of the Fetus and Newborn Infant*, 5th ed., Remington JS, and Klein JO, eds. Philadelphia: WB Saunders, 1217–1247.

52. Murray PR, et al. 1998. *Medical Microbiology*, 3rd ed. St Louis: Mosby–Year Book.

53. Ish-Horowicz MR, McIntyre P, and Nade S. 1992. Bone and joint infections caused by multiply resistant *Staphylococcus aureus* in a neonatal intensive care unit. *Pediatric Infectious Disease Journal* 11(2): 82–87.

54. Wong M, et al. 1995. Clinical and diagnostic features of osteomyelitis occurring in the first three months of life. *Pediatric Infectious Disease Journal* 14(12): 1047–1053.

55. Haley RW, et al. 1995. Eradication of endemic methicillin-resistant *Staphylococcus aureus* infections from a neonatal intensive care unit. *Journal of Infectious Diseases* 171(3): 614–624.

56. Haley RW, and Bregman DA. 1982. The role of understaffing and overcrowding in recurrent outbreaks of staphylococcal infection in a neonatal special-care unit. *Journal of Infectious Diseases* 145(6): 875–885.

57. Stoll BJ, et al. 2002. Late-onset sepsis in very low birth weight neonates: The experience of the NICHD Neonatal Research Network. *Pediatrics* 110(2 part 1): 285–291.

58. Sohn AH, et al. 2001. Prevalence of nosocomial infections in neonatal intensive care unit patients: Results from the first national point-prevalence survey. *Journal of Pediatrics* 139(6): 821–827.

59. Isaacs D, Australasian Study Group for Neonatal Infections. 2003. A ten year, multicentre study of coagulase negative staphylococcal infections in Australasian neonatal units. *Archives of Disease in Childhood. Fetal and Neonatal Edition* 88(2): F89–F93.

60. Raimundo O, et al. 2002. Molecular epidemiology of coagulase-negative staphylococcal bacteraemia in a newborn intensive care unit. *Journal of Hospital Infection* 51(1): 33–42.

61. Brodie SB, et al. 2000. Occurrence of nosocomial bloodstream infections in six neonatal intensive care units. *Pediatric Infectious Disease Journal* 19(1): 56–65.

62. Canadian Pediatric Society, Infectious Diseases and Immunization Committee. 1994 (reaffirmed April 2002). Coagulase negative staphylococci as pathogens: Believe it or not? *Canadian Journal of Paediatrics* 1(2): 61–63. Available at www.cps.ca/English/statements/ID/id9403.htm.

63. Shigeoka AO, Santos JI, and Hill HR. 1979. Functional analysis of neutrophil granulocytes from healthy, infected, and stressed neonates. *Journal of Pediatrics* 95(3): 454–460.

64. Anderson DC, Hughes BJ, and Smith CW. 1981. Abnormal motility of neonatal polymorphonuclear leukocytes. Relationship to impaired redistribution of surface adhesion sites by chemotactic factor or colchicine. *Journal of Clinical Investigation* 68(4): 863–874.

65. Fallat ME, et al. 1998. Central venous catheter bloodstream infections in the neonatal intensive care unit. *Journal of Pediatric Surgery* 33(9): 1383–1387.

66. Fanaroff AA, et al. 1998. Incidence, presenting features, risk factors, and significance of late onset septicemia in very low birth weight infants. The National Institute of Child Health and Human Development Neonatal Research Network. *Pediatric Infectious Disease Journal* 17(7): 593–598.

67. Isaacs D, et al. 1996. Late-onset infections of infants in neonatal units. *Journal of Paediatrics and Child Health* 32(2): 158–161.

68. Maayan-Metzger A, et al. 2000. Clinical and laboratory impact of coagulase-negative staphylococci bacteremia in preterm infants. *Acta Paediatrica* 89(6): 690–693.

69. Benjamin DK Jr, et al. 2001. Bacteremia, central catheters and neonates: When to pull the line. *Pediatrics* 107(6): 1272–1276.

70. Gin AS, and Zhanel GG. 1996. Vancomycin-resistant enterococci. *Annals of Pharmacotherapy* 30(6): 615–624.

71. Craft AP, Finer NN, and Barrington KJ. 2000. Vancomycin for prophylaxis against sepsis in preterm neonates (Cochrane Review). In *The Cochrane Library*, Issue 3, 2003. Oxford: Update Software.

72. Van Houten MA, et al. 2001. Does the empiric use of vancomycin in pediatrics increase the risk for Gram-negative bacteremia? *Pediatric Infectious Disease Journal* 20(2): 171–177.

73. Mullett MD, Cook EF, and Gallagher R. 1998. Nosocomial sepsis in the neonatal intensive care unit. *Journal of Perinatology* 18(2): 112–115.

74. Karlowicz MG, et al. 2002. Central venous catheter removal versus in situ treatment in neonates with coagulase-negative staphylococcal bacteremia. *Pediatric Infectious Disease Journal* 21(1): 22–27.

75. Maas A, et al. 1998. Central venous catheter–related bacteremia in critically ill neonates: Risk factors and impact of a prevention program. *Journal of Hospital Infection* 40(3): 211–224.

76. Kilbride HW, et al. 2003. Implementation of evidence-based potentially better practices to decrease nosocomial infections. *Pediatrics* 111(4 part 2): e519–e533.

77. Centers for Disease Control and Prevention. 2002. Guidelines for the prevention of intravascular catheter–related infections. *MMWR* 51(RR-10): 1–29.

78. Mermel LA. 2001. Guidelines for the management of intravascular catheter–related infections. *Clinical Infectious Diseases* 32(9): 1249–1272.

79. Teberg AJ, et al. 1987. Clinical manifestations of epidemic neonatal listeriosis. *Pediatric Infectious Disease Journal* 6(9): 817–820.

80. Pong A, and Bradley JS. 1999. Bacterial meningitis and the newborn infant. *Infectious Disease Clinics of North America* 13(3): 711–733.
81. Bromiker R, et al. 2001. Neonatal bacteremia: Patterns of antibiotic resistance. *Infection Control and Hospital Epidemiology* 22(12): 767–770.
82. Harris JS, and Goldmann DA. 2001. Infections acquired in the nursery: Epidemiology and control. In *Infectious Diseases of the Fetus and Newborn Infant*, 5th ed., Remington JS, and Klein JO, eds. Philadelphia: WB Saunders, 1371–1418.
83. Baltimore RS, et al. 2001. Early-onset neonatal sepsis in the era of Group B streptococcal prevention. *Pediatrics* 108(5): 1094–1098.
84. Chen KT, et al. 2001. No increase in rates of early-onset neonatal sepsis by non–Group B Streptococcus or ampicillin-resistant organisms. *American Journal of Obstetrics and Gynecology* 185(4): 854–858.
85. Sinha A, Yokoe D, and Platt R. 2003. Intrapartum antibiotics and neonatal invasive infections caused by organisms other than Group B Streptococcus. *Journal of Pediatrics* 142(5): 492–497.
86. Nambiar S, and Singh N. 2002. Change in epidemiology of health care–associated infections in a neonatal intensive care unit. *Pediatric Infectious Disease Journal* 21(9): 839–842.
87. Stoll BJ, et al. 2002. Changes in pathogens causing early-onset sepsis in very-low-birth-weight infants. *New England Journal of Medicine* 347(4): 240–247.
88. American Academy of Pediatrics. 2000. *Red Book: Report of the Committee on Infectious Diseases*, 25th ed. Elk Grove Village, Illinois: AAP, 212–214, 241–247, 266–272, 501–506.
89. Cleary TG, Guerrant RL, and Pickering LK. 2001. Microorganisms responsible for neonatal diarrhea. In *Infectious Diseases of the Fetus and Newborn Infant*, 5th ed., Remington JS, and Klein JO, eds. Philadelphia: WB Saunders, 1249–1326.
90. Unhanand M, et al. 1993. Gram-negative enteric bacillary meningitis: A twenty-one year experience. *Journal of Pediatrics* 122(1): 15–21.
91. Long SS, and Klein JO. 2001 Bacterial infections of the urinary tract. In *Infectious Diseases of the Fetus and Newborn Infant*, 5th ed., Remington JS, and Klein JO, eds. Philadelphia: WB Saunders, 1035–1046.
92. Adler JL, et al. 1970. Nosocomial colonization with kanamycin-resistant Klebsiella pneumoniae, types 2 and 11, in a premature nursery. *Journal of Pediatrics* 77(3): 376–385.
93. Karlowicz MG, Buescher ES, and Surka AE. 2000. Fulminant late-onset sepsis in a neonatal intensive care unit, 1988–1997, and the impact of avoiding empiric vancomycin therapy. *Pediatrics* 106(6): 1387–1390.
94. Szanton VL. 1957. Epidemic of salmonellosis: A 30 month study of 80 cases of *Salmonella Oranienburg* infection. *Pediatrics* 20(5): 794–808.
95. Aserkoff B, and Bennett JV. 1969. Effect of antibiotic therapy in acute salmonellosis on the fecal excretion of salmonellae. *New England Journal of Medicine* 281(12): 636–640.
96. Dixon JMS. 1965. Effect of antibiotic treatment on duration of excretion of *Salmonella typhimurium* by children. *British Medical Journal* 5474: 1343–1345.
97. Neill MA, et al. 1991. Failure of ciprofloxacin to eradicate convalescent fecal excretion after acute salmonellosis: Experience during an outbreak in health care workers. *Annals of Internal Medicine* 114(3): 195–199.
98. Doran TI. 1999. The role of *Citrobacter* in clinical disease of children. Review. *Clinical Infectious Diseases* 28(2): 384–394.
99. Brook I. 1990. Bacteremia due to anaerobic bacteria in newborns. *Journal of Perinatology* 10(4): 351–356.
100. Krohn MA, et al. 1991. Vaginal Bacteroides species are associated with an increased rate of preterm delivery among women in preterm labor. *Journal of Infectious Diseases* 164(1): 88–93.
101. McDonald HM, et al. 1991. Vaginal infections and preterm labor. *British Journal of Obstetrics and Gynaecology* 98(5): 427–435.
102. Johnson S, and Gerding DN. 1998. *Clostridium difficile*–associated diarrhea. *Clinical Infectious Diseases* 26(5): 1027–1034. (Comment in *Clinical Infectious Diseases*, 1999, 28[4]: 936–937.)
103. Sherertz RJ, and Sarubbi FA. 1982. The prevalence of *Clostridium difficile* and toxin in a nursery population: A comparison between patients with necrotizing enterocolitis and an asymptomatic group. *Journal of Pediatrics* 100(3): 435–439.
104. Centers for Disease Control and Prevention. 1998. Neonatal tetanus—Montana 1998. *MMWR* 47(43): 928–930.
105. Centers for Disease Control and Prevention. 2001. *National Overview of Sexually Transmitted Diseases, 2000*. Atlanta: U.S. Department of Health and Human Services, Centers for Disease Control and Prevention, September. Available at www.cdc.gov/std/stats/2000NatOverview.htm.
106. Gutman LT. 2001. Gonococcal infections: Epidemiology and control. In *Infectious Diseases of the Fetus and Newborn Infant*, 5th ed., Remington JS, and Klein JO, eds. Philadelphia: WB Saunders, 1199–1216.
107. Diener B. 1981. Cesarean section complicated by gonococcal ophthalmia neonatorum. *Journal of Family Practice* 13(5): 739, 743–744.
108. Nickerson CW. 1973. Gonorrhea amnionitis. *Obstetrics & Gynecology* 42(6): 815–817.
109. Cassell GH, Waites KB, and Crouse DT. 2001. Mycoplasmal infections. In *Infectious Diseases of the Fetus and Newborn Infant*, 5th ed., Remington JS, and Klein JO, eds. Philadelphia: WB Saunders, 733–767.
110. Waites KB, et al. 1988. Chronic *Ureaplasma urealyticum* and *Mycoplasma hominis* infections of central nervous system in preterm infants. *Lancet* 1(8575-8576): 17–21.
111. Cassell GH, Waites KB, and Crouse DT. 1991. Perinatal mycoplasmal infections. *Clinics in Perinatology* 18(2): 241–262.
112. Gannon H. 1993. *Ureaplasma urealyticum* and its role in neonatal lung disease. *Neonatal Network* 12(3): 13–18.
113. Shepard MC. 1954. The recovery of pleuropneumonia-like organisms from Negro men with and without nongonococcal urethritis. *American Journal of Syphilis, Gonorrhea, and Venereal Diseases* 38: 113–124.
114. Dinsmoor MJ, Ramamurthy RS, and Gibbs RS. 1989. Transmission of genital mycoplasmas from mother to neonate in women with prolonged membrane rupture. *Pediatric Infectious Disease Journal* 8(8): 483–487.
115. Sanchez PJ, and Regan JA. 1988. *Ureaplasma urealyticum* colonization and chronic lung disease in low birth weight infants. *Pediatric Infectious Disease Journal* 7(8): 542–546.
116. Hillier SL, et al. 1991. Microbiologic causes and neonatal outcomes associated with chorioamnion infection. *American Journal of Obstetrics and Gynecology* 165(4 part 1): 955–961.
117. Gilbert GL. 1996. Chlamydial and mycoplasmal infections. *Seminars in Neonatology* 1(2): 119–125.
118. Wang EE, et al. 1993. *Ureaplasma urealyticum* and chronic lung disease of prematurity: Critical appraisal of the literature on causation. *Clinical Infectious Diseases* 17(supplement 1): S112–S116.
119. Cassell GH, et al. 1988. Association of *Ureaplasma urealyticum* infection of the lower respiratory tract with chronic lung disease and death in very-low-birth-weight infants. *Lancet* 2(8605): 240–245.
120. Dyke MP, et al. 1993. *Ureaplasma urealyticum* in a neonatal intensive care population. *Journal of Paediatrics and Child Health* 29(4): 295–297.
121. Izraeli S, et al. 1991. Genital mycoplasmas in preterm infants: Prevalence and clinical significance. *European Journal of Pediatrics* 150(11): 804–807.
122. Payne NR, et al. 1993. New prospective studies of the association of *Ureaplasma urealyticum* colonization and chronic lung disease. *Clinical Infectious Diseases* 17(supplement 1): S117–S121.
123. Waites KB, Crouse DT, and Cassell GH. 1993. Systemic neonatal infection due to *Ureaplasma urealyticum*. *Clinical Infectious Diseases* 17(supplement 1): S131–S135.

124. Ollikainen J, et al. 1993. *Ureaplasma urealyticum* cultured from brain tissue of preterm twins who died of intraventricular hemorrhage. *Scandinavian Journal of Infectious Diseases* 25(4): 529–531.

125. Likitnukul S, et al. 1986. Role of genital mycoplasmas in young infants with suspected sepsis. *Journal of Pediatrics* 109(6): 971–974.

126. Starke JR, and Smith MHD. 2001. Tuberculosis. In *Infectious Diseases of the Fetus and Newborn Infant*, 5th ed., Remington JS, and Klein JO, eds. Philadelphia: WB Saunders, 1179–1197.

127. Centers for Disease Control and Prevention. 2001. *Reported Tuberculosis in the United States, 2000*. Atlanta: Department of Health and Human Services, Centers for Disease Control and Prevention, August. Available at www.cdc.gov/nchstp/tb/surv/surv2000/default.htm.

128. Centers for Disease Control and Prevention. 2001. *Sexually Transmitted Disease Surveillance 2000 Supplement, Chlamydia Prevalence Monitoring Project Annual Report 2000*. Atlanta: U.S. Department of Health and Human Services, Centers for Disease Control and Prevention, November. Available at www.cdc.gov/std/chlamydia2000/ct2000.pdf.

129. Schachter J, and Grossman M. 2001. Chlamydia. In *Infectious Diseases of the Fetus and Newborn Infant*, 5th ed., Remington JS, and Klein JO, eds. Philadelphia: WB Saunders, 769–778.

130. Hess DL. 1993. Chlamydia in the neonate. *Neonatal Network* 12(3): 9–12.

Notes

CHAPTER 5

Neonatal Viral and Fungal Infections

Susan Givens Bell, MS, RNC

Neonatal viral infections—respiratory syncytial virus, influenza, and others—have a significant impact on the neonatal intensive care patient. Viral illness can prolong the length of stay, increase the cost of hospitalization, complicate chronic respiratory or cardiovascular illness, or even result in death. The blood-borne viruses, human immunodeficiency virus (HIV) and hepatitis, confer a lifetime of health-related issues on infants who acquire these diseases perinatally. Fungal infections, often the consequence of antibiotic therapy for suspected or proved bacterial infection, also may result in prolonged hospital stay, increased expense, and possibly death.

NEONATAL VIRAL INFECTIONS

Respiratory Syncytial Virus
Etiology and Epidemiology

Respiratory syncytial virus (RSV) is a large, enveloped, single-stranded RNA virus of the family Paramyxoviridae, genus Pneumovirus. The two major strains, A and B, circulate concurrently during seasonal outbreaks from October through April in temperate climates. The clinical and epidemiologic significance of serotype variation are not known.[1,2]

RSV is the primary cause of bronchiolitis and pneumonia in infants and children less than two years of age. In addition, RSV is a common cause of nosocomial viral infections. The incubation period from time of exposure to first symptoms is two to eight days. Most infants will have symptoms in four to six days. Viral shedding usually occurs for three to eight days, but young infants may shed virus for up to four weeks. The duration of viral shedding is most likely related to the severity of the illness and the immunologic integrity of the infant.[1,2]

RSV has earned its reputation as the most important respiratory virus in infants and young children for several reasons. First, it is omnipresent and highly contagious. The only source of RSV infection is humans. Transmission occurs by close or direct contact with contaminated secretions. The virus can survive for several hours on nonporous surfaces and for 30 minutes or more on the hands.[1,3] RSV can be spread by droplet contamination during sneezing, coughing,

FIGURE 5-1 ◆ X-ray of infant at six months of age in the acute stage of active RSV pneumonia.

The changes of hyperinflation with areas of atelectasis are marked.

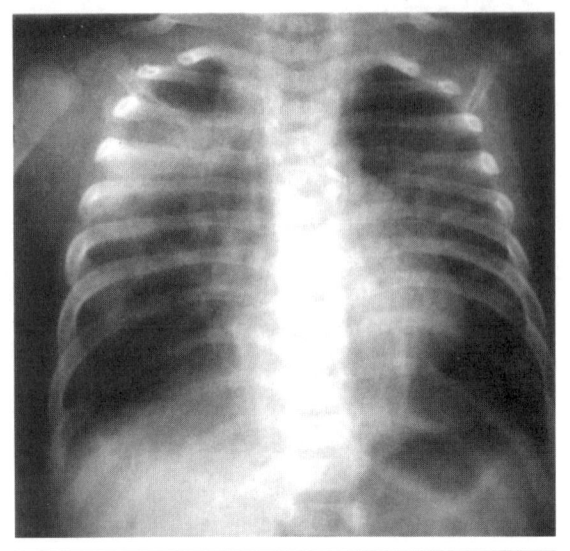

From: Kirpalani H, et al. 1999. The chest. In *Imaging of the Newborn Baby*, Kirpalani H, Mernagh J, and Gill G, eds. Philadelphia: Churchill Livingstone, 33. Reprinted by permission.

suctioning, or endotracheal intubation. The hands are also a common source of inoculation with RSV. The portal of entry is usually the nose or eye, with subsequent spread to the upper, then the lower respiratory tract. Second, the virus prefers the respiratory tracts of very young infants and children less than three years of age. This preference appears to be primarily immunologic in nature. Most people over the age of three years have RSV neutralizing antibodies that help combat infection.[3] Neonatal intensive care patients at particularly high risk for nosocomial RSV infection are those who are extremely premature and those with bronchopulmonary dysplasia (BPD), congenital heart disease (CHD), or immunodeficiency.[1] The severity of the illness is generally inversely proportional to age.[3] Third, immunity to RSV is brief and incomplete; therefore, there is the opportunity for reinfection throughout life.[1,2]

Clinical Manifestations and Diagnosis

In the first few weeks of life, infants (particularly preterm infants) with RSV present with lethargy, irritability, and poor feeding, occasionally accompanied by apneic episodes. Respiratory symptoms are minimal.[1] In older infants, upper respiratory tract symptoms including cough, pharyngitis, and rhinitis are early manifestations. Several days after the onset of the initial symptoms, lower respiratory tract symptoms such as wheezing, tachypnea, cyanosis, and retractions are seen in more than half the previously healthy infants with RSV. Most patients have a fever. Pneumonia is the most common manifestation of lower respiratory tract infection. Interstitial or alveolar infiltrates on chest radiograph are diagnostic findings of pneumonia. Other radiographic findings may include atelectasis or hyperinflated lung fields (Figure 5-1). Wheezing is a diagnostic sign of bronchiolitis.[2]

Rapid laboratory diagnosis can be made on nasal secretions using either latex agglutination immunofluorescence assay (IFA) or enzyme-linked immunosorbent assay (ELISA). Viral cultures and polymerase chain reaction (PCR) may be performed in some facilities.[2,3] Breton compared the accuracy of two RSV specimen collection methods. The researcher suggests that because the nasal wash method is likely to be less traumatic for the infant, it be the preferred procedure for RSV specimen collection.[4] The nasal wash method consists of instilling 3–5 drops of normal saline into one nostril and then aspirating the nasal contents with a plastic bulb catheter designed to go no farther than the top of the nostril. The nasopharyngeal method consists of instilling 3–5 drops of normal saline into one nostril, then using an 8 or 10 French suction catheter (a 5 or 6 French catheter should be used on smaller, premature infants) and mechanical suction to aspirate secretions from the nasopharynx by applying gentle suction as the catheter is slowly removed. Laboratory test results for RSV showed no significant difference between the two methods.

Treatment and Prevention

Treatment for RSV is primarily supportive. Oxygen is administered to correct hypoxia. Mechanical ventilation is provided for those infants in acute respiratory failure. Adequate hydration helps to thin respiratory secretions. Antibiotics are not used unless secondary bacterial infection is present. Contact precautions are maintained for the duration of the illness. Cohorting of infected infants helps prevent the spread of the disease.

Antiviral therapy. Ribavirin (Virazole), a broad-spectrum antiviral agent, is the only drug approved by the U.S. Food and Drug Administration (FDA) for treatment of RSV in infants. Its mechanism of action is inhibition of messenger RNA transcription and viral protein synthesis. Ribavirin is aerosolized and delivered as small particles to facilitate its reaching the lower respiratory tract. A drying chamber is used to prevent "rain out," or condensation on the tubing. The drug can be delivered via oxygen hood, oxygen tent, or ventilator. Infants receive the medication for 12–20 hours per day for one to seven days.[1,2,5]

The use of ribavirin remains controversial. One concern is the high cost of the drug relative to its benefits. Ribavirin moderately decreases viral load.[6,7] Following ribavirin therapy, patients demonstrate mild improvement in illness score. (A 0 [baseline] to 5 [respiratory failure] score determined by changes from baseline of percent oxygen saturation, respiratory rate, and retractions and adventitial sounds.[8]) They also exhibit higher PaO_2 and higher oxygen saturation. Studies have not demonstrated improved mortality rates or significant reduction in length of hospitalization following treatment with ribavirin.[8–11] However, these results may be due to inadequate sample size.[9–11] Another area of controversy is safety. Because ribavirin is aerosolized for administration, there is concern for the safety of health care workers who treat infants receiving it. Their major complaints have been eye irritation, especially in contact lens wearers, and headache. These effects were reported as mild and resolved when exposure to the drug was discontinued.[12] Concern regarding reproductive and teratogenic toxicities has also been expressed. There have been reports of teratogenicity in several animal species, but not in primates.[13–15] The exact risk in humans is not known; however, there have been no reports of birth defects in infants with *in utero* ribavirin exposure.[16] Despite this, it is recommended that pregnant health care workers and family members avoid direct patient contact and medication preparation during ribavirin therapy.[17]

Because of concerns regarding cost versus benefit, safety issues, and variable clinical efficacy, consideration of ribavirin therapy should be limited to infants with the following characteristics:[18–24]

- Infants with risk factors for severe RSV illness:
    Congenital heart disease (including pulmonary hypertension)
    Bronchopulmonary dysplasia
    Cystic fibrosis
    Other chronic lung disease
    Previously healthy premature infants
    Infants <6 weeks of age
- Infants who have a high risk of mortality from RSV infection or who have prolonged RSV illness, including those with underlying immunosuppressive disorders or therapy:
    Acquired immunodeficiency syndrome
    Severe combined immunodeficiency syndrome
    Organ transplantation
- Infants who are severely ill (with or without mechanical ventilation). Useful criteria for determining severity of illness include:
    Arterial blood gas determinations
    Clinical response to other therapies

- Hospitalized patients who have an increased risk for progressing from a mild to a more severe course:
    - Infants <6 weeks of age
        - Infants with underlying medical conditions: Multiple congenital anomalies
        - Certain neurologic disorders (e.g., cerebral palsy)
        - Certain metabolic diseases (e.g., myasthenia gravis)

Bronchodilators. There is also debate regarding the efficacy of bronchodilators in infants with RSV. Derish and associates evaluated maximum expiratory flow at functional residual capacity (V_{max}FRC), a pulmonary function test to assess small-airway function, in 25 infants with acute respiratory failure caused by RSV bronchiolitis. The sample contained 12 infants born at term with no past medical problems and 13 infants with a history of prematurity and/or cardiac or pulmonary disease. The mean postconceptional age of the infants was 45.2 weeks; the mean chronological age was 9.2 weeks. At the time of the RSV illness, the infants born prematurely were older chronologically than were the infants born at term. The results of the study revealed a significant improvement in mean V_{max} FRC in this patient sample. However, only 3 patients had an increase into the normal range for age. In addition, 3 patients demonstrated a significant decrease in V_{max} FRC. Based on these findings, the researchers recommend a trial of bronchodilators for any infant with acute respiratory failure associated with RSV. They assert that clinical efficacy of bronchodilators for RSV, measured as duration of oxygen and ventilator requirements, remains to be seen.[25]

Corticosteroids. Corticosteroids have not been shown to be beneficial in the treatment of RSV.[1,5]

Immunotherapy. Other studied therapeutic approaches include the use of polyclonal and monoclonal antibody products with high titers against RSV. RSV immune globulin (RSVIG) has been found safe and effective in reducing viral load in patients with established RSV infection, but not in decreasing length of hospitalization.[3,26] Similar findings were noted with the monoclonal antibody product palivizumab (Synagis). The product is safe and does reduce viral concentration in deep tracheal secretions.[27,28] However, there was no significant difference between the treatment group and the control group when length of hospital stay, admission to the intensive care unit (ICU), number of days in the ICU, days of supplemental oxygen, and days of mechanical ventilation were examined.[28]

During RSV season, control of nosocomial outbreaks can be complicated by the presence of infected infants, staff, and visitors. The AAP suggests the following measures: (1) laboratory screening of patients for RSV, (2) cohorting of infected patients and staff, (3) exclusion of visitors with respiratory infections, and (4) exclusion of staff with RSV or other respiratory illnesses from caring for infants at high risk for RSV.[1]

Immunoprophylaxis. Both polyclonal and monoclonal antibody products have been studied for use as prophylaxis against RSV infection. RSV-IGIV (RespiGam), a polyclonal antibody product, has been shown to reduce the incidence of RSV in infants with a history of chronic lung disease (CLD) or prematurity or both. In addition, total days of RSV hospitalization and overall respiratory hospitalization were also decreased in this population.[29] The dose of RSV-IGIV is 750 mg/kg (15 ml/kg) given intravenously once a month beginning at the onset of and continuing throughout RSV season.[1] The primary complication of RSV-IGIV administration is related to fluid volume, particularly for patients with CLD. This can be managed by reducing the infusion rate and/or administering diuretics.[29] Disadvantages of RSV-IGIV include

TABLE 5-1 ◆ AAP Recommendations for Use of RSV-IGIV and Palivizumab

Infants and children less than two years of age who have CLD and have required medical management for their CLD within 6 months of the anticipated RSV season.

Infants born at or before 32 weeks gestation without CLD or who do not meet the preceding guideline should be considered based on their gestational age and their chronological age at the start of RSV season:

    Infants born at or before 28 weeks gestation may benefit from RSV immunoprophylaxis up to 12 months of age.

    Infants born between 29 and 32 weeks gestation may benefit from RSV immunoprophylaxis up to 6 months of age.

RSV-IGIV and palivizumab should not be used in patients with cyanotic heart disease. However, infants with CLD or prematurity who meet the preceding criteria and who have asymptomatic acyanotic heart disease (e.g., patent ductus arteriosis or ventricular septal defect) may benefit from RSV immunoprophylaxis. Note that neither RSV-IGIV nor palivizumab is FDA approved for patients with CHD.

Neither RSV-IGIV nor palivizumab has been studied for prophylactic or therapeutic use in immunocompromised patients. This patient group may benefit, however, from RSV immunoprophylaxis. Providers may consider substituting RSV-IGIV during the RSV season for those patients already receiving intravenous immune globulin monthly.

The need for and efficacy of RSV immunoprophylaxis in high-risk hospitalized infants during a nosocomial outbreak has not been studied.

    RSV immunoprophylaxis should begin at the onset of the season and stop at the end of the season. There are regional differences in the timing of RSV season. Providers should consult with their local health department to determine an optimal schedule.

    Immunizations. The measles-mumps-rubella and varicella vaccines should be deferred for 9 months after the last RSV-IGIV dose. Palivizumab does not interfere with the immune response to vaccines. (For more on immunizations, see Appendix E.)

Adapted from: American Academy of Pediatrics. 2000. Respiratory syncytial virus. In *Red Book: Report of the Committee on Infectious Diseases*, 25th ed., Pickering L, ed. Elk Grove Village, Illinois: American Academy of Pediatrics, 483–487; and American Academy of Pediatrics, Committee on Infectious Diseases and Committee of Fetus and Newborn. 1998. Prevention of respiratory syncytial virus infections: Indications for the use of palivizumab and update on the use of RSV-IGIV. *Pediatrics* 102(5): 1211–1216.

the need for monthly IV access, the time required for infusion (several hours for the 15 ml/kg volume), and the possible risk of transmission of blood-borne pathogens because RSV-IGIV is derived from human blood.[3]

The humanized RSV monoclonal antibody palivizumab (Synagis) has been shown effective for RSV prophylaxis in infants born at or before 35 weeks gestation or those who had CLD. Patients who received palivizumab prophylaxis had fewer RSV hospital days, fewer days with supplemental oxygen, fewer days with moderate or severe lower respiratory illness, and a lower incidence of ICU admissions. There was no significant difference in the need for mechanical ventilation, incidence of otitis media, or non-RSV respiratory hospitalizations.[30] Palivizumab does not reduce non-RSV respiratory hospitalizations because the monoclonal antibody is specific only to RSV, differentiating it from the polyclonal antibody preparation.[3,30]

The dose of palivizumab is 15 mg/kg, given by intramuscular (IM) injection monthly during RSV season. The IM injection has clear advantages over RSV-IGIV. There is no need for IV access, no concerns over fluid volume, and the time required to administer the antibody is reduced significantly. Palivizumab has been judged safe and effective for RSV prophylaxis. Potential adverse reactions include injection site erythema, swelling, pain, and bruising. Mild to moderate elevation of aspartate aminotransferase (AST) was seen in study subjects, but the levels were comparable in both the treatment and placebo groups.[30]

Despite some of the advantages of palivizumab over RSV-IGIV, specific considerations could favor the latter over the former. For example, RSV-IGIV immunoprophylaxis has been shown to decrease the rate of hospitalization for non-RSV respiratory illnesses; palivizumab has not.[31]

The AAP recommends the use of RSV-IGIV and palivizumab in the groups listed in Table 5-1.

An essential aspect of RSV prevention is parent and caregiver education. Preventive measures that are discussed during discharge teaching include eliminating exposure to cigarette smoke, limiting exposure to settings in which the risk of contagion is high (e.g., day care, malls, and grocery stores), especially during RSV season, and the importance of handwashing.[31]

Influenza

Etiology and Epidemiology

The influenza viruses comprise the Orthomyxoviridae family. There are three antigenic types: A, B, and C.[32,33] Because infection with influenza type C usually causes only mild respiratory illness or is asymptomatic and does not cause epidemics, it will not be discussed further. Type A influenza strains can be subclassified by two antigens, hemagglutinin (H) and neuraminidase (N). Human infection is caused by three immunologically distinct hemagglutinin subtypes (H_1, H_2, and H_3) and two neuraminidase subtypes (N_1 and N_2).

Immunity is determined by specific antibodies to these antigens.[33] Antigen immunity, especially to the hemagglutinin subtypes, decreases the risk of infection and lessens the severity of illness if infection does occur. However, infection with one subtype of the influenzavirus offers minimal if any protection against other subtypes.[34]

An antigenic drift, or *minor* variation, in subtypes occurs almost annually in influenza A and B. This drift can increase individuals' susceptibility to infection by a type of influenza with which they have previously been infected or against which they have been immunized. Antigenic shift, a *major* change in the predominant strain in either antigen, occurs at intervals of ten or more years. Antigenic shift has been observed only in influenza A. Antigenic shifts in the circulating viruses cause widespread epidemics.[33]

Transmission of influenza occurs through direct contact with an infected individual, by large droplet infection, or from articles recently contaminated with nasopharyngeal secretions. During influenza season, school-aged children have the highest occurrence of infection. Secondary spread to other family members is common.[33] Nosocomial influenza infection has been reported in the NICU.[35]

In temperate climates, outbreaks occur during the winter, usually peaking between late December and early March. Within a community, an epidemic generally peaks within two weeks of onset and lasts a minimum of four to eight weeks. It is not unusual for two or three strains of influenza to circulate in a community, resulting in a prolonged influenza season of three months or more.[33,36]

The incubation period for influenza is one to three days. An individual is most infectious 24 hours before the onset of symptoms and during the peak period of symptoms. Viral shedding in the nasal secretions is highest during the first 72 hours and usually stops seven days after the onset of symptoms, but may last longer in young children or immunodeficient individuals.[33]

Clinical Manifestations and Diagnosis

Neonates with influenza often present with a sepsis-like syndrome including symptoms such as lethargy, poor feeding, petechiae, shock, and apnea. There may be lower respiratory tract disease as well. Infants with CLD are likely to experience pulmonary complications such as bronchitis or pneumonia. Secondary bacterial infection may also occur. Denuded respiratory tract epithelium and poor mucociliary transport enhance the potential for bacterial invasion.[37]

Influenza A can be reliably diagnosed using rapid enzyme-linked and immunofluorescent techniques to check for the presence of virus in nasopharyngeal secretions. These techniques are not reliable for influenza B, however.[37] If viral cultures are performed, a nasopharyngeal swab or aspirate should be obtained in the first 72 hours of illness, during the height of viral shedding. Results are generally available in two to six days.[21] The complete blood count (CBC) may reveal leukopenia but is often normal. Common findings on chest radiographs include peribronchial infiltrates, hyperexpansion, segmental or lobar atelectasis, and hilar adenopathy. Interstitial infiltrates and effusions are indicative of secondary bacterial infection.[37]

Treatment and Prevention

Supportive care is the mainstay of influenza management. Energy conservation and adequate hydration are essential. The nurse can decrease environment stimulation to promote rest. Initiation of minimal handling may be necessary, depending upon how the infant responds to care. The degree of illness determines whether the neonate can continue enteral feedings. If they are continued, tube feedings may be necessary if bottle or breast feeding proves too tiring because of increased respiratory effort. Neonates with a lower respiratory infection may require supplemental oxygen, continuous positive airway pressure, or intubation and mechanical ventilation.[37]

Droplet precautions are initiated and maintained for the duration of the illness. Cohorting neonates with influenza helps prevent the spread of infection.

Good handwashing and immunization are the keys to influenza prevention. Neonates and infants under six months of age are not eligible for the influenza vaccine. The Centers for Disease Control and Prevention recommends that the following groups receive influenza immunization:[36]

- Women who will be in their second or third trimesters during the influenza season
- Physicians, nurse practitioners, nurses, respiratory therapists, and others who provide care for neonates
- Family members of hospitalized neonates

Annual immunization beginning at six months of age for infants who fall into high-risk groups—infants with bronchopulmonary dysplasia or hemodynamically significant cardiac disease, those receiving aspirin to prevent clotting for cardiac surgical grafts (aspirin increases the risk for post–viral infection Reye's syndrome), those with HIV infection, sickle cell anemia, and other hemoglobinopathies, and infants on immunosuppressive therapy[32,35]—should be discussed during discharge teaching. Optimal timing of vaccination is October through mid-November. Many hospital-based employee health services offer the vaccine free to employees.

Further measures to prevent nosocomial influenza include:

- *Restricting visitation.* Exclude any family members with signs of respiratory illness. If sibling visitation is allowed, carefully screen all children, especially those of school age.
- *Screening caregivers.* Employees with respiratory illness should not care for patients for the duration of their illness.

An alternative measure for influenza prevention is chemoprophylaxis with amantadine or rimantadine. These medications are not approved for use in children less than one year of age, but they can be administered to unimmunized, exposed individuals who provide care to high-risk patients. Two new drugs approved in 1999 for the treatment of acute uncomplicated influenza are zanamivir and oseltamivir. Neither is approved for prophylaxis. Zanamivir is approved for individuals 12 years of age and older, and oseltamivir is approved for those 18 years of age and older.[38] These medications may be helpful in reducing time loss from work for health care workers and time away from their infants for family members. None of these medications is a substitute for prevention through yearly vaccination.

FIGURE 5-2 ◆ Neonatal varicella: generalized crusted papules.

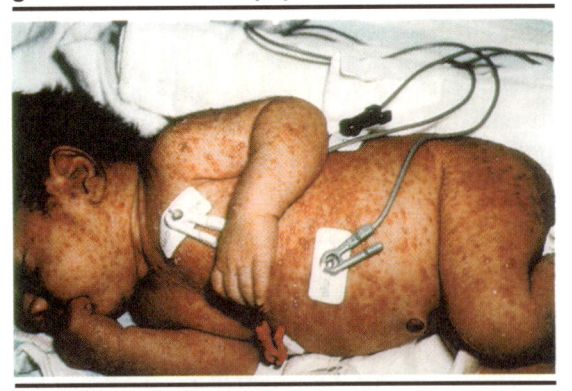

From: Friedlander SF, and Bradley JS. 2001. Viral infections. In *Textbook of Neonatal Dermatology*, Eichenfield LF, Frieden IJ, and Esterly NB, eds. Philadelphia: WB Saunders, 209. Reprinted by permission.

Postnatally Acquired Varicella

Etiology and Epidemiology

The varicella-zoster virus (VZV) is a member of the Herpesviridae subfamily alpha herpes virus. Primary infection with VZV results in chickenpox. Reactivation of the latent form, which persists after primary infection, results in herpes zoster, or "shingles." *In utero* exposure to VZV can result in zoster development early in life without the infant's ever having had extrauterine varicella. Varicella-zoster is a highly contagious virus. Winter and early spring are the most common times for outbreaks. Humans are the only source of infection. Viral transmission occurs by direct contact with individuals with varicella or zoster. Transmission may also occasionally occur by airborne spread from respiratory secretions and, rarely, from zoster lesions.[39] Nosocomial infections in newborn nurseries are rare.[2,39]

An individual is most contagious 1 to 2 days prior to and shortly after the onset of the rash. The incubation period is 10 to 21 days after exposure. Administration of varicella-zoster immune globulin (VZIG) prolongs the incubation period for up to 28 days. In the neonate born to a mother with active varicella, neonatal infection can develop between days 1 and 16 of life. The interval from onset of rash in the mother to onset of rash in the neonate is usually 9 to 15 days.[39]

Clinical Manifestations and Diagnosis

Clinical manifestations of chickenpox include mild fever and a generalized pruritic, vesicular rash (Figure 5-2).[39] The rash associated with herpes simplex virus (HSV) is indistinguishable from that of chickenpox. Therefore, any infant presenting with disseminated vesicular lesions should be cultured to evaluate for HSV. Enteroviruses can cause vesicular lesions, although they rarely do. Some noninfectious dermatological lesions, such as contact dermatitis and incontinentia pigmenti, may also be confused with chickenpox.[2]

Neonates are at risk for severe infection with pneumonia if the mother develops varicella five days before to two days after delivery (Figure 5-3).[37] The neonatal fatality rate associated with this time frame is as high as 30 percent.[39] Exposed healthy term neonates whose mothers have had chickenpox at some point prior to pregnancy generally have mild illness because maternal VZV IgG antibodies were passively transmitted to them during the third trimester.[2]

In addition to pneumonia, chickenpox may also be complicated by bacterial superinfection, thrombocytopenia, arthritis, hepatitis, encephalitis, meningitis, or glomerulonephritis.

Diagnosis is usually made based on history of exposure and clinical presentation. However, because of the importance of distinguishing HSV from chickenpox, immunofluorescent staining of vesicular scrapings using monoclonal antibodies is indicated. Although lumbar puncture (LP) is not discussed as part of the routine diagnostic evaluation, clearly, if meningitis is suspected, an LP would be performed. The cerebral spinal fluid (CSF) is collected in the usual manner and placed in viral culture medium in the microbiology lab.

Treatment and Prevention

Antiviral agents. Intravenous acyclovir is indicated for term neonates with central nervous system (CNS) involvement or pneumonia related to a varicella infection. The dose is 10 mg/kg/dose every 8 hours.[40] The dosing interval for neonates <34 weeks gestation is longer, every 12 hours, and the clinician may consider further increasing the dosing interval to every 24 hours for extremely premature neonates. Specific recommendations for dosing in the presence of renal failure are not available for infants less than six months of age; therefore, dosing intervals may be increased based on clinical judgment and by following renal and hepatic function.[41] Acyclovir is administered over 1 hour on a syringe pump.[31] Additional care is supportive. Pulmonary complications may necessitate intubation and mechanical ventilation.[42]

Isolation. In diagnosed or potential VZV infections, both airborne and contact precautions are initiated using the following guidelines:[39]
- Patients with varicella
    - Minimum of 5 days after the onset of the rash
    - Maintained for as long as the rash remains vesicular
- Exposed, susceptible patients
    - From 8 to 21 days after the onset of the rash in the index patient
    - Extended to 28 days if the exposed patient received VZIG
- Hospitalized neonates born to mothers with varicella
    - Until 21 days of age
    - Until 28 days of age if VZIG was given

FIGURE 5-3 ◆ This infant died at 12 days of life after developing disseminated varicella from a mother who manifested active skin lesions one week before delivery.

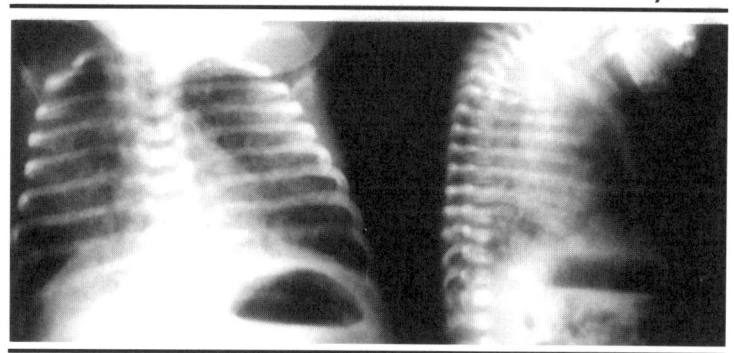

From: Manson D. 2002. Diagnostic imaging of neonatal pneumonia. In *Radiological Imaging of the Neonatal Chest*, Donoghue V, ed. New York: Springer-Verlag, 69. Reprinted by permission.

Immunoprophylaxis. VZIG should be given to the following infants exposed to chickenpox:[39]
- Newborns whose mothers had onset of chickenpox within five days before or within two days after delivery
- Hospitalized premature neonates ≥28 weeks gestation whose mothers have no history of chickenpox or who are seronegative for varicella
- Hospitalized premature neonates <28 weeks gestation regardless of maternal history

VZIG should be given within 96 hours of exposure. The dose is 125 units/10 kg, with a minimum dose of 125 units; fractional doses are not recommended. VZIG is given IM. It should never be administered intravenously.[43]

The following are other strategies to control the spread of varicella after hospital exposure:[30]
- Discharge all exposed susceptible patients as soon as possible.
- Isolate all exposed susceptible patients from day 8 to day 21 after exposure to the index patient. Hospital exposure for varicella is defined as being in the same two- to four-bed room or adjacent beds in a large ward, face-to-face contact with an infectious staff

member or patient, or a visit by a person deemed contagious. For neonates, exposure includes onset of varicella in the mother within five days prior to through two days after delivery. If the exposed patient received VZIG, continue isolation until day 28.

- Identify exposed, susceptible staff and restrict them from patient care from day 8 until day 21 after exposure to the index patient. Restrictions should continue until day 28 if the staff member received VZIG.

Immunization. Routine varicella immunization is not recommended prior to 12 months of age. Siblings and adult family members who are not immune to varicella should receive routine vaccination. Postexposure vaccination is recommended when an exposed individual over 12 months of age is not immune. Immunization given within three days and perhaps up to five days following exposure may prevent or modify illness. Health care staff who fall into this category should not participate in patient care from days 8 to 21 (day 28 if also given VZIG) following exposure.[44–46]

Enteroviruses

Etiology and Epidemiology

There are four categories of enteroviruses—poliovirus plus three categories of non-polioviruses: Coxsackievirus, echovirus, and the numbered, unclassified enteroviruses. Enteroviruses are small, single-stranded RNA viruses of the Picornaviridae (*pico* = "small," RNA = ribonucleic acid) family.[47–49] This section focuses on the nonpolioviruses.

Nonpoliovirus Enteroviruses

There are 23 Group A Coxsackieviruses (types A1–A22, A 24), 6 Group B Coxsackieviruses (types B1–B6), 31 echoviruses (types 1–9, 11–27, and 29–33), and 4 numbered, unclassified enteroviruses (types 68–71). Humans are the only host for enteroviruses, which are spread by fecal-oral and respiratory routes.[49] Neonatal infection can be acquired during birth or from an infected caregiver after birth. Nosocomial infections have been reported.[47,50]

The echoviruses and Group B Coxsackieviruses are the predominant enteroviruses implicated in neonatal disease. Infection occurs in 20–50 percent of infants whose mothers were ill within the week prior to delivery. Severity of neonatal illness is related to the severity of the maternal illness at the time of delivery and to the infant's postnatal age at the time of onset of infection. Neonates <10 days of age are at highest risk for severe infection as the result of an immature immune response and lack of specific maternal IgG antibody.[47] Young children have the highest attack rate. Other factors that contribute to Enterovirus infection are low socioeconomic status, poor hygiene, and a tropical climate. A summer-fall season pattern is observed in temperate climates. This seasonal pattern is less evident or nonexistent in tropical regions. The incubation period is three to six days. Viral shedding can occur in the absence of clinical illness. Fecal shedding and transmission can occur for several weeks after the onset of symptoms. Respiratory viral shedding generally lasts a week or less.[49]

Clinical Manifestations and Diagnosis

Neonates with Enterovirus infection present with a sepsis-like picture that is essentially indistinguishable from bacterial or fungal sepsis.[2,47] Symptomatic neonates present with fever, irritability, lethargy, poor feeding, poor perfusion, abdominal distention, macular or maculopapular rash (Figure 5-4),[50] and jaundice. Manifestations of severe enteroviral infection include myocarditis with or without encephalitis, hepatitis, necrotizing enterocolitis, disseminated intravascular coagulation (DIC), and pneumonia.[2,47,51–53] Disseminated herpes simplex manifested as pneumonia, hepatitis, and DIC is indistinguishable from disseminated Enterovirus infection.[2]

FIGURE 5-4 ◆ Fine erythematous rash associated with enterovirus infection.

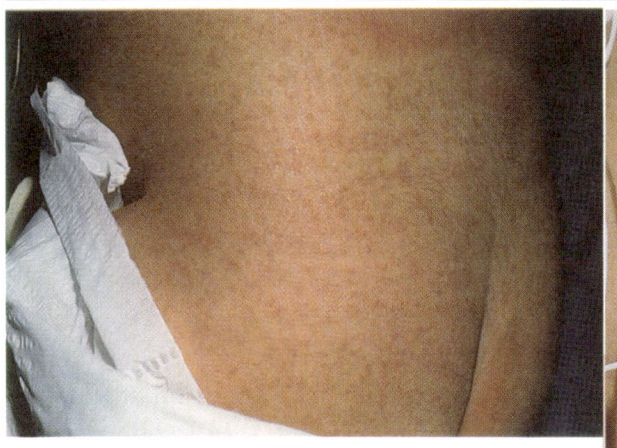

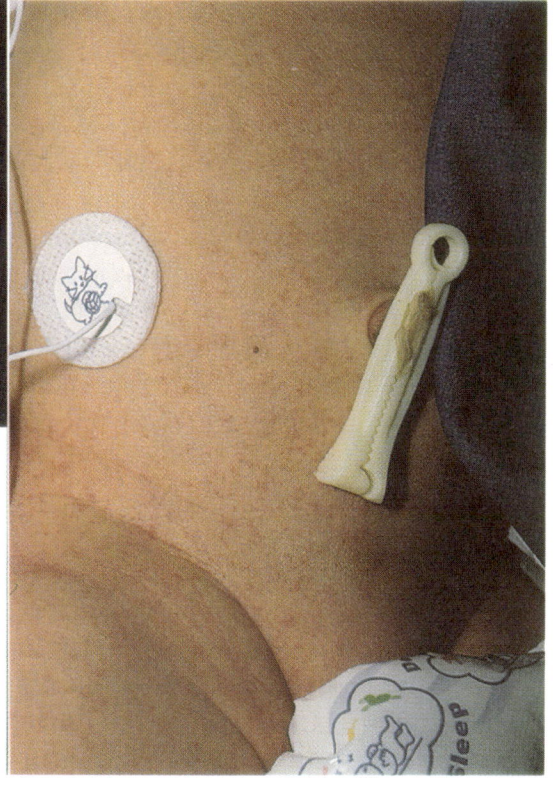

From: Friedlander SF, and Bradley JS. 2001. Viral infections. In *Textbook of Neonatal Dermatology*, Eichenfield LF, Frieden IJ, and Esterly NB, eds. Philadelphia: WB Saunders, 216. Reprinted by permission.

Survival following neonatal Enterovirus infection has been reported as 75–100 percent.[50,54] However, long-term sequelae may include hepatic, cardiac, and CNS dysfunction, depending on the system(s) affected by the disease.[55] Death related to Enterovirus infection is often caused by hepatic failure related to echoviruses or myocarditis associated with the Group B Coxsackieviruses.[51]

Diagnosis of an Enterovirus infection is accomplished by cell culture of throat, stool, and/or rectal swab specimens. If CNS involvement is suspected, CSF specimens may also be obtained. Specimens should be maintained at 4°C (39.2°F). Proper handling of the specimen is very important to ensure adequate viral recovery.[49] Cultures for Enterovirus have a sensitivity of 65–75 percent and take three to ten days for results.[56] Results from polymerase chain reaction for Enterovirus infection are available within 24 hours.[57] Rotbart and associates and Ahmed and colleagues both found 100 percent sensitivity when PCR was used to diagnose enteroviral meningitis.[56,58] Blood, throat, and urine specimens for PCR have sensitivities of 92 percent, 95 percent, and 77 percent, respectively.[56] Rapid diagnosis with highly sensitive Enterovirus PCR testing has many advantages. First, it enhances the recognition of infants with Enterovirus infection. Clear diagnosis of febrile Enterovirus infection will broaden our current understanding of these illnesses as well as their long-term consequences. Second, accurate diagnosis of viral illness with PCR will decrease the use of unnecessary antibiotics.[58,59]

Treatment and Prevention

The focus of treatment for Enterovirus infections is supportive. Respiratory and cardiovascular support may be necessary in the severely ill neonate. Hepatic involvement may affect clotting factors, and the neonate may require transfusion with blood products. Contact precautions are indicated in addition to standard precautions.

No specific antiviral therapy exists for the treatment of enteroviruses in neonates.

Intravenous immunoglobulin has been used prophylactically in an attempt to prevent spread of infection during a nursery outbreak. In a small study, researchers found that prophylactic IGIV containing viral neutralizing antibodies to a specific circulating Enterovirus did not prevent spread of the virus in the nursery, but it did decrease the risk for symptomatic infection by 14 percent.[60] IGIV has shown promise in reducing viremia and viruria in actual neonatal infections. Using IGIV lots preselected for high titers for frequently circulating Enterovirus and for serotypes that are particularly virulent may heighten the therapeutic benefit.[55,61] Large random clinical studies are needed to confirm the efficacy of immunotherapy.

Good handwashing and standard precautions are the core of preventing Enterovirus infections. There are no vaccines against the nonpoliovirus enteroviruses. Two factors contribute to the lack of impetus for vaccine development: (1) the multiple number of antigenic types of enteroviruses and (2) the mild and self-limiting nature of enteroviral infection in most populations.[51]

BLOOD-BORNE PERINATAL VIRAL INFECTIONS

Human Immunodeficiency Virus

Etiology and Epidemiology

HIV infection is caused by cytopathic human retroviruses—human immunodeficiency virus type 1 (HIV-1) and human immunodeficiency virus type 2 (HIV-2). In the U.S., HIV-1 is more common. HIV-2 is more common in West Africa than it is elsewhere in the world. HIV attacks T helper CD4+ lymphocytes, monocytes, and macrophages. CNS cells, such as glial cells, are at risk for invasion by HIV as well. Retroviruses are able to integrate into a target cell genome as proviruses. As the target cell replicates, the viral genome is copied; the virus therefore persists for the infected person's lifetime.[62]

The only known reservoir for HIV is humans. Monkeys, however, have viruses that are related to HIV. The virus can be isolated from a variety of body fluids, but only blood, semen, cervical secretions, and breast milk have been implicated in the transmission of HIV.[62]

Perinatal transmission of HIV from mother to child is the number one cause of HIV infection in children under 15 years of age. Acquired immune deficiency syndrome (AIDS) is responsible for the death of close to three million children globally. There are one million children currently living with HIV. In 1998, one in ten newly infected HIV patients was a child. Africa accounts for only 10 percent of the world's population, yet nine out of ten infants infected with HIV are born in this region.[63]

Women of childbearing age are one of the fastest growing groups of HIV-infected patients. Worldwide, approximately 12 million women of childbearing age are infected with HIV.[63] Vertical transmission of HIV can occur at three times: (1) *in utero* (primarily late in pregnancy); (2) during birth, with exposure to infected maternal blood and cervical secretions; and (3) via breastfeeding.[63,64] The proportion of transmissions that occurs during each of these time frames is unknown.[65] Unless preventive measures are initiated during pregnancy (see "Prevention and Treatment"), the infant of an infected mother has a 15–25 percent risk of acquiring HIV in industrialized countries and a 25–35 percent risk in developing nations. The difference in risk is primarily the result of the fact that breastfeeding is both more common and more prolonged in developing countries.[63]

The actual mechanism of maternal-to-child HIV transmission is not clear. One hypothesis is that it occurs when there is cutaneous or mucosal contact with free virions or HIV-infected cells in the amniotic fluid, cervical and vaginal secretions, and breast milk.[66] Several variables that affect vertical transmission of HIV are described in the literature, leading to the conclusion that vertical HIV transmission is multifactorial. Table 5-2 summarizes the findings of various research studies on vertical transmission of HIV.[67–72]

Clinical Manifestations and Diagnosis

Infants infected with HIV perinatally generally remain asymptomatic during the first few months of life. Estimated median age of onset of symptoms is three years. However, the number of perinatally infected infants who remain symptom free for more than five years has increased since 1993. This rise probably reflects diagnosis and treatment of HIV-infected women during pregnancy and in labor and treatment of their newborn infants.[62]

The infant's immune system is not only immature, but naïve as well. Thus, expression of HIV in this population has features that distinguish it from the disease in older children and adults.[61] During the neonatal period, the infant is usually clinically normal. Children infected with HIV are classified according to three parameters: clinical status, immunologic status, and infection status (Tables 5-3–5-5). Placement in a specific classification should have prognostic significance. Once given a specific classification, a child cannot be moved to a less severe category, even if his clinical or immunologic status improves.[73] Infection status is established by diagnostic testing as described below.[73,74]

The infant's immature immune system likely has difficulty containing the viral infection. This is evidenced by the pattern of HIV-1 RNA levels during the first two years of life. Shearer and associates found that, at birth, RNA levels are generally low (<10,000 copies/ml), and then there is a rapid rise (>100,000 copies/ml) within 1 to 2 months. Subsequently, levels fall until at least 24 months of age. This decline may be indicative of an immune process related to the maturity of the child. Infants with rapid disease progression tended to have higher HIV-1 RNA levels at birth and throughout most of the first two years of life. The pattern just described, however, was consistent in infants with early onset of symptoms and those with late infection. This pattern persisted regardless of the rate at which the disease progressed.[75]

Signs of HIV infection in infants are often nonspecific. Hepatosplenomegaly with associated lymphadenopathy may be an early sign of infection. Other common presenting features of HIV infection during the first year of life include oral candidiasis, failure to thrive, and failure to meet developmental milestones.[64] *Pneumocystis carinii* pneumonia is the most frequent indicator of HIV infection in children less than one year of age. Initial pneumonia infection usually occurs between three and six months of age.[76]

Early diagnosis is essential. There are implications for decisions regarding initiation of prophylactic and therapeutic medication as well as short- and long-term medical care for these infants.[64] Standard HIV testing using the ELISA and Western blot are not useful during the neonatal period and infancy. Maternal HIV antibodies received by the fetus via the placenta may persist for at least 18 months. PCR and HIV culture are the preferred methods of testing infants born to HIV-positive mothers.[64,73] However, HIV antigen may also be used to detect HIV. Table 5-6 outlines the diagnostic process for HIV in children.

Infants born to HIV-positive mothers should have either an HIV culture or a PCR performed at 1 month of age. Culture or PCR will identify approximately 30–50 percent of infected neonates. If the detection test is negative, it should be repeated at 4–6 months of age. A positive detection test is presumptive for HIV infection, but a second diagnostic test using the same or one of the other two detection methods should be done for confirmation. Infants younger than 18 months who develop an

TABLE 5-2 ◆ Factors for Vertical Transmission of HIV: Summary of Research Findings

Reference	Variables	Number of Subjects	Results
Duliège et al. 1995[68]	Birth order, delivery route, and concordance in transmission in twins	115 twin pairs born to HIV-infected mothers	HIV infection occurred in 35% of vaginally born "A" twins, 16% of cesarean-delivered "A" twins, 15% of vaginally born "B" twins, and 8% of the "B" twins born by cesarean section. Twenty percent of the twin pairs were discordant for infection. In these cases, the "A" twin was more likely to be infected than the "B" twin.
Minkoff et al. 1995[67]	Duration of rupture of membranes; Maternal immune status	127 infants	There is a correlation between duration of rupture of membranes (≥4 hours) and transmission of HIV in women with lower $CD4^+$ counts.
Sperling et al. 1996[69]	Maternal viral load; Zidovudine treatment	402 mother-infant pairs	Rate of transmission in the ZDV group = 7.6% and in the placebo group = 22.6%. In the placebo group, a high viral load at study entry or delivery or a positive viral culture increased the risk of transmission. Transmission occurred at a wide range of HIV-1 RNA levels in both groups.
Thea et al. 1997[70]	Maternal viral load at delivery	51 women who gave birth to infants infected with HIV-1 and 54 nontransmitting women	High maternal viral load increases the risk of HIV transmission in the absence of AIDS and advanced immunosuppression.
Mandelbrot et al. 1998[71]	Mode of delivery in the presence of zidovudine prophylaxis	2,834 singleton children born to HIV-infected mothers	Transmission risk is lower following elective cesarean section than after vaginal delivery or emergency cesarean section.
European Collaborative Study 1999[72]	Maternal RNA load; Race; Zidovudine use during pregnancy; Mode of delivery; Maternal AIDS by time of delivery; Premature delivery; Maternal drug use during pregnancy; Time since maternal diagnosis; Maternal $CD4^+$ count; Duration of rupture of membranes	373 mothers of children enrolled in the European Collaborative Study	The following factors are independently associated with transmission risk: Transmission increases with increased RNA levels. (There was no threshold below which transmission did not occur.) Elective cesarean section was associated with significantly lower transmission rates. Premature delivery (<37 weeks) was associated with an increased risk of transmission.

TABLE 5-3 ♦ Clinical Categories for Children with HIV Infection

Category N: Not Symptomatic

Children who have no signs or symptoms considered to be the result of HIV infection or who have only one of the conditions listed in Category A.

Category A: Mildly Symptomatic

Children with two or more of the conditions listed below but none of the conditions listed in Categories B and C.

- Lymphadenopathy (≥0.5 cm at more than two sites; bilateral = one site)
- Hepatomegaly
- Splenomegaly
- Dermatitis
- Parotitis
- Recurrent or persistent upper respiratory infection, sinusitis, or otitis media

Category B: Moderately Symptomatic

Children who have symptomatic conditions other than those listed for Category A or C that are attributed to HIV infection. Examples of conditions in clinical Category B include but are not limited to the following:

- Anemia (hemoglobin <8 gm/dl), neutropenia (absolute neutrophil count <1,000/mm^3), or thrombocytopenia (platelets <100,000/ mm^3) persisting ≥30 days
- Bacterial meningitis, pneumonia, or sepsis (single episode)
- Candidiasis, oropharyngeal (thrush), persisting >2 months in children >6 months of age
- Cardiomyopathy
- Cytomegalovirus infection, with onset before 1 month of age
- Diarrhea, recurrent or chronic
- Hepatitis
- HSV stomatitis, recurrent (more than two episodes within 1 year)
- HSV bronchitis, pneumonitis, or esophagitis with onset before 1 month of age
- Herpes zoster (shingles) involving at least two distinct episodes or more than one dermatome
- Leiomyosarcoma
- Lymphoid interstitial pneumonia or pulmonary lymphoid hyperplasia complex
- Nephropathy
- Nocardiosis
- Persistent fever (lasting >1 month)
- Toxoplasmosis, onset before 1 month of age
- Varicella, disseminated (complicated chickenpox)

Category C: Severely Symptomatic

Children with conditions or symptoms other than or along with those listed in Category A or B. Examples of conditions in clinical Category C include:

- Serious bacterial infections, multiple or recurrent (i.e., any combination of at least two culture-confirmed infections within a 2-year period) of the following types: septicemia, pneumonia, meningitis, bone or joint infection, or abscess of an internal organ or body cavity (excluding otitis media, superficial skin or mucosal abscesses, and indwelling catheter–related infections)
- Candidiasis, esophageal or pulmonary (bronchi, trachea, lungs)
- Coccidioidomycosis, disseminated (at a site other than or in addition to the lungs or cervical or hilar lymph nodes)
- Cryptococcosis, extrapulmonary
- Cryptosporidiosis or isosporiasis with diarrhea persisting >1 month
- Cytomegalovirus disease with onset of symptoms at age >1 month (at site other than liver, spleen, or lymph nodes)
- Encephalopathy (at least one of the following progressive findings present for at least 2 months in the absence of concurrent illness other than HIV infection that could explain the findings): (1) failure to attain or loss of developmental milestones or loss of intellectual ability, verified by standard developmental scale or neuropsychological tests; (2) impaired brain growth or acquired microcephaly demonstrated by head circumference measurements or brain atrophy demonstrated by computerized tomography or magnetic resonance imaging (serial imaging is required for children <2 years of age); (3) acquired symmetric motor deficit manifested by two or more of the following: paresis, pathological reflexes, ataxia, and gait disturbance
- Herpes simplex virus infection causing a mucocutaneous ulcer that persists for >1 month; or bronchitis, pneumonitis, or esophagitis for any duration affecting a child >1 month of age
- Histoplasmosis, disseminated (at a site other than or in addition to the lungs or cervical or hilar lymph nodes)
- Kaposi's sarcoma
- Lymphoma, primary, in brain

(continued on next page)

TABLE 5-3 ◆ Clinical Categories for Children with HIV Infection (continued)

Category C: Severely Symptomatic (cont.)	
Lymphoma, small, noncleaved cell (Burkitt's) or immunoblastic (or large cell) lymphoma of B-cell or unknown immunologic phenotype	Salmonella (nontyphoid) septicemia, recurrent
	Toxoplasmosis of the brain with onset at >1 month of age
Mycobacterium tuberculosis, disseminated or nonpulmonary	Wasting syndrome in the absence of a concurrent illness other than HIV infection that could explain the following findings: (1) persistent weight loss >10% of baseline or (2) downward crossing of at least two of the following percentile lines on the weight-for-age chart (e.g., 95th, 75th, 50th, 25th, 5th) in a child ≥1 year of age or (3) <5th percentile on weight-for-height chart on two consecutive measurements ≥30 days apart *plus* chronic diarrhea (i.e., at least two loose stools per day for ≥30 days) or documented fever (for ≥30 days, intermittent or constant)
Mycobacterium, other species or unidentified species, disseminated (at a site other than or in addition to the lungs, skin, or cervical or hilar lymph nodes)	
Mycobacterium avium complex or *Mycobacterium kansasii*, disseminated (at site other than or in addition to the lungs, skin, or cervical or hilar lymph nodes)	
Pneumocystis carinii pneumonia	
Progressive multifocal leukoencephalopathy	

Adapted from: Centers for Disease Control and Prevention. 1994. Revised classification system for human immunodeficiency virus infection in children less than 13 years of age. *MMWR* 43(RR-12): 1–10; and Centers for Disease Control and Prevention. 1987. Revision of the CDC surveillance case definition for acquired immunodeficiency syndrome. *MMWR* 36(supplement 1): 1–15.

AIDS-defining illness (Table 5-7) are considered to have HIV infection even in the absence of positive virologic testing.[62]

HIV infection can be excluded if a child has had two negative virologic tests both of which were performed when the child was 4 months of age or older. Follow-up serologic testing is important to rule out HIV infection or seroconversion. Two negative enzyme immunoassay (EIA) tests performed between 6 and 18 months of age or one negative EIA performed after 18 months of age excludes the diagnosis of HIV infection. Because maternal antibodies sometimes take longer than 18 months to clear the child's circulation, some experts suggest that final EIA testing be completed at 24 months of age.[62]

Prevention and Treatment

Worldwide, there are three strategies for preventing vertical transmission of HIV: (1) prevention of HIV infection in women of childbearing age; (2) family planning services and pregnancy termination, where legal and desired by the woman; (3) a course of antiretroviral drugs for the pregnant HIV-positive woman and her child and avoidance of breastfeeding.[63,77,78]

Antiretroviral therapy. In a double-blind, placebo-controlled, randomized study, Conner and associates found zidovudine (ZDV) given to the mother during pregnancy and then to the infant beginning at 8–12 hours of age reduced the risk of vertical transmission of HIV from 25 percent in the placebo group to 8 percent in

TABLE 5-4 ◆ Immunologic Categories Based on Age-Specific CD4⁺ T-Lymphocyte Counts and Percent of Total Lymphocytes

	Age of Child		
Immunologic Categories	<12 Months	1–5 Years	6–12 Years
1: No evidence of suppression	≥1,500 μl ≥25%	≥1,000 μl ≥25%	≥500 μl ≥25%
2: Evidence of moderate suppression	750–1,499 μl 15–24%	500–999 μl 15–24%	200–499 μl 15–24%
3: Severe suppression	<750 μl <15%	<500 μl <15%	<200 μl <15%

From: Centers for Disease Control and Prevention. 1994. Revised classification system for human immunodeficiency virus infection in children less than 13 years of age. *MMWR* 43(RR-12): 4.

TABLE 5-5 ♦ Pediatric HIV Classifications

Immunologic Categories	Clinical Categories			
	N: No Signs/Symptoms	A: Mild Signs/Symptoms	B:* Moderate Signs/Symptoms	C:* Severe Signs/Symptoms
1: No evidence of suppression	N1	A1	B1	C1
2: Evidence of moderate suppression	N2	A2	B2	C2
3: Severe suppression	N3	A3	B2	C3

Note: Children whose HIV infection status is not confirmed are classified by using the above grid with a letter E (for perinatally exposed) placed before the appropriate classification code (e.g., EN2). For definitions of the criteria for identifying a child's clinical category, see Table 5-3. For guidelines for identifying a child's immunologic category, see Table 5-4.

* Both category C and lymphoid interstitial pneumonitis in category B are reportable to state and local health departments as acquired immunodeficiency syndrome.

From: Centers for Disease Control and Prevention. 1994. Revised classification system for human immunodeficiency virus infection in children less than 13 years of age. *MMWR* 43(RR-12): 2.

---

the zidovudine group. The subjects of the study were HIV-positive pregnant women between 14 and 34 weeks gestation with CD4+ T-lymphocyte counts >200 cells/mm^3 who had not received any antiretroviral medications during their pregnancy. The medication protocol (AIDS Clinical Trial Group [ACTG] Protocol 076) for the study was as follows:[77]

- **Pregnancy.** Beginning between 14 and 34 weeks gestation, 100 mg ZDV PO five times a day
- **Labor and delivery.** 2 mg/kg ZDV IV bolus over one hour, followed by 1 mg/kg continuous IV infusion until delivery
- **Postnatal (infant).** 2 mg/kg/dose ZDV syrup PO every 6 hours, beginning 8–12 hours after birth, until six weeks of age. (*Note:* For infants who cannot tolerate oral ZDV, IV zidovudine 1.5 mg/kg/dose is given every 6 hours.[79])

Subsequently, the U.S. Public Health Service established recommendations for ZDV use to prevent perinatally acquired HIV infection in patients who meet the ACTG Protocol 076 clinical criteria as well as in those patients whose clinical situations are different. The recommendations were most recently updated in 2003 and are summarized in Table 5-8.[79]

Under ideal circumstances, treatment of the perinatally exposed infant begins *in utero* or, alternatively, follows the recommendations provided in one of the scenarios presented in Table 5-8. Perinatal ZDV therapy has not been associated with premature birth or adverse fetal growth (anthropometric measurements have been normal), and no specific minor or major anomaly clusters have been seen.[77] The only side effect observed in term infants treated with zidovudine is a mild transient anemia that reaches nadir at 6 weeks of age. The anemia resolves without treatment by 12 weeks of age.[77] In a study by Capperelli and colleagues, preterm infants with gestational ages of 29.7 ± 3 weeks (range 24–34.7) were observed to have anemia (hemoglobin ≤8.9 gm/dl), neutropenia (absolute neutrophils count ≤750/mm^3), and thrombocytopenia (≤75,000/mm^3). The scope of the study did not include observation of the resolution of these adverse hematologic events. Forty-five percent of the subjects received a transfusion to treat anemia, and 26 percent of the subjects received erythropoietin.[80]

A baseline CBC should be obtained at birth; CBCs should be repeated at 4 and 6 weeks of age to evaluate the progression of the anemia; and a follow-up CBC should be performed at 12 weeks of age to assess for resolution of the anemia. Premature infants, those with blood

TABLE 5-6 ◆ Diagnosis of HIV Infection in Children

Diagnosis: HIV Infected

(a) A child <18 months of age who is known to be HIV seropositive or born to an HIV-infected mother and who:

has positive results on two separate determinations (excluding cord blood) from one or more of the following HIV detection tests:
- HIV culture
- HIV polymerase chain reaction
- HIV antigen (p24)

or

meets criteria for AIDS diagnosis based on the 1987 AIDS surveillance case definition[74]

(b) A child ≥18 months of age born to an HIV-infected mother, or any child infected by blood, blood products, or other known modes of transmission (e.g., sexual contact) who:

is HIV-antibody positive by repeated reactive EIA and confirmatory test (e.g., Western blot or immunofluorescence assay [IFA])

or

meets any of the criteria in (a) above

Diagnosis: Perinatally Exposed (Prefix E)

A child who does not meet the criteria above who:

is HIV seropositive by EIA and confirmatory test (e.g., Western blot or IFA) and is <18 months of age at the time of the test

or

has unknown antibody status, but was born to a mother known to be infected with HIV

Diagnosis: Seroreverter (SR)

A child who is born to an HIV-infected mother and who:

has been documented as HIV-antibody negative (i.e., two or more negative EIA tests performed at 6–18 months of age or one negative EIA test after 18 months of age)

and

has had no other laboratory evidence of infection (has not had two positive viral detection tests, if performed)

and

has not had an AIDS-defining condition

From: Centers for Disease Control and Prevention. 1994. Revised classification system for human immunodeficiency virus infection in children less than 13 years of age. *MMWR* 43(RR-12): 3.

---

group incompatibilities, and those with anemia at birth require more frequent monitoring.[79,81]

Immediate care of the newborn of an HIV-positive mother consists of a routine physical and neurologic examination. Most infants born to HIV-positive mothers are term and asymptomatic. The nurse, however, must be alert to other potential medical problems, such as the effects of maternal substance abuse or signs of concurrent congenital infection.

Initiation of multidrug antiretroviral therapy in infants who have not previously received antiretroviral therapy has shown promise.[82] Additional clinical trials to assess the efficacy of early aggressive treatment with three or four antiretroviral medications have also shown potential for long-term suppression of viral replication.[83,84] Researchers are examining viral, immunologic, and clinical responses to this treatment strategy. Monotherapy with ZDV is recommended only for those infants with indeterminate HIV status during the first six weeks of life, to prevent perinatal infection. If infants are identified as HIV positive while receiving zidovudine chemoprophylaxis, they should be changed to a combination antiretroviral drug regimen.[85]

Antiretroviral therapy is ideally initiated in infants <12 months of age, as soon as the diagnosis is confirmed. Because infants are at high risk for disease progression, therapy is initiated regardless of clinical status, immunologic status, or viral load. Data regarding the efficacy of this method in neonates are not available. In addition, there is limited information on dosing of antiretroviral agents in the neonatal population. Table 5-9 summarizes the information currently available on antiretroviral agents. Regardless of when therapy is initiated, the ability and willingness of the infant's caregiver(s) to comply with the regimen must be assessed. Resistance to antiretroviral drugs develops rapidly if drug concentrations fall below therapeutic ranges.

TABLE 5-7 ♦ AIDS-Defining Illnesses in Children without Laboratory Evidence of HIV Infection

Candidiasis of the esophagus, trachea, bronchi, or lungs

Extrapulmonary cryptococcosis

Cryptosporidiosis with diarrhea persisting >1 month

Cytomegalovirus disease of an organ other than the liver, spleen, or lymph nodes in a person >1 month of age

Herpes simplex virus causing mucocutaneous ulcers that persist >1 month or bronchitis, pneumonia, or esophagitis for any duration affecting a person >1 month of age

Kaposi's sarcoma in a person <80 years of age

Primary lymphoma of the brain affecting a person <60 years of age

Lymphoid interstitial pneumonia and/or pulmonary lymphoid hyperplasia affecting a child <13 years of age

Disseminated *Mycobacterium avium* complex or *Mycobacterium kansasii* disease at a site other than or in addition to the lungs, skin, or cervical or hilar lymph nodes

Pneumocystis carinii pneumonia

Progressive multifocal leukoencephalopathy

Toxoplasmosis of the brain affecting a patient >1 month of age

Adapted from: Centers for Disease Control and Prevention. 1987. Revision of the CDC surveillance case definition for acquired immunodeficiency syndrome. MMWR 36(1S): 1S–15S.

Insufficient therapeutic levels may result either from inadequate dosing or from compliance issues.[85]

Breastfeeding. The AAP is a staunch supporter of breastfeeding. However, it does recommend that women who are HIV infected must be counseled not to breastfeed or to provide their milk for the nutrition of any infant. This recommendation applies to the U.S., where safe alternatives to breastfeeding are available and where infectious disease and malnutrition are not a major cause of infant mortality.[86]

In developing countries, the breastfeeding issue is more complicated. Breastfeeding has improved infant mortality rates by protecting newborns and children against a variety of illnesses, including diarrheal illness and pneumonia. However, the World Health Organization (WHO) and the Joint United Nations Programme on HIV/AIDS (UNAIDS) estimate the risk of HIV transmission via breastfeeding at 15 percent. Thus, in 1998, these organizations issued guidelines for HIV and infant feeding. The key to these guidelines is empowerment of women to make informed choices based on their own circumstances. To make an informed decision about infant feeding and other aspects of HIV, women and their partners, whenever possible, must have access to confidential counseling and HIV testing. According to the guidelines, it is important to promote breastfeeding in HIV-negative women and those of unknown status. Appropriate alternatives to breastfeeding, commercial formula or home-prepared formula, should be available and affordable in adequate amounts for HIV-positive women.[87,88]

***Pneumocystis carinii* pneumonia prophylaxis.** As noted earlier, initial infection with PCP usually occurs in infants with perinatally acquired HIV at 3–6 months of age.[76] In children <12 months of age, the onset of PCP is often acute and carries a poor prognosis. Prenatal or early neonatal identification of exposure to HIV allows for early initiation of PCP prophylaxis. The drug of choice and recommended regimen for PCP prophylaxis is trimethoprim/sulfamethoxazole (TMP-SMX): 150 mg TMP/m²/day with 750 mg SMX/m²/day PO in divided doses twice a day, three times per week on consecutive days.[89] Acceptable alternative dosing schedules for TMP-SMX and alternative drug regimens are outlined in Table 5-10. Before PCP prophylaxis is started, a baseline CBC with differential and platelet count should be obtained and then followed monthly.

Infants born to HIV-positive mothers are started on PCP prophylaxis at four to six weeks of age regardless of CD4⁺ count (CD4⁻ count is not used to establish the need for *Pneumocystis carinii* pneumonia [PCP] prophylaxis in

TABLE 5-8 ◆ Recommendations for the Use of Antiretroviral Drugs to Reduce Perinatal HIV Transmission

Clinical Scenario	Recommendations*
Scenario 1 HIV-infected pregnant women who have not received prior antiretroviral therapy	HIV-1-infected pregnant women must receive standard clinical, immunologic, and virologic evaluation. Recommendations for initiation and choice of antiretroviral therapy should be based on the same parameters used for persons who are not pregnant, although known and unknown risks and benefits of such therapy must be considered and discussed. The three-part ZDV chemoprophylaxis regimen should be recommended for all HIV-infected pregnant women to reduce the risk of perinatal transmission. The combination of ZDV chemoprophylaxis with additional antiretroviral drugs for treatment of HIV infection should be (1) discussed with the woman; (2) recommended for infected women whose clinical, immunologic, and virologic status indicates the need for treatment; or (3) recommended for infected women whose HIV-1 RNA is >1,000 copies/ml regardless of clinical or immunologic status. Women who are in the first trimester of pregnancy may consider delaying initiation of therapy until after 10–12 weeks gestation.
Scenario 2 HIV-infected women receiving antiretroviral therapy during the current pregnancy	HIV-1-infected women receiving antiretroviral therapy in whom pregnancy is identified after the first trimester should continue therapy. ZDV should be a component of the antenatal antiretroviral treatment regimen after the first trimester whenever possible. Women receiving antiretroviral therapy in whom pregnancy is recognized during the first trimester should be counseled regarding the benefits and potential risks of antiretroviral administration during this period, and continuation of therapy should be considered. If therapy is discontinued during the first trimester, all drugs should be stopped and reintroduced simultaneously to avoid the development of resistance. ZDV administration is recommended for the pregnant woman during the intrapartum period and for the newborn—regardless of the antepartum antiretroviral regimen.
Scenario 3 HIV-infected women in labor who have had no prior therapy.†	Several effective regimens are available for women in labor who have had no prior therapy. 1. Intrapartum IV ZDV followed by 6 weeks of ZDV for the neonate. Mother: 2 mg/kg IV bolus, followed by continuous infusion of 1 mg/kg/hour until delivery. Neonate: ZDV 2 mg/kg PO every 6 hours for 6 weeks. 2. Oral ZDV and lamivudine (3TC) during labor, followed by 1 week of oral ZDV-3TC for the neonate. Mother: ZDV 600 mg PO at onset of labor, then 300 mg PO every 3 hours until delivery and 3TC 150 mg PO at onset of labor, then 150 mg PO every 12 hours until delivery. Neonate: ZDV 4 mg/kg PO every 12 hours and 3TC 2 mg/kg PO every 12 hours for 7 days. 3. Nevirapine—a single dose at the onset of labor and a single dose for the neonate at 48–72 hours of age. Mother: 200 mg PO. Neonate: 2 mg/kg PO. or 4. Two-dose nevirapine regimen in combination with intrapartum IV ZDV and a single dose of nevirapine and 6 weeks of ZDV for the neonate. Mother: ZDV 2 mg/kg IV bolus, followed by continuous infusion of 1 mg/kg/hour until delivery and nevirapine 200 mg PO single dose at onset of labor. Neonate: ZDV 2 mg/kg PO every 6 hours for 6 weeks and nevirapine 2 mg/kg PO single dose at 48–72 hours of age. In the immediate postpartum period, the woman should have appropriate assessments (e.g., CD4+ count and HIV-1 RNA copy number) to determine whether antiretroviral therapy is recommended for her own health.

(continued on next page)

TABLE 5-8 ♦ Recommendations for the Use of Antiretroviral Drugs to Reduce Perinatal HIV Transmission (continued)

Clinical Scenario	Recommendations*
Scenario 4 Infants born to mothers who received no antiretroviral therapy during pregnancy or the intrapartum period	The 6-week neonatal ZDV component of the ZDV chemoprophylactic regimen should be discussed with the mother and offered for the newborn.
	ZDV should be initiated in the infant as soon as possible after delivery—preferably within 12–24 hours of birth.‡
	Some clinicians may choose to use ZDV in combination with other antiretroviral drugs, particularly if the mother has or is suspected of having ZDV-resistant virus. However, the efficacy of this approach for prevention of transmission is unknown, and appropriate dosing regimens for neonates are incompletely defined.
	In the immediate postpartum period, the woman should have appropriate assessments (e.g., CD4+ count and HIV-1 RNA copy number) to determine whether antiretroviral therapy is recommended for her own health.

Note: The current adult dosing regimen for zidovudine is 200 mg three times a day or 300 mg two times a day and is an acceptable alternative to 100 mg five times a day.[79]
Recommended ZDV dosing for infants <35 weeks gestation at birth is 1.5 mg/kg IV or 2 mg/kg PO every 12 hours, advancing to every 8 hours at 2 weeks of age if ≥30 weeks gestation at birth or at 4 weeks of age if <30 weeks gestation at birth.[80] Specific dosing schedules for premature infants have not be established for lamivudine or nevirapine.

* Discussion of treatment options and recommendations should not be coercive, and the final decision regarding the use of antiretroviral drugs is the responsibility of the woman. A decision to not accept treatment with ZDV or other drugs should not result in punitive action or denial of care. Use of ZDV should not be denied to a woman who wishes to minimize exposure of the fetus to other antiretroviral drugs and who therefore chooses to receive only ZDV during pregnancy to reduce the risk of perinatal transmission.

† Up to 70 percent of perinatal transmission may occur during the intrapartum period; therefore, in theory, the administration of ZDV during labor, followed by the 6-week regimen for the neonate, may be efficacious in the prevention of HIV in the infant.[64]

‡ If postexposure prophylaxis is started after 2 days of age, it is not likely to be efficacious in preventing vertical transmission of HIV. Additionally, infection is already established in most infants by 14 days of age.[79]

Adapted from: Public Health Service Task Force. 2003. Recommendations for the use of antiretroviral drugs in pregnant HIV-infected women for maternal health and interventions to reduce perinatal HIV-1 transmission in the United States. Rockville, Maryland: AIDSinfo, 35–36. Available at http://aidsinfo.nih.gov/guidelines/perinatal/archive%5CPER—061603.pdf.

HIV-exposed infants less than one year of age). Those identified as HIV exposed after six weeks of age begin PCP prophylaxis immediately upon identification. Infants under four weeks of age should not receive PCP prophylaxis because they are at low risk for PCP infection, and sulfa drugs interfere with bilirubin metabolism.[89] In addition, zidovudine and sulfa drugs administered concurrently can exacerbate ZDV-associated anemia.[81] Therefore, infants on ZDV therapy should begin PCP prophylaxis at six weeks of age, when they have completed the ZDV course.

Prevention of other opportunistic infections. In addition to PCP, there are 19 microorganisms that cause opportunistic infection in HIV-infected individuals. The U.S. Public Health Service and the Infectious Diseases Society of America have published a set of guidelines for the prevention of opportunistic infections in persons with HIV infection.[90]

Issues to discuss as part of teaching in anticipation of discharge from the nursery or the NICU, as well as issues for future consideration, include the following:

- Pets

    Any pet with diarrheal illness should be seen by a veterinarian and examined for Cryptosporidium, Salmonella, and Campylobacter.

    When obtaining a new pet, avoid animals less than six months of age (or less than one year for cats). Avoid purchasing

TABLE 5-9 ♦ Dosing of Antiretroviral Agents in Neonates

Category	Medication	Neonatal Dosage
Nucleoside/nucleotide analog reverse transcriptase inhibitor (NRTI/NtRTI)	Didanosine (dideoxyinosine, ddI) [Videx]	Infants <90 days of age: 50 mg/m^2 every 12 hours PO
	Lamivudine (3TC) [Epivir]	Infants <30 days of age: 2 mg/kg twice a day PO
	Stavudine (d4T) [Zerit]	Under evaluation in Pediatric AIDS Clinical Trial Group protocol 332
	Zalcitabine (ddC) [Hivid]	Unknown
	Zidovudine (ZDV, AZT) [Retrovir]	Premature infants: Infants <35 weeks gestation at birth: 1.5 mg/kg IV or 2 mg PO every 12 hours from birth to 2 weeks of age; then, if ≥30 weeks gestation at birth, 2 mg/kg every 8 hours at 2 weeks of age or at 4 weeks of age if <30 weeks gestation at birth
		Term neonates: 2 mg/kg every 6 hours PO or 1.5 mg/kg every 6 hours IV
Nonnucleoside reverse transcriptase inhibitor (NNRTI)	Delavirdine (DLV) [Rescriptor]	Unknown
	Efavirenz (DMp-266, EFV) [Sustiva]	Unknown
	Nevirapine (NVP) [Viramune]	Through 2 months of age: Under study in Pediatric AIDS Clinical Trial Group protocol 356: 5 mg/kg or 120 mg/m^2 once daily for 14 days; then 120 mg/m^2 every 12 hours for 14 days; then 200 mg/m^2 every 12 hours PO
Protease inhibitor (PI)	Indinavir [Crixivan]	Unknown (Because of its side effect of hyperbilirubinemia, it should not be given to neonates until further information is available.)
	Nelfinavir [Viracept]	Under study in Pediatric AIDS Clinical Trial Group protocol 353: 40 mg/kg PO every 12 hours
	Ritonavir [Norvir]	Under study in Pediatric AIDS Clinical Trial Group protocol 354 (single-dose pharmacokinetics)
	Saquinavir [Invirase]	Unknown

Note: The most current information on antiretroviral agents in neonatal and pediatric populations is available at http://AIDSinfo.nih.gov.

Adapted from: The Working Group on Antiretroviral Therapy and Medical Management of HIV-Infected Children. 2003. Guidelines for the use of antiretroviral agents in pediatric HIV infection, 32–49. Available at www.AIDSinfo.nih.gov.

animals from pet stores, shelters, and breeding facilities because hygiene conditions vary in those facilities.

Wash hands after handling pets, especially before eating or handling food.

Cat ownership increases the risk for toxoplasmosis and Bartonella infection.

Clean litter box daily, preferably by someone who is HIV negative and not pregnant, and wash hands immediately after cleaning the box to decrease the risk for toxoplasmosis.

To decrease the risk for toxoplasmosis, keep cats indoors, do not allow them to hunt, and do not feed them raw or undercooked meat.

Avoid activities that may lead to a cat scratch or bite, to reduce the risk for Bartonella

TABLE 5-10 ◆ Acceptable Alternative Regimens for PCP Prophylaxis for Infants ≥4 Weeks of Age*

Medication	Schedule
TMP-SMX	150 mg TMP/m^2/day with 750 mg SMX/m^2/day PO as a single daily dose three times per week on consecutive days
	150 mg TMP/m^2/day with 750 mg SMX/m^2/day PO divided bid and administered seven days per week
	150 mg TMP/m^2/day with 750 mg SMX/m^2/day PO divided bid and administered three times per week on alternate days
Dapsone (if TMP-SMX is not tolerated)	2 mg/kg (not to exceed 100 mg) PO once daily

* ZDV and sulfa drugs administered concurrently can exacerbate ZDV-associated anemia.[81] Therefore, infants on ZDV therapy should begin PCP prophylaxis at 6 weeks of age, when they have completed the ZDV course.

Adapted from: Centers for Disease Control and Prevention. 1995. 1995 revised guidelines for prophylaxis against *Pneumocystis carinii* pneumonia for children infected with or perinatally exposed to human immunodeficiency virus. MMWR 44(RR-4): 1–11.

infection. Wash scratches and bites immediately, and do not allow cats to lick a human's open cuts or wounds.

Flea control is essential in preventing Bartonella infection.

Avoid contact with reptiles to decrease the risk for salmonellosis.

Wear gloves when cleaning aquariums to reduce the risk of infection with *Mycobacterium marinum*.

Avoid contact with exotic animals, such as nonhuman primates.

Avoid contact with young farm animals, especially calves and lambs, to prevent cryptosporidiosis.

- Food- and water-related exposures

Avoid raw or undercooked eggs, poultry, meat, and seafood, as well as unpasteurized dairy products. These items may contain enteric pathogens. Poultry and meat should be cooked to an internal temperature of 165°F (73.8°C). Produce should be washed thoroughly.

Knives, cutting boards, counters, and hands that have been in contact with raw food should be washed thoroughly.

To avoid listeriosis, ready-to-eat foods such as hot dogs and cold cuts from delicatessens should be heated to steaming before eating.

Do not drink from or swim in lakes or rivers to avoid cryptosporidiosis and giardiasis.

It is not necessary to boil water for formula preparation unless there is a community "boil water" advisory.

Tuberculosis prevention and detection. Maternal tuberculosis (TB) status is ideally established during pregnancy. This is the recommendation of the American Academy of Pediatrics, Committee on Pediatric AIDS. Even if it were not, however, maternal TB status, as well as the status of other household members, should be assessed before the infant is discharged from the nursery or NICU. The presence of maternal hematogenous dissemination of TB requires evaluation of the infant for congenital TB. The infant should be separated from the mother or any other household contact with active pulmonary TB until the person is no longer contagious.[81] Infant exposure to a person with contagious TB requires that the newborn be skin tested for tuberculosis and have a chest radiograph. Even if the results of the initial skin test are negative, the infant is started on TB prophylaxis with isoniazid for 3 months A follow-up skin test is performed after 3 months of prophylaxis. If the skin test is negative, isoniazid may be discontinued. If the skin test is positive, indicated by induration of ≥5 mm, the infant is then continued on isoniazid for a total of at least 6 months. For HIV-infected infants, isoniazid therapy is continued for 12 months.[81,91]

Monitoring of hematologic and immunologic parameters. The AAP recommends the following tests for HIV-exposed neonates during the first four months of life:[81]

- **Birth.** CBC with differential (baseline; also used to follow zidovudine-associated anemia), PCR for HIV DNA and/or viral culture for HIV
- **Four weeks of age.** CBC with differential, PCR for HIV DNA and/or viral culture for HIV, T-cell profile
- **Six weeks of age.** CBC with differential (baseline for beginning PCP prophylaxis)
- **Two months of age.** CBC with differential
- **Four months of age.** CBC with differential, PCR for HIV DNA and/or viral culture for HIV, quantitative immunoglobulins

Immunizations. Routine immunizations for HIV-exposed infants begin on the same schedule as for nonexposed infants. Hepatitis B vaccine is given at birth, four weeks of age, and six months of age. Diphtheria-tetanus-acellular pertussis (DTaP) and *Haemophilus influenzae* (Hib) are given at two, four, and six months of age. Inactivated polio vaccine (IPV) is given at two and four months of age. The third dose of IPV may be given as early as six months of age. HIV-infected infants or infants living with an HIV-infected person should receive an initial influenza vaccine at six months of age, then yearly.[81,90] (For more information on immunizations, see Appendix E.)

Family support. A diagnosis of HIV infection can be overwhelming. In some cases, the first time the mother is aware of her own status is when her infant is diagnosed. Social services are necessary to assess the needs of the family and their infant. Depending on the mother's circumstances, placement of the infant in foster care or with another family member may be necessary.

Viral Hepatitis

Six types of hepatitis virus have been identified: A, B, C, D, E, and G. These viruses vary in their relevance to perinatal illness. Each is considered separately here.

Hepatitis A

Etiology and epidemiology. Hepatitis A (HAV) is a member of the Picornaviridae family. The primary route of transmission is fecal-oral. Hepatitis A infection is endemic in developing countries. In the U.S., there are periodic outbreaks among specific populations, particularly Native Americans (including Alaskan natives) and certain Hispanic and Hasidic communities. Major sources of HAV are personal contact, child daycare centers, international travel to endemic areas, food- or water-borne outbreaks, sexual contact between males, and intravenous drug use. Nosocomial outbreaks can occur in the nursery as the result of viral shedding from an infected, asymptomatic neonate.[92] The index patient may be infected by vertical transmission, blood transfusion, or some undetermined cause.[93–97] Staff and family members may become infected through contact with the index patient. Subsequently, other neonates may become infected through contact with infected staff.[94] Although vertical transmission does not appear to be a significant problem, there may be increased risk of infection if maternal HAV occurs less than two weeks prior to delivery.[98] Transfusion-related HAV and vertical transmission are rare.[93] Adults probably shed virus for only two weeks, but infected neonates may shed HAV for several months.[99] The average incubation period is 25 to 30 days, with a range of 15 to 50 days.[92]

Clinical manifestations and diagnosis. Neonates with hepatitis A are usually asymptomatic. HAV infection in infants is usually recognized when hospital staff or other caregivers who are infected due to inadequate handwashing present with clinical HAV infection after providing care for the neonate.[96,100] The adult caregiver will have abrupt onset of symptoms including fever, malaise, jaundice, anorexia, and nausea. The symptomatic infant will have only mild, nonspecific symptoms without jaundice. Although the illness generally lasts several weeks, prolonged or relapsing illness may persist for as long as six months. Fulminant HAV infection is rare. Hepatitis A infection does not result in chronic illness.[92]

Diagnosis of HAV is made using serologic tests for HAV-specific IgM and IgG. The presence of IgM indicates current or recent illness. Serum IgM is present at the onset of HAV infection. IgM usually disappears within four months, but may persist for at least six months. Shortly after the appearance of IgM, anti-HAV IgG is detectable. A past infection is indicated by the presence of anti-HAV IgG in the absence of HAV-IgM.[92]

Treatment and prevention. Treatment is supportive. Contact precautions are initiated for one week after the onset of symptoms. The key to prevention of transmission from infected neonates to other neonates and health care workers is good hygiene and good handwashing. Postexposure administration of immune globulin to nonvaccinated contacts provides protection against HAV through passive transfer of antibody. Ig should be given as soon as possible after exposure, but not more than two weeks after the last exposure. To prevent HAV infection in the neonate whose mother is infected less than two weeks before or after delivery, Ig administration may be considered. In addition to preventing infection in the neonate, Ig administration also prevents potential transmission of the virus to others who have contact with the infant.[100,101] Vaccination against HAV is not routine, but is recommended for certain groups of individuals: children two years of age and older who live in countries or communities with high endemic rates and/or periodic outbreaks of HAV infection, men who have sex with men, illegal-drug users, individuals with specific occupational risks (e.g., handling HAV-infected primates, research laboratory settings), individuals with clotting-factor disorders, and those with chronic liver disease.[86,90]

Hepatitis B

Etiology and epidemiology. The hepatitis B virus (HBV) is a DNA-containing hepadnavirus from the family Hepadnaviridae. It has three important structural components: surface antigen (HBsAg), core antigen (HBcAg), and e antigen (HBeAg).[102,103] Hepatitis B is transmitted by HBsAg-positive blood or body fluids, including wound exudates, semen, cervical secretions, and saliva. The highest concentration of virus is found in blood and serum; saliva has the lowest concentration. Transmission can occur via transfusion of blood and blood products, sharing or reuse of unsterilized syringes and needles, percutaneous or mucous-membrane exposure to blood and body fluids, sexual contact (homosexual or heterosexual), and perinatally. Transfusion-related transmission is rare in countries that routinely screen blood donors and practice viral inactivation of blood products. HBV can survive on inanimate objects for at least one week. Percutaneous contact such as a needlestick or a broken skin contact with a contaminated object can result in HBV infection.[102]

In parts of the world with low endemicity, such as most areas of the U.S., Canada, Western Europe, Australia, and southern South America, infection occurs primarily in adolescents and adults. Approximately 5–8 percent of the population in these regions has been infected; 0.2–0.9 percent are chronic carriers of HBV. However, there are regions of high endemicity in these countries, including Alaskan natives and inner-city groups. Up to 90 percent of the adult

TABLE 5-11 ◆ The Four Stages of Hepatitis B Virus Infection

Stage	Viral Replication	HBV Laboratory Markers	Immune Response	Time Period	Disease Process
1	Active	HBsAg: positive Antibody to HBsAg: negative HBV DNA: strongly positive Antibody to HBcAg: positive HBeAg: positive Antibody to HBeAg: negative AST, ALT: normal	Immune tolerance and incubation	Possibly decades for those infected as neonates	No symptoms of illness
2	Active	HBsAg: positive Antibody to HBsAg: negative HBV DNA: positive Antibody to HBcAg: positive HBeAg: positive Antibody to HBeAg: negative AST, ALT: elevated	Immune response develops or improves Cytokine stimulation Direct cell lysis Inflammatory process	Acute infection: 3–4 weeks Chronic infection: 10 or more years	Symptomatic hepatitis Progression to cirrhosis
3	End of active replication	HBsAg: positive Antibody to HBsAg: negative HBV DNA: negative* Antibody to HBcAg: positive HBeAg: negative Antibody to HBeAg: positive AST, ALT: normal	Patient remains HBsAg positive, most likely due to integration of the S gene into the hepatocyte genome	Indefinite	Infection cleared Resolution of symptoms
4	None	HBsAg: negative Antibody to HBsAg: positive HBV DNA: negative† Antibody to HBcAg: positive HBeAg: negative Antibody to HBeAg: positive AST, ALT: normal		Indefinite	Unlikely to be reinfected or have a reactivated infection

Note: In summary, individuals with acute infection will have circulating HBsAg, anti-HBc, and HBeAg. In chronic infection, both HBsAg and anti-HBc are present. The presence of anti-HBe in HBsAg carriers confers a lower risk for transmission. Individuals with resolved HBV will test positive for anti-HBs and anti-HBc. The presence of only anti-HBs indicates immunity via HBV vaccine.[102,104]

* HBV DNA may remain detectable in some patients using PCR methods.

† HBV DNA is not detectable by any method.

Adapted from: Lee WM. 1997. Hepatitis B virus infection. *New England Journal of Medicine* 337(24): 1733–1745; and American Academy of Pediatrics. 2000. Hepatitis B. In *Red Book: Report of the Committee on Infectious Diseases*, 25th ed., Pickering L, ed. Elk Grove Village, Illinois: American Academy of Pediatrics, 289–302.

population in these endemic areas have been infected. Of these adults, 8–15 percent are chronically infected. In these pocket areas of high endemicity, new infections occur primarily in infants and children under five years of age. Geographic regions that are highly endemic are China, Southeast Asia, Eastern Europe, the Central Asian republics, most of the Middle East, Africa, the Amazon basin, certain Caribbean islands, and the Pacific islands.

Hepatitis B infection in the remainder of the world is of intermediate endemicity, with 2–7 percent of the population having chronic carrier status.[102] Worldwide, there are more than 350 million chronic carriers of HBV. Many of these individuals will die from either chronic liver disease, such as cirrhosis, or primary hepatocellular carcinoma.[102]

Vertical transmission of hepatitis B occurs in infants born to HBsAg-positive mothers. In the majority of cases, transmission occurs around the time of delivery, when the infant is exposed to contaminated maternal secretions. Without preventive measures, 90 percent of these infants will go on to become chronic carriers if the mother is also HBeAg positive.[105,106] The exact mechanism by which infants born to HBsAg- and HBeAg-positive mothers become carriers is unclear. There is a high incidence of prematurity (35 percent) in mothers with HBV during pregnancy, regardless of infection status in the neonate.[98] If vertical transmission does not occur, infants born to HBsAg-positive mothers are still at risk for horizontal transmission during the first five years of life. The immaturity of the neonate's immune system most likely plays a role, making it unable to clear HBV. Neither HBV nor the surface antigen crosses the placenta, but both anti-HBc (antibody to the core antigen) and HBeAg do. These may interfere with the developing immune response.[99,102]

The incubation period for acute infection averages 120 days, with a range of 45–160 days.[102]

Clinical manifestations and diagnosis. Clinical manifestations of HBV infection range from asymptomatic seroconversion to fulminant fatal hepatitis. Young children, including neonates, are generally asymptomatic and are not jaundiced, but occasionally a neonate will present with clinical hepatitis and jaundice.[99,100,102] There are reports in the literature of infants with fulminant hepatitis, including one who received appropriate immunoprophylaxis.[107] Fulminant hepatitis B in young infants manifests with feeding difficulties, irritability, jaundice due to elevated total and direct bilirubin, coagulopathy, elevated alanine aminotransferase (ALT), and hypoglycemia.[108]

Many chronic carriers develop progressive liver disease at some point in their lives, usually as young or middle-aged adults. The immune system begins to attack infected hepatocytes, liver enzyme levels become elevated, and the inflammatory pattern associated with chronic hepatitis is observed.[99,102]

Both serologic antigen tests and assays for antibody detection are commercially available. In addition, testing for quantitative serum HBV DNA is available by PCR or branched-chain DNA. It is helpful to consider the four stages of HBV infection when evaluating the various antigen and antibody test results. The first two stages occur during the viral replication phase. Stages 3 and 4 comprise the integrative phase during which most infected cells are cleared, replication ceases, and antibody to HBsAg is present, signaling the development of full immunity to the virus.[104] The life cycle of HBV is summarized in Table 5-11.

Treatment and prevention. There is no specific treatment for acute HBV infection. For infants born to HBsAg-positive mothers, standard precautions are initiated, and the infant is bathed to remove maternal blood and secretions. Infants who acquire chronic infection at birth are at increased risk for serious liver disease, including primary hepatocellular carcinoma, at a young age. The age of onset of chronic illness is not described, however, the risk for chronic infection is inversely related to age at time of acute infection. Follow-up testing for hepatic complications is essential, but the frequency of testing and indications for specific tests have not been established. Infants and children with serum transaminase levels greater than twice normal, elevated α-fetoprotein concentration, or an abnormal abdominal ultrasound are referred to a gastroenterologist for management.[102]

During the Conference on Global Disease Elimination and Eradication in February 1998, hepatitis B was named as a candidate viral disease for elimination or eradication. In 1991, the World Health Organization called for all nations to include HBV vaccine in their national immunization programs. So far, about 100 countries have complied. One barrier for many of the poorer countries is the expense of the vaccine. Some of its cost is being defrayed by regional vaccine purchases. HBV eradication will require immunization for several generations.[105,109,110]

Routine immunization. Term and premature infants weighing ≥2,000 gm at birth born to HBsAg-negative mothers receive the first dose of hepatitis B vaccine by two months of age. The initial dose may be administered in the immediate newborn period. The second dose is administered at least one month after the first. The third and final dose is given at least four months after the second dose, but not before six months of age.[102,111]

The ideal time to begin hepatitis B vaccine in premature neonates weighing <2,000 gm born to HBsAg-negative mothers is not clear. The current recommendation is to delay immunization until the infant weighs 2,000 gm or until two months of age.[91] Losonsky and associates reassessed this recommendation. They evaluated response to hepatitis B vaccine in 118 premature infants (born at <37 weeks gestation) in three weight categories: <1,000 gm, 1,000–1,500 gm, and >1,500 gm. Each infant was given recombinant hepatitis B vaccine during the first week of life, at one to two months of age, and at six to seven months of age. The researchers found that after two doses of vaccine, the seroprotection rate was low regardless of weight. Infants with birth weights <1,000 gm were the poorest responders. After three doses of vaccine, the seroprotection rate improved with weight. Infants with the lowest birth weights had the lowest response rate. Ninety-six percent of the infants who weighed >1,700 gm at birth achieved protective antibody levels following three doses of vaccine. The researchers also found that poor weight gain in the first six months of life and steroid administration in the first few months of life were associated with inadequate immune response to early hepatitis B immunization in premature infants. These results support the current recommendation to delay initiation of hepatitis B immunizations in premature infants.[112]

Single-antigen preservative-free (thimerosal-free) hepatitis B vaccine should be used in children less than six months of age, with priority given to newborn infants. As of March 28, 2000, both Recombivax HB, pediatric (Merck) and Engerix-B, pediatric/adolescent (SmithKline Beecham Biologicals) are preservative-free. Thimerosal is no longer used in any of the pediatric hepatitis B vaccines licensed in the U.S. Children who were not immunized against hepatitis B as infants, who missed doses, or who were given doses earlier than recommended should be immunized between 11 and 12 years of age.[111] Children in high-risk groups should not wait until 11–12 years of age for immunization. They should be immunized as soon as it is recognized that immunizations were missed.[102]

Immunoprophylaxis for infants born to HBsAg-positive mothers. All infants born to HBsAg-positive mothers should receive postexposure immunoprophylaxis with hepatitis B immune globulin (HBIG) and hepatitis B vaccine within 12 hours of birth. The dose of HBIG is 0.5 ml given IM. Hepatitis B vaccine is given concurrently at a different site. This dosage includes premature infants regardless of birth weight. However, for those weighing <2,000 gm at birth, this dose of hepatitis B vaccine is not counted as one of the three required in the childhood immunization schedule.[102]

Immunoprophylaxis for infants born to mothers with unknown HBsAg status. Serologic testing for HBsAg in all pregnant women is essential to identify infants who require immediate immunoprophylaxis following delivery. However, not all mothers are tested, for reasons that can include lack of prenatal care. Infants born to mothers whose status is not known should receive a dose of hepatitis B vaccine within 12 hours of delivery. Blood should be drawn to determine maternal HBsAg status. If the mother is HBsAg positive, the infant should receive HBIG as soon as possible, but no later than one week of age.[111]

Breastfeeding. There appears to be no increased risk of maternal-to-child transmission of HBV via breastfeeding.[102] All mothers, regardless of HBsAg status, who desire to breastfeed their infants should be encouraged and supported. This is particularly true in developing countries, where there are many potential problems associated with bottle feeding.[99,102,113]

Immunization for health care workers. It is strongly recommended that health care workers receive immunization against HBV. Two IM injections are given four weeks apart, followed by a third dose five months later. A nonimmune health care worker who experiences percutaneous or mucous-membrane exposure to HBsAg-positive blood or body fluids should receive HBIG within seven days of exposure. The hepatitis B vaccine series is also initiated at this time. If the hepatitis B series is not initiated, the health care worker should receive a second dose of HBIG one month after the first dose.[114]

Hepatitis C

Etiology and epidemiology. Hepatitis C virus (HCV) is a small, lipid-enveloped, single-stranded RNA virus of the Flaviviridae family. There are numerous HCV genotypes, and although infection can be experimentally reproduced in chimpanzees, humans are the only known host.[115,116]

Globally, it is estimated that as many as 170 million people may be HCV infected. Prevalence varies from region to region as well as within specific geographic areas. The lowest prevalence rates of antibody to HCV (anti-HCV), less than 2.5 percent, are among most populations in Africa, the Americas, Europe, and Southeast Asia. The western Pacific areas have average prevalence rates of 2.5–4.9 percent. In the Middle East, however, prevalence rates range from 1 percent to 12 percent.[116]

Risk factors for HCV vary as well. In developed countries, exposure to blood or blood products from HCV-infected individuals is the most common mode of transmission. In countries where blood donors are screened and those at risk for HCV infection are eliminated from the donor pool, the risk of infection via transfusion is reduced significantly. However, current serologic tests fail to detect anti-HCV in approximately 5 percent of infected donors. Other risk factors include treatment for hemophilia with blood products made before 1987, intravenous drug use, chronic hemodialysis, high-risk sexual practices (e.g., multiple sex partners), and medical or dental procedures performed with inadequately sterilized instruments.[115–117] Risk factors in developing countries include transfusion with unscreened blood or with blood products that have not undergone viral inactivation; contaminated needles; ritual circumcision or scarification with unsterilized objects; any activity that causes a break in the skin, such as bloodletting as part of traditional medicine, tattooing, and ear and body piercing; and intravenous drug use.[116]

Vertical transmission of HCV does occur. The risk of mother-to-child transmission is around 5 percent, with transmission occuring at delivery. However, for infants born to mothers who are coinfected with HCV and HIV, the risk of vertical transmission increases to

14 percent and 17 percent based on detection in the mother of anti-HCV and of HCV RNA, respectively.[118-124] It has been suggested that the increased risk of perinatal HCV transmission in the presence of HIV coinfection in the mother may be related to a high HCV viral load associated with immunodeficiency.[125,126] The role of delivery method in perinatal transmission of HCV is not clear. There have been studies that report decreased transmission rates among infants delivered by cesarean section[122,127] Other studies have had too few mothers delivered by cesarean section to fully explore the role of delivery in perinatal HCV transmission.[118,128,129] The role of breastfeeding in the transmission of HCV is unclear as well. Some references state that maternal-to-child transmission is not associated with breastfeeding.[115,116] However, there are reports in the literature of possible transmission of HCV during breastfeeding. But the number of infants in these reports is small, and the difference in HCV infection among bottle-fed and breastfed infants did not reach statistical significance.[128,130] Large-scale studies that include determination of viral titers in the breast milk are needed to further clarify this matter.[127]

Clinical manifestations and diagnosis. The incubation period for HCV infection is two weeks to six months, with an average of six to seven weeks.[115] Vertical infection may occur *in utero*, as evidenced by presence of HCV RNA immediately after birth[131] or at the time of delivery.[128] This incubation period is applicable to neonates infected during delivery.

Maternal HCV infection does not appear to affect the course of pregnancy. Infants infected with HCV are usually asymptomatic. There are no reports of fulminant hepatitis in infants born to HCV-infected mothers.[100] Generally, vertically acquired HCV infection cannot be clinically detected, although there are serologic, virologic, and biochemical markers of disease.[132,133] These are described below.

The diagnosis of HCV in infants born to HCV-positive mothers is based on either the presence of specific, nonmaternal IgG beyond 18 months of age or the detection of HCV RNA by PCR on two separate occasions or both.[132,134] Timing of these tests is important from the point of view of both accuracy and cost-effectiveness. A negative serum antibody test (anti-HCV) at any age almost always excludes infection.[135] However, there have been case reports in the literature of children with and without HIV coinfection who are HCV carriers with nondetectable anti-HCV levels.[125,132] An accurate diagnosis based on serologic studies alone can be made by 18 months of age. By this time, maternal antibodies are no longer detectable.[135] Hepatitis C virus RNA-PCR can be performed immediately after birth; however, because of the low sensitivity of PCR in the newborn, a negative result offers little useful information. Because of the relatively high cost of PCR testing, it is prudent to delay it until four weeks of age. If the HCV RNA-PCR is negative at this time, the infant is probably not infected. However, a confirmatory anti-HCV serologic test at 18 months of age is recommended.[135] If the HCV RNA-PCR test is positive at 1 month of age, the probability of infection in an infant born to an HIV-negative mother is 73 percent. This probability rises to 90 percent if the mother is HIV positive.[125] As mentioned, a second PCR is needed to establish the presence of HCV infection. The National Institutes of Health recommends performance of HCV RNA tests on two occasions between 2 and 6 months of age.[136] Gibb and colleagues suggest that the virologic diagnosis of HCV infection should be confirmed with a serologic test at 12 to 15 months of age.[125]

Alanine aminotransferase is the biochemical marker used to follow perinatal HCV infection. The European Paediatric Hepatitis C Virus Infection Network studied 104 perinatally HCV infected children for a mean of four years. Serum

ALT levels, considered elevated if the ALT concentration was greater than 1.5 times normal for age, were followed in 87 percent of the children. The researchers found that ALT levels were high during the first two years of life and then declined significantly. Among individual children, ALT levels fluctuated widely with either persistent or transient elevations. Mean ALT concentration peaked at four to six months of age and again at two years of age in this group of subjects. The researchers state, however, that ALT concentration may not be a consistent marker for HCV infection because 16 percent of the children in their study had ALT levels within normal range for age throughout the follow-up period.[132]

The researchers also evaluated viremia and antibody response over the study period. They found that the children fell into one of three categories. Hepatitis C virus RNA by PCR was present throughout the follow-up period in 52 percent of the subjects. Forty-two percent of the children had periods of intermittent viremia. In some samples, HCV RNA was below detectable levels. Finally, the remaining 6 percent of children had persistent anti-HCV after 18 months of age, but never had detectable HCV RNA. One child was transiently anti-HCV negative between the ages of 7 and 28 months and one between 6 and 22 months. The researchers suggest this was due to delayed antibody production. Four children positive for HCV RNA-PCR never developed antibodies to HCV. The remaining children all seroconverted and were positive for anti-HCV when last tested.[132]

The degree of liver damage associated with vertically acquired HCV infection appears to remain mild to moderate throughout childhood.[132,133] Among 20 children who underwent liver biopsy for persistently elevated ALT levels and persistent viremia, no single typical histologic finding was observed. The most frequent findings were steatosis and portal lymphoid aggregates. None of the children had severe liver damage.[132] The progression of liver disease into adulthood for those perinatally infected with HCV needs further exploration.

Treatment and prevention. Strategies to prevent vertical HCV transmission have not been clearly defined. The risks associated with breastfeeding and mode of delivery are ambiguous at this point.[115,116,118,122,127–129] The current recommendation for treatment of HCV infection in adults is combination therapy with ribavirin and pegylated interferon. Both ribavirin and interferon are contraindicated in pregnancy.[136] Researchers have suggested the possibility of using antiviral agents in protocols similar to those used to reduce vertical transmission of HIV.[128,136] Avoiding prolonged labor after rupture of membranes and avoiding fetal scalp electrodes may reduce perinatal transmission.[136]

Four of the children in the European Paediatric Hepatitis C Virus Infection Network study received interferon therapy with mixed results. One child received treatment for a year, resulting in normalization of ALT concentration. When treatment was stopped, there was a relapse, with rising ALT levels. Another child treated for one year was PCR negative 3, 6, and 10 months after initiation of therapy, but was PCR positive one day after therapy was discontinued. In the remaining two patients, the result seems to be positive. One child was HCV RNA negative 25 months after therapy was stopped. In the second child, HCV RNA was undetectable 39 and 52 months after the start of therapy. It is not clear if the child was continuing on therapy when testing was performed. The ages at which therapy was initiated in the children is not stated.[132]

Because most HCV infections are caused by percutaneous exposures, health care workers are at risk for acquisition of HCV infection. There is no vaccine to prevent HCV, and postexposure immunoprophylaxis with immune globulin and antiviral agents is not recommended. Health care workers should be educated about the potential for HCV infection. The Centers for Disease Control and Prevention makes the following recommendations for follow-up of occupational exposures:[137]

- For the source, perform anti-HCV testing.
- For the person exposed to an HCV-positive source
    Perform baseline testing for anti-HCV and ALT concentration.
    Perform follow-up testing at four to six months postexposure. If earlier diagnosis is desired, testing for HCV RNA may be done four to six weeks after exposure.
- Confirm all positive anti-HCV results by enzyme immunoassay using supplemental anti-HCV testing (e.g., recombinant immunoblot assay).[117,137]

The primary objective of global public health activities is the prevention of new cases of HCV infection. Priorities for prevention include the following:[116,117]

- Universal screening of blood, plasma, organ, tissue, and semen donors
- Viral inactivation of plasma-derived products
- Risk reduction counseling and services
- Medical management, as recommended, for adults with
    Persistently elevated ALT levels
    Detectable HCV RNA
    Liver biopsy with portal or bridging fibrosis or moderate or greater degrees of inflammation and necrosis
- Public and professional education

Goals for the future include cost containment for therapeutic agents, development of efficacious and cost-effective therapies, and immunoprophylaxis. Vaccine development is difficult, however, because of the many different genotypes of HCV.[116]

Hepatitis D

Etiology and epidemiology. Hepatitis D virus (HDV) is a viral particle consisting of an HBsAg-coated RNA genome and delta protein antigen (HDAg). Hepatitis D virus is unable to produce infection without the presence of HBV.[138]

Infection with hepatitis D virus may occur at the same time as the initial HBV infection (coinfection), or it may occur as superinfection in an individual with chronic HBV infection.[107,138] In the presence of HBV, HDV is transmitted by blood and blood products, intravenous drug use, and sexual contact.[139] Vertical transmission from mother to fetus/neonate is rare.[138] The incidence, transmission, and significance of HDV infection in the neonate has not been elucidated.[98] Areas of high prevalence include southern Italy, parts of Eastern Europe, South America, Africa, and the Middle East. Despite the prevalence of HBV in the Far East, HDV is uncommon in that part of the world.[138]

The incubation period in cases of HDV coinfection is similar to that of hepatitis B, an average of 120 days, with a range of 45 to 160 days. For HDV superinfection, the incubation period is two to eight weeks based on findings in animal models. There is a chronic carrier state.[138]

Clinical manifestations and diagnosis. In incidences of superinfection with HDV, the rate of fulminant hepatitis and chronic hepatitis that progress to cirrhosis is higher than in cases of acute HBV infection. Clinical manifestations in coinfection coincide with those for HBV.[138]

Detection of HDAg in hepatic tissue or serum and IgM-specific antibody, along with positive tests for HBsAg and anti-HBc-IgM, is diagnostic for HDV/HBV coinfection. Acute superinfection is diagnosed by serologic evidence of HDAg and IgM-specific antibody (acute hepatitis D infection) and HBsAg and anti-HBc-IgG (chronic hepatitis B infection).

Chronic HDV infection is indicated by the serologic presence of delta virus IgG-specific antibody and seropositivity for HBsAg.[138]

Treatment and prevention. Treatment is supportive. Standard precautions are initiated. Prevention of HDV is the same as for HBV. Neither antiviral nor immunotherapy is available for HDV infection. Therefore, HBsAg carriers should diligently avoid situations that could place them at increased risk of superinfection.[103,107]

Hepatitis E

Etiology and epidemiology. Hepatitis E virus (HEV) is a nonenveloped single-stranded RNA virus.[103,140] Hepatitis E was formerly known as enterically transmitted non-A, non-B hepatitis.

Transmission of the hepatitis E virus occurs by the fecal-oral route. The infection has an epidemiology similar to that of HAV. Infection with HEV is more common in adults than in children. Mortality is low (1–3 percent) in most young adults, but there is a high case-fatality rate (15–25 percent) among pregnant women with third-trimester HEV infection. The pregnant woman may die several days after onset of fulminant hepatitis or show signs of recovery from severe hepatitis only to bleed to death during delivery. Either scenario often results in fetal loss as well. Mild HEV infection during pregnancy has also been suggested as the cause for spontaneous abortion and intrauterine demise. The pathophysiology of the increased mortality seen with perinatal HEV is not presently understood.[99,103,140–142]

Khuroo and associates found support for vertical transmission of HEV in a series of eight mothers and their infants. Five infants were positive for HEV RNA. These infants also had IgG anti-HEV in their blood from samples drawn at birth. This would be expected as the result of passive acquisition of maternal antibodies. However, the authors assert that persistence of IgG in follow-up samples to six months of age demonstrates that these antibodies are also the result of an immune response by the infants.[143]

Parts of Asia, Africa, and Mexico are noted to have HEV epidemics or sporadic outbreaks. A contaminated water source is the usual cause. Fecal viral shedding and viremia last for at least two weeks. The incubation period ranges from 15 to 60 days, with an average of 40 days. There is no progression to chronic disease.[140]

Clinical manifestations and diagnosis. Infection with HEV is acute. Symptoms include jaundice due to elevated direct bilirubin, malaise, fever, anorexia, abdominal pain, and arthralgia.[140] The infants in the study by Khuroo and associates showed varying manifestations. Only one was jaundiced at birth; that infant also had an elevated serum ALT level. Four other infants also had elevated serum ALT levels, but were not jaundiced. This suggests anicteric hepatitis. Two infants were hypothermic and hypoglycemic. Both died within 24 hours of delivery. The authors suggest that these deaths may have been related to fetal metabolic disturbances resulting from severe maternal liver disease. Postmortem liver biopsy on one of these infants showed massive hepatic necrosis.[143]

Diagnosis of HEV infection may be achieved by serologic testing for anti-HEV antibodies and identification of viral-like particles in stool specimens by electron microscopy.[87,92] Viral RNA can also be identified in stool and serum by PCR.[140]

Treatment and prevention. Treatment is supportive. Contact and standard precautions are initiated for the hospitalized patient. Good sanitation and avoidance of potentially contaminated food and water are the best means of prevention.[140]

Immune globulins produced in the West have not been shown effective in preventing infection. The prophylactic efficacy of immune globulin prepared from donors in endemic areas is not known.[144] Experimental vaccines have shown promise in animal models.[145] Because HEV occurs predominately in poorer countries, however, major vaccine manufacturers have limited financial incentive for commercial development of a vaccine.

Hepatitis G

Etiology and epidemiology. First identified in 1995, hepatitis G virus (HGV) is a single-stranded RNA virus with worldwide distribution.[146,147] Hepatitis G virus belongs to the Flaviviridae family and is distantly related to HCV.[148] Interestingly, a strain of HGV, HGBV, was discovered in the 1960s and named for the surgeon (GB) from whom it was originally derived. The surgeon developed hepatitis, and his serum caused hepatitis in tamarins, a species of small primate. There are three different HGBV agents. HGBV-A and HGBV-B seem to be tamarin viruses; HGBV-C is a human virus. Hepatitis G and HGBV-C have amino acid sequences that are 95 percent homologous and thus are considered strains of the same virus.[149] In addition, HGV has a 27 percent homology with HCV.[150]

Hepatitis G infection is found in both adults and children throughout the world. In the U.S., 1.5 percent of blood donors are positive for HGV. Among adults with chronic HBV or HCV infection, 10–20 percent also are infected with HGV.[150] There is evidence of parenteral transmission of HGV infection because of the high incidence among hemodialysis patients and intravenous drug users.[146] Hepatitis G infection may be transmitted by organ transplantation. The presence of HGV infection among homosexual and bisexual individuals indicates the possibility of sexual transmission as well.[150] Vertical transmission to the fetus/newborn does occur and is associated with high viral titers in the mother.[150–154] In one study of 20 infants born to HGV RNA-positive mothers, 75 percent were found to be HGV RNA positive at a median age of 12 months. In each of these infants, at least one sample drawn at a younger age was analyzed for confirmation and to determine onset of viremia.[154] Breastfeeding does not appear to contribute to HGV transmission. Breast milk samples from 15 HGV RNA-positive women were tested by PCR. No HGV RNA was detected in any of the samples regardless of the level of viremia in the mother.[155] Finally, neonatal transfusion-related HGV infection has been reported in the literature. The serum from 251 infants who had received blood products during the neonatal period was analyzed for HGV infection. The analysis was performed at a mean interval of 37 months (range 10–70 months) posttransfusion. Hepatitis G virus RNA was detected in 19 (7.6 percent) of the patients.[156] The incubation period is unknown.[150]

Clinical manifestations and diagnosis. Infection with HGV appears to be asymptomatic. Hepatitis G virus may very well be a benign passenger of other viruses. Experts wonder if perhaps it was named among the hepatitis viruses prematurely. Often HCV and HGV—and less often HBV and HGV—are found together in the serum. ALT levels in those with HCV and HGV coinfection run parallel to those of HCV, not HGV, infection. Hepatitis G virus infection has no obvious effect on clinical outcome.[147,149]

Palomba and associates examined vertical transmission of HGV in women with HCV and HIV infection. They found that although most of the infants developed persistent HGV infection, none had clinical or biochemical evidence of liver disease. Some of these children have been followed for more than 7 years. They continue to be symptom free and without biochemical evidence of liver disease.[153] Fourteen of the 19 children with transfusion-related HGV infection were followed for a mean of 15 years. Four of the 14 showed persistent HGV infection, but no clinical signs of liver diseases. Liver function tests remained within normal range for age.[156]

Serologic markers for HGV infection are anti-HGV and anti-HGV-E2. Presence of anti-HGV indicates recent or past HGV infection.[157] As with antibody levels with other viral infections, timing of testing of the infant is a consideration to allow for clearance of maternal antibodies. This usually occurs around 18 months of age. Anti-HGV-E2 is the antibody to recombinant envelope protein, and its presence is often associated with viral clearance.[157] Hepatitis G virus RNA can be detected by reverse transcriptase polymerase chain reaction (RT-PCR).[157] Timing of neonatal or infant testing is not described in the literature. Because of the distance relationship between HGV and HCV, PCR testing at 1–2 months of age and again at 6 months of age seems reasonable.

Treatment and prevention. No treatment for HGV infection is required except that necessary for any coinfection. Prevention of vertical transmission is aimed at educating adults, especially women of childbearing age, to avoid situations that place them at risk for infection (e.g., intravenous drug use). Presently, HGV seems to be a harmless virus. However, because its discovery is so recent, the long-term consequences of perinatally acquired persistent or chronic infection are not known.

NEONATAL FUNGAL INFECTIONS

The incidence of nosocomial fungal infections in the NICU has increased over the years, especially as we care for infants who require more invasive procedures and prolonged hospitalization.[158,159] Candida and Malassezia species are implicated in neonatal fungal infections.

Candida

Etiology and Epidemiology

The most common cause of neonatal fungal infections is Candida species. There are more than 150 species of Candida. *C. albicans* causes the majority of Candida infections in the NICU. Other species reported in the literature and observed in practice include *C. parapsilosis*, *C. glabrata (Torulopsis glabrata)*, *C. tropicalis*, and *C. guilliermondii (Pichia guilliermondii)*.[158,160–162]

Candida species are present on the skin and in the mouth, the gastrointestinal (GI) tract, and the vagina of healthy persons. If a pregnant woman is infected with vulvovaginal candidiasis, the newborn may acquire the organism *in utero* or during vaginal delivery. Candida appears to cause ascending infection and is capable of penetrating intact amniotic membranes. Despite this, congenital candidiasis is rare.[163] The organism is most commonly acquired postnatally.

Children at highest risk for nosocomial Candida infection include premature, low birth weight neonates, those who have undergone cardiothoracic surgery, and those requiring admission to the intensive care unit.[164] Other risk factors associated with Candida infection are described in the literature. Infection with HIV or the presence of other immune deficiencies also increases an individual's susceptibility to Candida infections.[160]

In a study assessing nosocomial infections in the NICU, researchers found that the incidence of Candida infection increased proportionately to a decrease in birth weight. Fifteen percent of infants weighing <1 kg at birth developed Candida infections, compared with 7 percent and 4 percent for infants with birth weights of 1–1.5 kg and >1.5 kg, respectively. The researchers also looked at other variables, such as ventilatory support, central venous and arterial catheters, and antibiotics. These were regarded as acute variables if they were present at the time of sepsis. The total number of days a particular variable was applicable deemed it a summary variable. Evaluating only Candida sepsis as the outcome in relation to birth weight and the acute and summary variable, the researchers noted that the acute variables of ventilatory support and the presence of a central venous catheter, along with the summary variable of antibiotic administration, were significant risk factors for Candida sepsis. In fact, extended use of antibiotics to treat premature infants for suspected, not proved, sepsis was associated with an increased likelihood of subsequent blood culture–positive sepsis, particularly Candida sepsis.[165]

Another multicenter study examined risk factors for colonization with Candida species. The researchers found that the prevalence of Candida colonization was 23 percent (486 out of 2,157 NICU admissions). Fourteen percent of the infants were colonized with *C. albicans*, 7 percent with *C. parapsilosis*, and the remainder with other Candida species. Using multiple logistic regression analysis, adjusting for length of stay, birth weight <1,000 grams, and gestational age <32 weeks, the researchers evaluated for risk factors associated with the two most prominent Candida species. Essentially, they found that the sicker the neonate, the higher the risk. The use of third-generation cephalosporins was also found to be a risk factor for both *C. albicans* and *C. parapsilosis*. Infants with central venous catheters and those who received intravenous lipid infusions were at increased risk for *C. albicans*. The use of histamine$_2$ blockers was found to be an independent risk factor for *C. parapsilosis*. Delivery by cesarean section was protective against colonization with *C. albicans*. The researchers found several variables that were not associated with colonization with Candida species, including premature rupture of membranes, gender, maternal antibiotics, intubation, frequency of intubation, steroid administration, antibiotic administration other than third-generation cephalosporins, and surgical procedures.[166]

Characteristics of the preterm neonate contribute to the pathophysiology of fungal infections. Host factors include immature skin structure and disruption of cutaneous barriers.[167] Furthermore, preterm infants are relatively immunodeficient. The premature infant processes fewer T cells, there is a decreased number of neutrophils when compared to adults, and the function of the neutrophils present is diminished.[168] Saiman and associates assert the importance of GI colonization in the pathogenesis of Candida sepsis.[169] Factors that most likely contribute to loss of normal GI flora and allow for fungal overgrowth include treatment with third-generation cephalosporins and delayed enteral feedings. The histamine$_2$ blockers may also alter the gastrointestinal environment and promote the colonization of Candida species.[166] Although not evaluated in their study, Saiman and colleagues also suggest that colonization of the skin or respiratory tract may contribute to infection with Candida.[166]

In another study, researchers found that prolonged hospitalization related to the presence of major congenital anomalies was a risk factor for the development of Candida in infants weighing >2.5 kg at birth.[162] Saiman and colleagues also explored the horizontal transmission of Candida species from the hands of health care workers. They proposed that increased

FIGURE 5-5 ◆ White plaques of oral candidiasis (thrush).

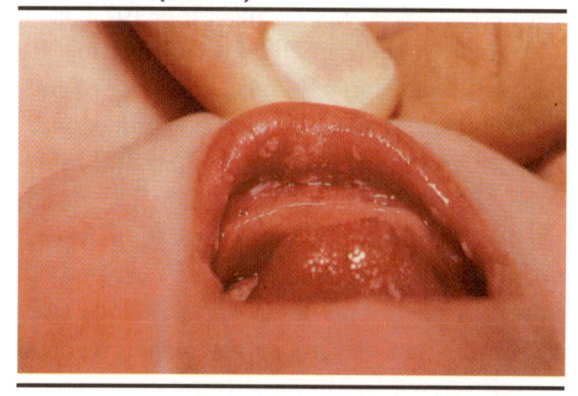

From: Pong AL, and McCuaig CC. 2001. Fungal infections, infestations, and parasitic infections in neonates. In *Textbook of Neonatal Dermatology*, Eichenfield LF, Frieden IJ, and Esterly NB, eds. Philadelphia: WB Saunders, 225. Reprinted by permission.

FIGURE 5-6 ◆ Congenital candidiasis: diffuse, erythematous, pustular eruption.

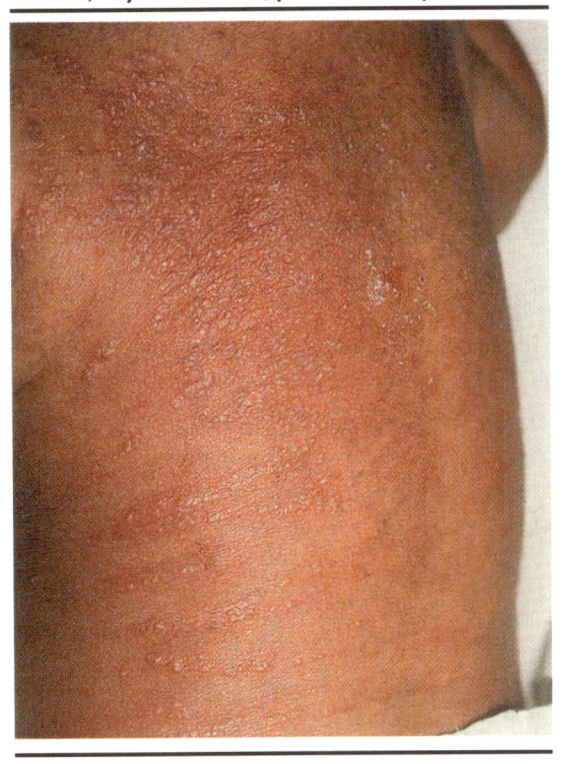

From: Pong AL, and McCuaig CC. 2001. Fungal infections, infestations, and parasitic infections in neonates. In *Textbook of Neonatal Dermatology,* Eichenfield LF, Frieden IJ, and Esterly NB, eds. Philadelphia: WB Saunders, 224. Reprinted by permission.

FIGURE 5-7 ◆ Palmar pustules associated with congenital candidiasis.

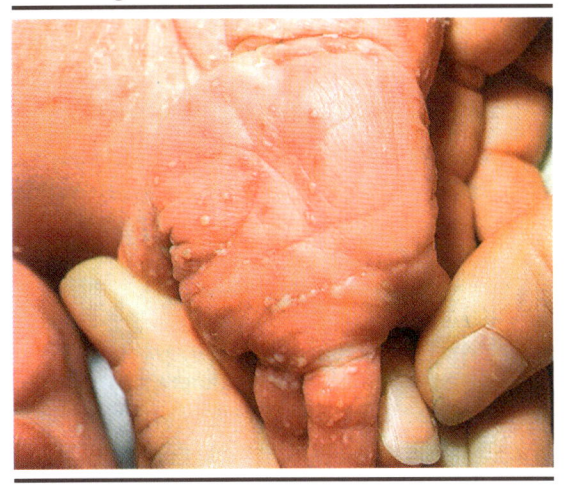

From: Pong AL, and McCuaig CC. 2001. Fungal infections, infestations, and parasitic infections in neonates. In *Textbook of Neonatal Dermatology,* Eichenfield LF, Frieden IJ, and Esterly NB, eds. Philadelphia: WB Saunders, 224. Reprinted by permission.

colonization, particularly with *C. parapsilosis*, was associated with increased handling of sicker infants by health care workers.[166]

Clinical Manifestations and Diagnosis

Mucocutaneous Candida infection in the neonatal period presents as oral thrush or lesions of the gluteal folds, neck, groin, and axillae. Oral candidiasis typically appears as whitish patches on the tongue and on the gingival and buccal mucosa (Figure 5-5). It can be distinguished from formula residual by the inability of the caregiver to wipe the patches from the oral surfaces. The neonate who is taking enteral feedings by nipple may refuse to suck. This reticence is most likely the result of discomfort associated with candidiasis. On the skin, candidiasis appears as diffuse, scaling dermatitis or an erythematous pustular rash, often with satellite lesions (Figure 5-6).[170]

Congenital cutaneous candidiasis presents with scaling lesions, erythematous papules, and pustules at birth. The rash may progress to bullous lesions. The head, trunk, extremities, and intertriginous areas are usually involved. A hallmark of congenital cutaneous candidiasis is palmar and plantar pustules (Figure 5-7).[163,167]

Symptoms of systemic congenital candidiasis reported in the literature include elevated white blood cell (WBC) count with a left shift of the WBC differential; hyperglycemia; and other signs associated with sepsis, such as poor perfusion, metabolic acidosis, and worsening respiratory distress.[163]

Invasive nosocomial candidiasis can involve any organ or anatomic site.[160] Signs and symptoms are indistinguishable from those observed in bacterial sepsis, including apnea, bradycardia, temperature instability, shock, diffuse maculopapular rash, glucose instability, glucosuria, metabolic acidosis, thrombocytopenia, and leukopenia. Candida infection may also have orthopedic manifestations, including osteomyelitis and osteoarthritis.[171] Candida infection can progress rapidly to death.[160]

Diagnosis of mucocutaneous candidiasis is generally made by clinical signs. Scrapings of cutaneous lesions can be prepared with 10 percent potassium hydroxide (KOH) to document the presence of budding yeast and pseudohyphae.[160,170]

Invasive candidiasis is diagnosed by cultures (e.g., urine, blood, CSF).[160] The urinary tract is the most frequent site of infection. A catheterized or suprapubic urine specimen is obtained for KOH (a rapid screening tool) and culture. If intravascular catheters are present, blood cultures are obtained from these lines, as well as from a peripheral site. In the absence of a central line, some clinicians obtain blood cultures from two peripheral sites. The rationale for two peripheral cultures is to improve the chance of microorganism recovery. Unfortunately, blood cultures can be falsely negative. New tests, including rapid, noninvasive tests for antigens in serum and urine and molecular probes, are under investigation and may facilitate diagnosis of Candida infections.[172]

Treatment and Prevention

Oral candidiasis is treated with nystatin oral suspension, 100,000 units/ml, 1 ml for premature infants and 2 ml for term infants. The oral mucosa is swabbed every six hours. Treatment is continued for three days after the mouth is clear of lesions.[173] If the infant is breastfeeding, the mother may have cutaneous candidiasis on her nipples. Topical treatment with nystatin oral suspension is effective treatment.

Skin lesions are treated with topical creams or ointments. Nystatin is usually effective and the least expensive of the available creams and ointments.[160] The topical cream or ointment is applied four times a day and is continued for three days after all the lesions have cleared.[173] Moist lesions often found in the creases of the groin and neck can be treated with nystatin powder. The powder is applied four times a day and is continued until the area has dried.

Amphotericin B is the drug of choice for treating systemic Candida infections.[160] The initial dose is 0.25–0.5 mg/kg given IV over 2–6 hours. The maintenance dose is 0.5–1 mg/kg given IV over 2–6 hours every 24–48 hours. Dose reduction is not necessary for infants with renal impairment; however, should serum creatinine increase >0.4 mg/dl during therapy, the dose is held for two to five days. Therapy may last for four to six weeks, depending on the severity of the illness. Amphotericin B is nephrotoxic, causing injury to the tubular epithelium that results in urinary potassium losses, decreased sodium reabsorption, and renal tubular acidosis. Hematologic side effects include anemia and thrombocytopenia. Phlebitis may occur at the infusion site. Serum electrolytes, creatinine, blood urea nitrogen (BUN), and CBC should be monitored at least every other day.[173]

An alternative to amphotericin B is liposomal amphotericin B, a preparation of amphotericin B incorporated into unilamellar liposomes. (See Chapter 8 for more information on liposomal amphotericin B, including dosing.) Another alternative to amphotericin B is fluconazole, which has been shown to be effective in the treatment of systemic Candida infections in neonates.[174,175] In addition, fluconazole produced few side effects.[174] Fluconazole may be administered IV or PO. An initial loading dose of 12 mg/kg is given. Subsequent doses of 6 mg/kg are given IV over 30–60 minutes or PO.[173,176] Dose frequency is based on gestational and postnatal age. Renal function (urine output, serum creatinine, and BUN) is monitored during fluconazole therapy. Elevation of transaminases has been associated with fluconazole administration, so AST and ALT should be monitored as well. The CBC is followed for eosinophilia.[173]

In cases of severe systemic infection or if there is CNS involvement, flucytosine is given concurrently with amphotericin B or fluconazole.[160,173] The dose is 12.5–37.5 mg/kg/dose every six hours PO. Because this medication is given PO, gastrointestinal status should be followed closely. Renal function is monitored as well. Laboratory monitoring includes twice-weekly CBC and platelet count and periodic AST and ALT.[173]

Prevention of colonization and infection with Candida species in the neonate is a challenge. Prolonged use of broad-spectrum antibiotics should be minimized as much as possible. Scrupulous care of central vascular catheter sites is imperative.[160] The importance of good hand-washing before and after patient contact cannot be overemphasized.

In 2001, Kaufman and associates explored the efficacy of fluconazole prophylaxis against fungal colonization and infection in extremely low birth weight premature neonates. Based on pharmacokinetic studies in premature infants, the neonates received fluconazole intravenously six weeks using the following dosing schedule:[177]

- 3 mg/kg every third day (every 72 hours) during weeks 1 and 2
- 3 mg/kg every other day (every 48 hours) during weeks 3 and 4
- 3 mg/kg every day (every 24 hours) during weeks 5 and 6

The results of the study are promising. The researchers found that fluconazole prophylaxis was effective in preventing fungal infections in extremely low birth weight premature neonates. Additionally, there were no adverse effects and resistance to fluconazole was not noted.[177]

Malassezia

Etiology and Epidemiology

The genus of lipophilic yeast, Malassezia, includes *M. furfur*, *M. pachydermatis*, and *M. sympodailis*. There are reports in the literature of both *M. furfur* and *M. pachydermatis* causing nosocomial infections in neonates.[178–181] *M. furfur* infection is associated with low birth weight and administration of IV fat emulsion.[180] In one study of neonates with *M. pachydermatis* infection, risk factors included severe illness in low birth weight infants and the presence of arterial catheters for more than nine days.[178]

Skin colonization with *M. furfur* is a normal event that occurs in neonates regardless of health status.[181] *M. pachydermatis* likely is introduced to the nursery on health care providers' hands after colonization by contact with their pet dogs. *M. pachydermatis* is associated with canine otitis externa.[178] The portal of entry for Malassezia species into the bloodstream from the skin is most likely indwelling intravenous catheters.[181]

Clinical Manifestations and Diagnosis

Symptoms of Malassezia fungemia are often indistinguishable from those of bacteremia. The neonate presents with fever, apnea, bradycardia, and pneumonitis. A CBC may reveal thrombocytopenia.[182] The diagnosis is made by blood cultures, looking specifically for Malassezia species. A request for the microbiology lab to look specially for Malassezia is included in the order for the culture. *M. furfur* does not grow on routine culture. It should be cultured in an oil-enriched medium.[183] Urine and skin cultures may be obtained as well.

Treatment and Prevention

Treatment for *M. furfur* consists of removing the central vascular catheter if present and temporarily stopping lipid therapy. *M. furfur* is often susceptible to antifungal agents, but antifungal therapy is usually unsuccessful unless the central line is removed. *M. furfur* is implicated in both adhesion of catheters to the vein wall and catheter occlusion.[184,185] Thrombi or fibrin sheaths may develop on the surface of the infected catheter.[184,186,187] Fungal infection may occur in conjunction with thrombus formation.[188] The combination of the fungus and thrombus acts like an abscess, making it difficult for the antifungal agent to reach the infection.[189] It has not been determined if antifungal therapy in addition to catheter removal is useful in treating positive *M. furfur* cultures from sites other than the blood.[182]

Treatment of *M. pachydermatis* infection is not discussed in the literature. Removal of central vascular catheters is probably an appropriate approach. Because *M. pachydermatis* is not obligately lipophilic, it may not be necessary to discontinue lipid infusions.

Handwashing before and after patient care is essential in preventing the spread of Malassezia species in the NICU. Intravascular catheters, especially those through which hyperalimentation is infused, must be managed using aseptic technique.[178–182]

Summary

Neonates can be infected with any of a number of viruses. A high index of suspicion based on a knowledge of seasonal variation in virus prevalence in a specific community can help the clinician with definitive diagnosis. Treatment for viral illness is generally supportive. Viral illnesses can have wide-ranging impact on the neonate, from increased length of hospitalization to death. The onus of prevention falls to the adult caregivers, both professionals and family members. Hand hygiene and immunization against specific viral illnesses are important keys to prevention of viral infections in neonates.

The year 2003 marked the 20th anniversary of the discovery of HIV-1. Over the past two decades, amazing progress has been made; thus, the quality of life for many persons with HIV has improved. For HIV-positive women, introduction of the protocol for zidovudine administration during pregnancy and labor, followed by administration of the drug to their infants, resulted in a significant decrease in vertical transmission of HIV. Research to find efficacious, cost-effective strategies to reduce the incidence of mother-to-child transmission of HIV is ongoing.

The effects of the hepatitis viruses vary. Three of them, HBV, HCV, and HEV, seem to have the greatest negative impact in the fetus and neonate. Vertically acquired HBV and HCV both have long-term sequelae for the neonate as a result of liver damage. Maternal HEV infection can result in fetal and neonatal loss.

Fungi are among the common causes of nosocomial infections in the neonatal intensive care unit. Colonization, which may occur at the time of delivery or during the first few days in the NICU, plays an important role in fungal infections. Neonatal infection, regardless of the offending organism, frequently results in increased length of hospital stay and increased cost of care. Outcomes for neonatal viral infections, blood-borne infections, and fungal infections range from no long-term sequelae to a lifetime of health-related issues and even death.

References

1. American Academy of Pediatrics. 2000. Respiratory syncytial virus. In *Red Book: Report of the Committee on Infectious Diseases*, 25th ed., Pickering L, ed. Elk Grove Village, Illinois: American Academy of Pediatrics, 483–487.
2. Keyserling HL. 1997. Other viral agents of perinatal importance: Varicella, parvovirus, respiratory syncytial virus, and enterovirus. *Clinics in Perinatology* 24(1): 193–211.
3. Rodriquez WJ. 1999. Respiratory syncytial virus infections in infants. *Seminars in Pediatric Infectious Diseases* 10(3): 161–181.
4. Brenton S. 1997. RSV specimen collection methods: Nasal vs nasopharyngeal. *Pediatric Nursing* 23(6): 621–622, 629.
5. DeVincenzo J. 1997. Prevention and treatment of respiratory syncytial virus infections. *Advances in Pediatric Infectious Disease* 13: 1–47.
6. Hall CB, et al. 1983. Aerosolized ribavirin treatment of infants with respiratory syncytial virus infection. A randomized double-blind study. *New England Journal of Medicine* 308(24): 1443–1447.
7. Hall CB, et al. 1985. Ribavirin treatment of respiratory syncytial virus infection in infants with underlying cardiopulmonary disease. *JAMA* 254(21): 3047–3051.
8. Groothius JR, et al. 1990. Early ribavirin treatment of respiratory syncytial viral infection in high risk children. *Journal of Pediatrics* 117(15): 792–798.

9. Taber L, et al. 1983. Ribavirin aerosol treatment of bronchiolitis associated with respiratory syncytial virus infections in infants. *Pediatrics* 72(5): 613–618.
10. Meert KL, et al. 1994. Aerosolized ribavirin in mechanically ventilated children with respiratory syncytial virus lower respiratory tract disease. A prospective double-blind, randomized trial. *Critical Care Medicine* 22(4): 566–572.
11. Smith DW, et al. 1991. A controlled trial of aerosolized ribavirin in infants receiving mechanical ventilation for severe respiratory syncytial virus infection. *New England Journal of Medicine* 325(1): 24–29.
12. Janai HK, et al. 1990. Ribavirin: Adverse drug reactions, 1986 to 1988. *Pediatric Infectious Disease Journal* 9(3): 209–211.
13. Kilham L, and Ferm VH. 1977. Congenital anomalies induced in hamster embryos with ribavirin. *Science* 195(4276): 413–414.
14. Kochhar DM, Penner JD, and Knedsen TB. 1980. Embryotoxic, teratogenic, and metabolic effects of ribavirin in mice. *Toxicology and Applied Pharmacology* 52(1): 99–112.
15. Hillyard IW. 1980. The preclinical toxicology and safety of ribavirin. In *Ribavirin: A Broad Spectrum Antiviral Agent*, Smith RA, and Kilpatrick W, eds. New York: Academic Press, 59–71.
16. Buck ML. 1997. Prevention and treatment of respiratory syncytial virus: The search for a cost-effective strategy. *Pediatric Pharmacotherapy* 3(10): 1–3.
17. Ito S, and Koren G. 1993. Exposure of pregnant women to ribavirin-contaminated air: Risk assessment and recommendations. *Pediatric Infectious Disease Journal* 12(1): 2–5.
18. American Academy of Pediatrics, Committee on Infectious Diseases. 1996. Reassessment of indications for ribavirin therapy in respiratory syncytial virus infections. *Pediatrics* 97(1): 137–140.
19. Navas L, et al. 1992. Improved outcome of respiratory syncytial virus infection in a high-risk hospitalized population of Canadian children. *Journal of Pediatrics* 121(3): 348–354.
20. Moler FW, et al. 1992. Respiratory syncytial virus morbidity and mortality estimates in congenital heart disease patients: A recent experience. *Critical Care Medicine* 20(10): 1406–1413.
21. Wang EEL, Law BJ, and Stephens D. 1995. Pediatric Investigators Collaborative Network on Infections in Canada (PICNIC) prospective study of risk factors and outcomes in patients hospitalized with respiratory syncytial viral lower respiratory tract infection. *Journal of Pediatrics* 126(2): 212–219.
22. Hall CB, et al. 1986. Respiratory syncytial viral infection in children with compromised immune function. *New England Journal of Medicine* 315(2): 77–81.
23. Moler FW, et al. 1996. Effectiveness of ribavirin in otherwise well infants with respiratory syncytial virus-associated respiratory failure. *Journal of Pediatrics* 128(3): 422–428.
24. Law BJ, Wang EE, and Stephens D. 1995. Ribavirin does not reduce hospital stay (LOS) in patients with respiratory syncytial virus (RSV) lower respiratory tract infection (LRTI). *Pediatric Research* 34: 110A.
25. Derish M, et al. 1998. Aerosolized albuterol improves airway reactivity in infants with acute respiratory failure from respiratory syncytial virus. *Pediatric Pulmonology* 26(1): 12–20.
26. Rodriquez WJ, et al. 1997. Respiratory syncytial virus (RSV) immune globulin intravenous therapy for RSV lower respiratory tract infection in infants and young children at high risk for severe RSV infection. *Pediatrics* 99(3): 454–461.
27. DeVincenzo JP, et al. 1998. Viral concentration in upper and lower respiratory secretions from respiratory syncytial virus (RSV) infected children treated with RSV monoclonal antibody (MEDI-493). *Pediatric Research* 43: 144A.
28. Saez-Llorens X, et al. 1998. Phase I/II, double-blind, placebo-controlled, multi-dose escalation trial of a human respiratory syncytial virus (RSV) monoclonal antibody (MEDI-493) in children hospitalized with RSV. *Pediatric Research* 43: 156A.
29. The PREVENT Study Group. 1997. Reduction of respiratory syncytial virus hospitalization among premature infants and infants with bronchopulmonary dysplasia using respiratory syncytial virus immune globulin prophylaxis. *Pediatrics* 99(1): 93–99.
30. The IMpact-RSV Study Group. 1998. Palivizumab, a humanized respiratory syncytial virus monoclonal antibody, reduces hospitalization from respiratory syncytial virus infection in high-risk infants. *Pediatrics* 102(3 part 1): 531–537.
31. American Academy of Pediatrics, Committee on Infectious Diseases and Committee of Fetus and Newborn. 1998. Prevention of respiratory syncytial virus infections: Indications for the use of palivizumab and update on the use of RSV-IGIV. *Pediatrics* 102(5): 1211–1216.
32. Centers for Disease Control and Prevention. 1999. Influenza. Available at www.cdc.gov/ncidod/diseases/flu/fluinfo.htm.
33. American Academy of Pediatrics. 2000. Influenza. In *Red Book: Report of the Committee on Infectious Diseases*, 25th ed., Pickering L, ed. Elk Grove Village, Illinois: American Academy of Pediatrics, 51–59.
34. Centers for Disease Control and Prevention. 1997. Prevention and control of influenza: Recommendations of the Advisory Committee on Immunization Practices (ACIP). *MMWR* 46(RR-9): 1–25.
35. Munoz FM, et al. 1999. Influenza A virus outbreak in a neonatal intensive care unit. *Pediatric Infectious Disease Journal* 18(9): 811–815.
36. Centers for Disease Control and Prevention. 1999. Prevention and control of influenza: Recommendations of the Advisory Committee on Immunization Practices (ACIP). *MMWR* 48(RR-4): 1–28.
37. Fete TJ, and Noyes B. 1996. Common (but not always considered) viral infections of the lower respiratory tract. *Pediatric Annals* 25(10): 577–584.
38. Centers for Disease Control and Prevention. 1999. Neuraminidase inhibitors for treatment of influenza A and B infections. *MMWR* 48(RR-14): 1–10.
39. American Academy of Pediatrics. 2000. Varicella-zoster infections. In *Red Book: Committee on Infectious Diseases*, 25th ed., Pickering L, ed. Elk Grove Village, Illinois: American Academy of Pediatrics, 624–638.
40. Zenk KE, Sills JH, and Koeppel RM. 2003. Acyclovir. *Neonatal Medications & Nutrition: A Comprehensive Guide*, 3rd ed. Santa Rosa, California: NICU INK, 11–12.
41. Young TE, and Mangum OB. 2003. *Neofax*, 16th ed. Raleigh, North Carolina: Acorn, 2–3.
42. Reynolds L, Struik S, and Nadel S. 1999. Neonatal varicella: Varicella zoster immunoglobulin (VZIG) does not prevent disease. *Archives of Disease in Childhood. Fetal and Neonatal Edition* 81(1): F69–F70.
43. Centers for Disease Control and Prevention. 1996. Prevention of varicella: Recommendations of the Advisory Committee on Immunization Practices (ACIP). *MMWR* 45(RR-11): 1–36.
44. Centers for Disease Control and Prevention. 1999. Prevention of varicella: Update recommendations of the Advisory Committee on Immunization Practices (ACIP). *MMWR* 48(RR-6): 1–5.
45. Beaver JH. 1999. National Immunization Program, Centers for Disease Control and Prevention. Personal communication. October 29.
46. Salzman MB, and Garcia C. 1998. Postexposure varicella vaccination in siblings of children with active varicella. *Pediatric Infectious Disease Journal* 17(3): 256–257.
47. Zaoutis T, and Klein JD. 1998. Enterovirus infections. *Pediatrics in Review* 19(6): 183–191.
48. American Academy of Pediatrics. 2000. Poliovirus infections. In *Red Book: Report of the Committee on Infectious Diseases*, 25th ed., Pickering L, ed. Elk Grove Village, Illinois: American Academy of Pediatrics, 465–470.

49. American Academy of Pediatrics. 2000. Enterovirus (nonpolio) infections. In *Red Book: Report of the Committee on Infectious Diseases*, 25th ed., Pickering L, ed. Elk Grove Village, Illinois: American Academy of Pediatrics, 236–238.

50. Jankovic B, et al. 1999. Severe neonatal Echovirus 17 infection during a nursery outbreak. *Journal of Pediatric Infectious Disease* 18(4): 393–394.

51. Rotbart H. 1998. Enteroviruses. In *Krugman's Infectious Diseases of Children*, 10th ed., Katz S, Gershon A, and Hotez P, eds. Philadelphia: Mosby-Year Book, 81–97.

52. American Academy of Pediatrics. 2000. Active and passive immunization. In *Red Book: Report of the Committee on Infectious Diseases*, 25th ed., Pickering L, ed. Elk Grove Village, Illinois: American Academy of Pediatrics, 1–81.

53. Modlin JF. 1996. Update on enterovirus infections in infants and children. *Advances in Pediatric Infectious Diseases* 12: 155–180.

54. Abzug MJ, Levin MJ, and Rotbart HA. 1993. Profile of enterovirus disease in the first two weeks of life. *Pediatric Infectious Disease Journal* 12(10): 820–824.

55. Abzug MJ, and Rotbart HA. 1999. Enterovirus infections of neonates and infants. *Seminars in Pediatric Infectious Diseases* 10(3): 169–176.

56. Rotbart H, et al. 1997. Diagnosis of enterovirus infection by polymerase chain reaction on multiple specimen types. *Pediatric Infectious Disease Journal* 16(4): 409–410.

57. van Vliet K, et al. 1998. Multicenter evaluation of the Amplicor enterovirus PCR test with cerebrospinal fluid from patients with aseptic meningitis. *Journal of Clinical Microbiology* 36(9): 2652–2657.

58. Ahmed A, et al. 1997. Clinical utility of the polymerase chain reaction for diagnosis of enteroviral meningitis in infancy. *Journal of Pediatrics* 131(3): 393–397.

59. Byington CL, et al. 1999. A polymerase chain reaction–based epidemiologic investigation of the incidence of nonpolio enteroviral infections in febrile and afebrile infants 90 days and younger. *Pediatrics* 103(3): e27.

60. Pasic S. 1997. Intravenous immunoglobulin prophylaxis in an Echovirus 6 and Echovirus 4 nursery outbreak. *Pediatric Infectious Disease Journal* 16(7): 718–720.

61. Abzug MJ, et al. 1995. Neonatal enterovirus infection: Virology, serology, and effects of intravenous immune globulin. *Clinical Infectious Diseases* 20(5): 1201–1206.

62. American Academy of Pediatrics. 2000. HIV infection. In *Red Book: Report of the Committee on Infectious Diseases*, 25th ed., Pickering L, ed. Elk Grove Village, Illinois: American Academy of Pediatrics, 325–350.

63. Joint United Nations Programme on HIV/AIDS (UNAIDS). 1999. Prevention of HIV transmission from mother to child: Strategic options. Geneva, Switzerland: UNAIDS, 5–19. Available at www.unaids.org/publications/documents/mtct/una9940e.pdf.

64. Kline MW. 1999. Vertically acquired human immunodeficiency virus infection. *Seminars in Pediatric Infectious Diseases* 10(3): 147–153.

65. Lindsay MK, and Nesheim SR. 1997. Human immunodeficiency virus infection in pregnant women and their newborns. *Clinics in Perinatology* 24(1): 161–180.

66. Van de Perre P. 1999. Mother-to-child transmission of HIV-1: The "all mucosal" hypothesis as a predominant mechanism of transmission. *AIDS* 13(9): 1133–1138.

67. Minkoff H, Burns DN, and Landesman S. 1995. The relationship of the duration of ruptured membranes to vertical transmission of the human immunodeficiency virus. *American Journal of Obstetrics and Gynecology* 173(2): 585–589.

68. Duliège A, et al. 1995. Birth order, delivery route, and concordance in the transmission of human immunodeficiency virus type 1 from mothers to twins. *Journal of Pediatrics* 126(4): 625–632.

69. Sperling RS, et al. 1996. Maternal viral load, zidovudine treatment, and the risk of transmission of human immunodeficiency virus type 1 from mother to infant. *New England Journal of Medicine* 335(22): 1621–1629.

70. Thea DM, Steketee RW, and Pliner V. 1997. The effect of maternal viral load on the risk of perinatal transmission of HIV-1. *AIDS* 11(4): 437–444.

71. Mandelbrot L, et al. 1998. Perinatal HIV-1 transmission: Interaction between zidovudine prophylaxis and mode of delivery in the French perinatal cohort. *JAMA* 280(1): 55–60.

72. The European Collaborative Study. 1999. Maternal viral load and vertical transmission of HIV-1: An important factor, but not the only one. *AIDS* 13(11): 1377–1385.

73. Centers for Disease Control and Prevention. 1994. Revised classification system for human immunodeficiency virus infection in children less than 13 years of age. *MMWR* 43(RR-12): 1–10.

74. Centers for Disease Control and Prevention. 1987. Revision of the CDC surveillance case definition for acquired immunodeficiency syndrome. *MMWR* 36(SU01): 1S–15S.

75. Shearer WT, et al. 1997. Viral load and disease progression in infants infected with human immunodeficiency virus type 1. *New England Journal of Medicine* 336(19): 1337–1342.

76. Simonds RJ, et al. 1993. Pneumocystis carinii pneumonia among U.S. children with perinatally acquired HIV infection. *JAMA* 270(4): 470–473.

77. Connor EM, et al. 1994. Reduction of maternal-infant transmission of human immunodeficiency virus type 1 with zidovudine treatment. *New England Journal of Medicine* 331(18): 1173–1180.

78. Simonds RJ, et al. 1998. Impact of zidovudine use on risk and risk factors for perinatal transmission of HIV. *AIDS* 12(3): 301–308.

79. Public Health Service Task Force. 2003. Recommendations for the use of antiretroviral drugs in pregnant HIV-1-infected women for maternal health and interventions to reduce perinatal HIV-1 transmission in the United States. Rockville, Maryland: AIDSinfo, 1–47. Available at www.AIDSinfo.nih.gov.

80. Capparelli EV, et al. 2003. Pharmacokinetics and tolerance of zidovudine in preterm infants. *Journal of Pediatrics* 142(1): 47–52.

81. American Academy of Pediatrics, Committee on Pediatric AIDS. 1997. Evaluation and medical treatment of the HIV-exposed infant. *Pediatrics* 99(6): 909–917.

82. Luzuriaga K, et al. 1997. Combination treatment with zidovudine, didanosine, and nevirapine in infants with human immunodeficiency virus type 1 infection. *New England Journal of Medicine* 336(19): 1343–1349.

83. Luzuriaga K, et al. 2000. Early therapy of vertical human immunodeficiency virus type 1 (HIV-1) infection: Control of viral replication and absence of persistent HIV-1-specific immune response. *Journal of Virology* 74(15): 6984–6991.

84. Rongkavilit C, et al. 2001. Pharmacokinetics of stavudine and didanosine coadministered with nelfinavir in human immunodeficiency virus–exposed neonates. *Antimicrobial Agents and Chemotherapy* 45(12): 3585–3590.

85. The Working Group on Antiretroviral Therapy and Medical Management of HIV-Infected Children. 2003. Guidelines for the use of antiretroviral agents in pediatric HIV infection. Available at www.AIDSinfo.nih.gov.

86. American Academy of Pediatrics, Committee on Pediatric AIDS. 1995. Human milk, breast feeding, and transmission of immunodeficiency virus in the United States. *Pediatrics* 96(5): 977–979.

87. Joint United Nations Programme on HIV/AIDS (UNAIDS). 1999. WHO, UNICEF, UNAIDS statement on current status of WHO/UNAIDS/UNICEF policy guidelines. Geneva, Switzerland: UNAIDS, 1–5. Available at www.unaids.org/publications/documents/mtct/mtctpolicy99.html.

88. Joint United Nations Programme on HIV/AIDS (UNAIDS). 1999. AIDS: 5 years since ICPD. Emerging issues and challenges for women, young people & infants. Geneva, Switzerland: INAIDS. Available at www.unaids.org/publications/documents/human/gender/newsletter.pdf.

89. Centers for Disease Control and Prevention. 1995. 1995 revised guidelines for prophylaxis against *Pneumocystis carinii* pneumonia for children infected or perinatally exposed to human immunodeficiency virus. *MMWR* 44(RR-4): 1–11.

90. Centers for Disease Control and Prevention. 2002. Guidelines for preventing opportunistic infections among HIV-infected persons—2002 Recommendation of the U.S. Public Health Service and the Infectious Diseases Society of America. *MMWR* 51(RR-8): 1–27.

91. American Academy of Pediatrics. 2000. Tuberculosis. In *Red Book: Report of the Committee on Infectious Diseases*, 25th ed., Pickering L, ed. Elk Grove Village, Illinois: American Academy of Pediatrics, 593–613.

92. American Academy of Pediatrics. 2000. Hepatitis A. In *Red Book: Report of the Committee on Infectious Diseases*, 25th ed., Pickering L, ed. Elk Grove Village, Illinois: American Academy of Pediatrics, 280–289.

93. Gelber SE, and Ratner AJ. 2002. Hospital acquired viral pathogens in the neonatal intensive care unit. *Seminars in Perinatology* 26(5): 345–356.

94. Noble RC, et al. 1984. Posttransfusion hepatitis a in a neonatal intensive care unit. *JAMA* 252(19): 2711–2715.

95. Klein BS, et al. 1984. Nosocomial hepatitis A: A multinursery outbreak in Wisconsin. *JAMA* 252(19): 2716–2721.

96. Watson JC, et al. 1993. Vertical transmission of hepatitis A resulting in an outbreak in a neonatal intensive care unit. *Journal of Infectious Diseases* 167(3): 567–571.

97. Rosenblum LS, et al. 1991. Hepatitis A outbreak in a neonatal intensive care unit: Risk factors for transmission and evidence of prolonged viral excretion among preterm infants. *Journal of Infectious Diseases* 164(3): 476–482.

98. Crumpacker CS. 2001. Hepatitis. In *Infectious Diseases of the Fetus and Newborn Infant*, 5th ed., Remington JS, and Klein JO, eds. Philadelphia: WB Saunders, 913–941.

99. Kane MA. 1997. Hepatitis viruses in the neonate. *Clinics in Perinatology* 24(1): 181–191.

100. Mast EE, and Alte MJ. 1999. Viral hepatitis A, B, and C in the newborn infant. *Seminars in Pediatric Infectious Diseases* 10(3): 201–207.

101. Centers for Disease Control and Prevention. 1999. Prevention of hepatitis A through active or passive immunization: Recommendation of the Advisory Committee on Immunization Practices. *MMWR* 48(12): 1–30.

102. American Academy of Pediatrics. 2000. Hepatitis B. In *Red Book: Report of the Committee on Infectious Diseases*, 25th ed., Pickering L, ed. Elk Grove Village, Illinois: American Academy of Pediatrics, 289–302.

103. Duff P. 1998. Hepatitis in pregnancy. *Seminars in Perinatology* 22(4): 277–283.

104. Lee WM. 1997. Hepatitis B virus infection. *New England Journal of Medicine* 337(24): 1733–1745.

105. World Health Organization. 1998 (revised October 2000). Hepatitis B. Fact Sheet WHO/204 1–5. Available at www.who.int/inffs/en/fact204.html.

106. Centers for Disease Control and Prevention. 2003. Hepatitis B Fact Sheet. Available at www.cdc.gov/ncidod/diseases/hepatitis/b/bfact.pdf.

107. Rosh JR, et al. 1994. Fatal fulminant hepatitis B in an infant despite appropriate prophylaxis. *Archives of Pediatric and Adolescent Medicine* 148(12): 1349–1351.

108. Freese D. 1993. Universal prenatal screening for hepatitis B. *Hepatitis B Coalition News* 3(1): 1–3. Available at www.immunize.org/catg.d/p2120.htm.

109. Fenner F. 1999. Candidate viral diseases for elimination or eradication. *MMWR* 48(SU01): 86–90.

110. Losos J. 1999. Report of the Workgroup on Viral Diseases. *MMWR* 48(SU01): 126–137.

111. Centers for Disease Control and Prevention. 2003. Recommended childhood and adolescent immunization schedule. *MMWR* 52(4): Q1–Q4.

112. Losonsky GA, et al. 1999. Hepatitis B vaccination of premature infants: A reassessment of current recommendations for delayed immunization. *Pediatrics* 103(2): e14.

113. Global Programme for Vaccines and Immunizations (GPV) and the Divisions of Child Health and Development (CHD), and Reproductive Health (Technical Support) (RHT), World Health Organization. 1996. Hepatitis B and breastfeeding. Division of Child Health and Development Update 22: 1–5. Available at www.who.int/child-adolescent-health/New_Publications/NUTRITION/updt-22.htm.

114. Centers for Disease Control and Prevention. 1997. Immunization of health-care workers: Recommendations of the Advisory Committee on Immunization (ACIP) and the Hospital Infection Control Practices Advisory Committee (HICPAC). *MMWR* 46(RR-18): 1–44.

115. American Academy of Pediatrics. 2000. Hepatitis C. In *Red Book: Report of the Committee on Infectious Diseases*, 25th ed., Pickering L, ed. Elk Grove Village, Illinois: American Academy of Pediatrics, 302–306.

116. World Health Organization. 1999. Global surveillance and control of hepatitis C. *Journal of Viral Hepatitis* 6(1): 35–47.

117. Centers for Disease Control and Prevention. 1998. Recommendations for prevention and control of hepatitis C virus (HCV) infection and HCV-related chronic disease. *MMWR* 47(RR-19): 1–39.

118. Lam JPH, et al. 1993. Infrequent vertical transmission of hepatitis C. *Journal of Infectious Diseases* 167(3): 572–576.

119. Manzini P, et al. 1995. Human immunodeficiency virus infection as a risk factor for mother-to-child hepatitis C virus transmission: Persistence of anti–hepatitis C virus in children is associated with the mother's immunoblotting pattern. *Hepatology* 21(2): 328–332.

120. Zucotti GV, et al. 1995. Effect of hepatitis C genotype on mother-to-infant transmission of virus. *Journal of Pediatrics* 127(2): 278–280.

121. Zanetti AR, et al. 1995. Mother-to-infant transmission of hepatitis C virus. Lombardy Study Group on Vertical HCV Transmission. *Lancet* 345(8945): 289–291.

122. Paccagnini S, et al. 1995. Perinatal transmission and manifestation of hepatitis C virus infection in a high-risk population. *Pediatric Infectious Disease Journal* 14(3): 195–199.

123. Cilla G, et al. 1992. Maternal-infant transmission of hepatitis C virus infection. *Pediatric Infectious Disease Journal* 11(5): 417.

124. Novati R, et al. 1992. Mother-to-child transmission of hepatitis C virus detected by nested polymerase chain reaction. *Journal of Infectious Diseases* 165(4): 720–723.

125. Gibb DM, et al. 2000. Mother-to-child transmission of hepatitis C virus: Evidence for preventable peripartum transmission. *Lancet* 356(9233): 904–907.

126. Thomas SL, et al. 1998. A review of hepatitis C virus (HCV) vertical transmission: Risk of transmission to infants born to mothers with and without HCV viraemia or human immunodeficiency virus infection. *International Journal of Epidemiology* 27(1): 108–117.

127. Tovo P, et al. 1997. Increased risk of maternal-infant hepatitis C virus transmission for women coinfected with human immunodeficiency virus type 1. *Clinical Infectious Diseases* 25(5): 1121–1124.

128. Tajiri H, et al. 2001. Prospective study of mother-to-infant transmission of hepatitis C virus. *Pediatric Infectious Disease Journal* 20(1): 10–14.

129. Papaevangelou V, et al. 1998. Increased transmission of vertical hepatitis C virus (HCV) infection to human immunodeficiency virus (HIV)-infected infants of HIV- and HCV-coinfected women. *Journal of Infectious Diseases* 178(4): 1047–1052.

130. Kumar RM, and Shahul S. 1998. Role of breast-feeding in transmission of hepatitis C virus to infants of HCV-infected mothers. *Journal of Hepatology* 178(2): 191–197.

131. Resti M, et al. 1998. Mother to child transmission of hepatitis C virus: Prospective study of risk factors and timing of infection in children born to women seronegative for HIV-1. *British Medical Journal* 17(7156): 437–441.

132. European Paediatric Hepatitis C Virus Infection Network, et al. 2000. Persistence rate and progression of vertically acquired hepatitis C infection. *Journal of Infectious Diseases* 181(2): 419–424.

133. Bortolotti F, et al. 1997. Hepatitis C virus infection and related liver disease in children of mothers with antibody to the virus. *Journal of Pediatrics* 130(6): 990–993.

134. Thomas SL, et al. 1997. Use of polymerase chain reaction and antibody tests in the diagnosis of vertically transmitted hepatitis C virus infections. *European Journal of Clinical Microbiology and Infectious Disease* 16(10): 711–719.

135. Dunn DT. 2001. Timing and interpretation of tests for diagnosing perinatally acquired hepatitis C virus infection. *Pediatric Infectious Disease Journal* 20(7): 715–716.

136. National Institutes of Health. 2002. Consensus Development Conference Statement, Management of Hepatitis C: 2002. 1–44. Available at http://consensus.nih.gov/cons/116/Hepc091202.pdf.

137. Centers for Disease Control and Prevention. 2001. Updated U.S. Public Health Service guidelines for the management of occupational exposures to HBV, HCV, and HIV and recommendations for post-exposure prophylaxis. *MMWR* 50(RR-11): 1–52.

138. American Academy of Pediatrics. 2000. Hepatitis D. In *Red Book: Report of the Committee on Infectious Diseases*, 25th ed., Pickering L, ed. Elk Grove Village, Illinois: American Academy of Pediatrics, 306–307.

139. Centers for Disease Control and Prevention. 2003. Hepatitis D (delta) virus modes of transmission. Available at www.cdc.gov/ncidod/diseases/hepatitis/slideset/hep_d/slide_3.htm.

140. American Academy of Pediatrics. 2000. Hepatitis E. In *Red Book: Report of the Committee on Infectious Diseases*, 25th ed., Pickering L, ed. Elk Grove Village, Illinois: American Academy of Pediatrics, 307–308.

141. Scharschmidt BF. 1995. Hepatitis E: A virus in waiting. *Lancet* 346(8974): 519–520.

142. Centers for Disease Control and Prevention. 2003. Hepatitis E—Clinical features. Available at www.cdc.gov/ncidod/diseases/hepatitis/slideset/hep_e/slide_2.htm.

143. Khuroo MS, Kamill S, and Jameel S. 1995. Vertical transmission of hepatitis E virus. *Lancet* 345(8956): 1025–1026.

144. Centers for Disease Control and Prevention. 2003. Prevention and control measures for travelers to HEV-endemic regions. Available at www.cdc.gov/ncidod/diseases/hepatitis/slideset/hep_e/slide_6.htm.

145. Tsarev SA, et al. 1994. Successful passive and active immunization of cynomolgus monkeys against hepatitis E. *Proceedings of the National Academy of Science* 91(21): 10198–10202.

146. Patrick CC. 1998. Hepatitis G virus. *Pediatric Infectious Disease Journal* 17(11): 1045–1046.

147. Kew MC, and Kassianides C. 1996. HGV: Hepatitis G virus or harmless G virus? *Lancet* 348(supplement 2): S10.

148. Linnen J, et al. 1996. Molecular cloning and disease association of hepatitis G virus: A transfusion-transmissible agent. *Science* 271(5248): 505–508.

149. Alter HJ. 1996. The cloning and clinical implication of HGV and HGBV-C. *New England Journal of Medicine* 334(23): 1536–1537.

150. American Academy of Pediatrics. 2000. Hepatitis G. In *Red Book: Report of the Committee on Infectious Diseases*, 25th ed., Pickering L, ed. Elk Grove Village, Illinois: American Academy of Pediatrics, 308–309.

151. Feucht H, et al. 1996. Vertical transmission of hepatitis G. *Lancet* 347(9001): 615–616.

152. Miura T, et al. 1998. Mother-to-child transmission of hepatitis G virus. *Pediatrics* 102(5): 1222–1223.

153. Palomba E, Bairo A, and Tovo P-A. 1999. High rate of maternal-infant transmission of hepatitis G virus in HIV-1 and hepatitis C virus–infected women. *Acta Paediatrica Scandinavica* 88(12): 1392–1395.

154. Wejstal R, et al. 1999. Perinatal transmission of hepatitis G virus (GB virus type C) and hepatitis C virus infections—A comparison. *Clinical Infectious Diseases* 28(4): 816–821.

155. Schroter M, et al. 2000. Detection of TT virus DNA and GB virus type C/hepatitis G virus RNA in serum and breast milk: Determination of mother-to-child transmission. Journal of Clinical Microbiology 38(2): 745–747.

156. Woelfe J, et al. 1998. Persistent hepatitis G virus infection after neonatal transfusion. *Journal of Pediatric Gastroenterology and Nutrition* 26(4): 402–407.

157. Moyer MS, and Jenson HB. 2002. Viral hepatitis. In *Pediatric Infectious Diseases, Principles and Practice*, 2nd ed., Jenson HB, and Baltimore RS, eds. Philadelphia: WB Saunders, 943–962.

158. Huang Y, et al. 1998. Association of fungal colonization and invasive disease in very low birth weight infants. *Pediatric Infectious Disease Journal* 17(9): 819–822.

159. Jarvis WR. 1996. The epidemiology of colonization. *Infection Control and Hospital Epidemiology* 17(1): 47–52.

160. American Academy of Pediatrics. 2000. Candidiasis. In *Red Book: Report of the Committee on Infectious Diseases*, 25th ed., Pickering L, ed. Elk Grove Village, Illinois: American Academy of Pediatrics, 198–201.

161. Stoll BJ, et al. 1996. Late-onset sepsis in very low birth weight neonates: A report from the National Institute of Child Health and Human Development Neonatal Research Network. *Journal of Pediatrics* 129(1): 63–71.

162. Rabalis GP, et al. 1996. Invasive candidiasis in infants weighing more than 2,500 grams at birth admitted to a neonatal intensive care unit. *Pediatric Infectious Disease Journal* 15(4): 348–352.

163. Pradeepkumar VK, Rajadurai VS, and Tan KW. 1998. Congenital candidiasis: Varied presentations. *Journal of Perinatology* 18(4): 311–316.

164. MacDonald L, Baker C, and Chenoweth C. 1998. Risk factors for candidemia in a children's hospital. *Clinical Infectious Diseases* 26(3): 642–645.

165. Mullett MD, Cook EF, and Fallagher R. 1998. Nosocomial sepsis in the neonatal intensive care unit. *Journal of Perinatology* 18(2): 112–115.

166. Saiman L, et al. 2001. Risk factor for *Candida* species colonization of neonatal intensive care unit patients. *Pediatric Infectious Disease Journal* 20(12): 1119–1124.

167. Rowen JL, et al. 1995. Invasive fungal dermatitis in the ≤1,000-gram neonate. *Pediatrics* 95(5): 682–687.

168. Bektas S, Goetze B, and Speer CP. 1990. Decreased adherence, chemotaxis and phagocytic activities of neutrophils from preterm neonates. *Acta Paediatrica Scandinavica* 79(11): 1031–1038.

169. Saiman L, et al. 2000. Risk factors for candidemia in neonatal intensive care unit patients. The National Epidemiology of Mycosis Survey study group. *Pediatric Infectious Disease Journal* 19(4): 319–324.

170. Westin WL, Lane AT, and Morelli JG. 1996. Skin diseases in newborns. In *Color Textbook of Pediatric Dermatology*, 2nd ed., Westin WL, Lane AT, and Morelli JG, eds. Philadelphia: Mosby-Year Book, 325–353.

171. Scarella A, et al. 1998. Liposomal amphotericin B treatment for neonatal fungal infections. *Pediatric Infectious Disease Journal* 17(2): 146–148.

172. Centers for Disease Control and Prevention. 2002. Candidiasis: Technical information. National Center for Infectious Disease, Division of Bacterial and Mycotic Diseases. Available at www.cdc.gov/ncidod/dbmd/diseaseinfo.

173. Young TE, and Mangum OB. 2003. *Neofax*, 16th ed. Raleigh, North Carolina: Acorn, 6, 30–33.

174. Driessen M, et al. 1996. Fluconazole vs. amphotericin B for the treatment of neonatal fungal septicemia: A prospective randomized trial. *Pediatric Infectious Disease Journal* 15(12): 1107–1112.

175. Wainer S, et al. 1997. Prospective study of fluconazole therapy in systemic neonatal fungal infection. *Pediatric Infectious Disease Journal* 16(8): 763–767.

176. Zenk KE, Sills JH, and Koeppel RM. 2003. Fluconazole. *Neonatal Medications & Nutrition: A Comprehensive Guide*, 3rd ed. Santa Rosa, California: NICU Ink, 252–253.

177. Kaufman D, et al. 2001. Fluconazole prophylaxis against fungal colonization and infection in preterm infants. *New England Journal of Medicine* 345(23): 1660–1666.

178. Welbel S, et al. 1994. Nosocomial *Malassezia pachydermatis* bloodstream infections in a neonatal intensive care unit. *Pediatric Infectious Disease Journal* 13(2): 104–108.

179. Chang H, et al. 1998. An epidemic of *Malassezia pachydermatis* in an intensive care nursery associated with colonization of health care workers' pet dog. *New England Journal of Medicine* 338(11): 706–711.

180. American Academy of Pediatrics. 2000. Fungal disease. In *Red Book: Report of the Committee on Infectious Diseases*, 25th ed., Pickering L, ed. Elk Grove Village, Illinois: American Academy of Pediatrics, 249–251.

181. Lemming JP. 1995. Neonatal skin as a reservoir of Malassezia species. *Pediatric Infectious Disease Journal* 14(8): 719–721.

182. American Academy of Pediatrics. 2000. *Malassezi furfur* invasive infections. In *Red Book: Report of the Committee on Infectious Diseases*, 25th ed., Pickering L, ed. Elk Grove Village, Illinois: American Academy of Pediatrics, 343.

183. Macon, M, et al. 1986. Methods for optimal recovery of *Malassezia furfur* from blood cultures. *Journal of Clinical Microbiology* 24(5): 696–700.

184. Kim EH, et al. 1993. Adhesion of percutaneously inserted silastic central venous lines to the vein wall associated with *Malassezia furfur* infection. *Journal of Parenteral and Enteral Nutrition* 17(5): 458–460.

185. Azimi PH. 1988. *Malassezia furfur*: A cause of occlusion of percutaneous central catheters in infants in the intensive care nursery. *Pediatric Infectious Disease Journal* 7(2): 100–113.

186. Powell DA, et al. 1984. Broviac-related *Malassezia furfur* sepsis in five infants receiving intravenous fat emulsions. *Journal of Pediatrics* 105(6): 987–990.

187. Weiner GM, et al. 1998. Successful treatment of neonatal arterial thromboses with recombinant tissue plasminogen activator. *Journal of Pediatrics* 133(1): 133–136.

188. Decker MD, and Edwards KM. 1988. Central venous catheter infections. *Pediatric Clinics of North America* 35(3): 579–612.

189. Lacey SR, et al. 1988. Successful treatment of Candida infected caval thrombosis in critically ill infants by low dose streptokinase infusion. *Journal of Pediatric Surgery* 23(12): 1204–1207.

NOTES

Notes

CHAPTER 6

Clinical and Laboratory Evaluation of Neonatal Infection

ELLEN TAPPERO, RNC, MN, NNP

Bacterial infections continue to be responsible for significant mortality and long-term morbidity in newborn infants.[1,2] If not treated in the early phases, bacterial infections in newborns can progress rapidly and can cause devastating consequences or death, even if appropriate antibiotic therapy is started later. Early identification of sepsis and prompt institution of appropriate therapy improve the outcome in neonatal infections. Unfortunately, neonatal infections can be difficult to recognize because the signs of bacterial infections are often nonspecific and may be clinically indistinguishable from those associated with noninfectious conditions. Another obstacle to diagnosing infection in the neonate relates to the large number of predisposing risk factors the newborn possesses. For this reason, many newborns are evaluated for sepsis and started on antibiotics to ensure that the rare case (1–2.5 cases per 1,000 live births) of early-onset bacterial infection is not overlooked.[3]

Despite considerable attention to the challenge over the past two decades, there is still no completely reliable way of rapidly diagnosing neonatal sepsis, making the diagnostic task a constant concern for those caring for newborns. The problem of identifying which newborns to work up and treat for sepsis has led investigators to evaluate many new adjunctive diagnostic tests. Finding the most reliable screening test for sepsis is receiving heightened emphasis as health care providers attempt to decrease the unnecessary use of antibiotics, minimize the development of resistant organisms, and reduce the length of hospital stays and medical costs.

INCIDENCE OF INFECTION

In the neonatal period, sepsis is estimated to affect 1–8 infants per 1,000 live births.[1,4–6] The risk of infection is inversely related to gestational age and birth weight, with infection three to ten times more prevalent in preterm than in term infants.[5,7] In one large study of 7,861 very low birth weight (VLBW) infants (<1,500 gm) by the National Institute of Child Health and Human Development (NICHD) Neonatal Research Network, early-onset sepsis (within 72 hours of age) with positive blood culture was uncommon, occurring at a rate of 19 per 1,000 live births (1.9 percent). Infants

6 Clinical and Laboratory Evaluation of Neonatal Infection

FIGURE 6-1 ♦ Pathways of ascending or intrapartum infections.

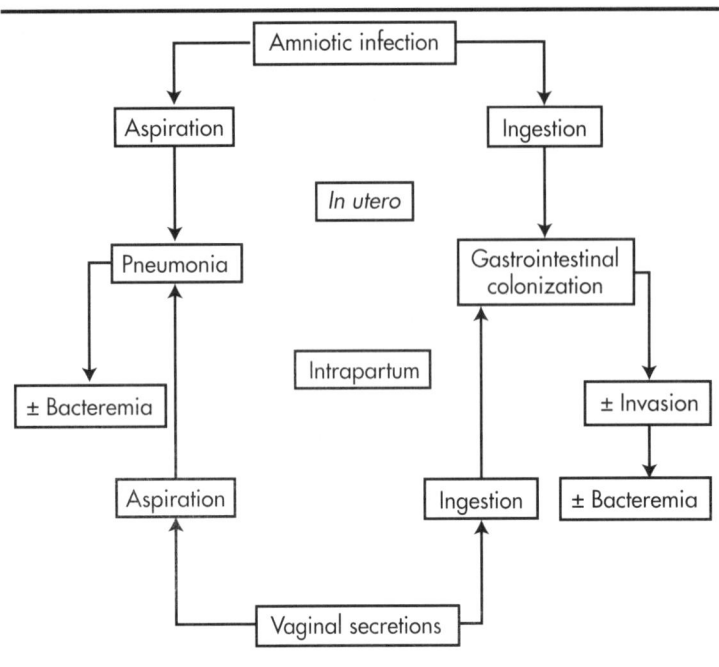

```
                    ┌─── Amniotic infection ───┐
                    ↓                          ↓
                Aspiration                 Ingestion
                    ↓           In utero        ↓
                Pneumonia                 Gastrointestinal
                    ↓                      colonization
                    ↓        Intrapartum        ↓
                ± Bacteremia               ± Invasion
                    ↑                          ↓
                Aspiration   Ingestion    ± Bacteremia
                    ↑            ↑
                    └─ Vaginal secretions ─┘
```

From: Stoll BJ. 2004. Infections of the neonatal infant. In *Nelson Textbook of Pediatrics*, 17th ed., Behrman RE, Kliegman RM, and Jenson HB, eds. Philadelphia: WB Saunders, 625. Reprinted by permission.

with clinical sepsis but negative blood cultures in this same VLBW group were estimated at an additional 47 percent.[1]

Technological advances in neonatal intensive care over the past few decades have permitted the survival of a population of VLBW infants who would not have lived in the past. Very low birthweight infants require prolonged hospitalization, increasing the risk for late-onset sepsis (occurring at >72 hours of age). Late-onset sepsis rates range from 10 to 32 percent, with the incidence increasing with lower gestational age and length of hospitalization.[7,8] In a recent study done by the NICHD Neonatal Research Network looking at the incidence of late-onset sepsis (occurring after three days of age) in VLBW infants, of the 6,215 infants who survived beyond three days, 21 percent had one or more episodes of blood culture–proven late-onset sepsis.[8]

Incidence rates vary from nursery to nursery and depend on the presence of conditions that predispose infants to bacterial infections.

Transmission of Infection

Sepsis in the newborn period may have been acquired prenatally across the placenta from the maternal bloodstream, or the infant may have been infected during labor. Transplacental transmission may occur at different times during gestation, with signs of sepsis present at birth or delayed for months or years. The most common transplacentally passed pathogens include viruses and the bacteria *Treponema pallidum* (syphilis) and *Listeria monocytogenes*. (For more information on intrauterine infections, see Chapter 3.)

Vertical transmission of infection from mother to infant may take place *in utero*, just before delivery, or during delivery (Figure 6-1). Neonatal bacterial infection usually follows exposure of the fetus to organisms colonizing the maternal genital tract. Ascending intra-amniotic infection followed by aspiration or inhalation of infected amniotic fluid can result in pneumonia or systemic neonatal infection, especially with rupture of amniotic membranes longer than 18 hours.

Neonatal infection acquired during vaginal delivery is also usually from bacteria colonizing the mother's genital tract (see Figure 6-1). Group B streptococci, *Escherichia coli* and other Gram-negative rods, *Haemophilus influenzae*, *L. monocytogenes*, and Enterococcus are the microorganisms predominately responsible for early-onset sepsis in the newborn.[1,3,5,9]

TABLE 6-1 ◆ Maternal Risk Factors for Early-Onset Sepsis in the Newborn

Maternal age <20 years
Elevated maternal white cell count or left shift
Prolonged duration of intrauterine monitoring
Previous stillbirth or spontaneous abortion
Group B streptococcal bacteriuria during pregnancy
Amnionitis and maternal fever
Fetal distress or neonatal depression
Premature rupture of membranes
Premature delivery
Low birth weight

Adapted from: Freij BJ, and McCracken GH. 1999. Acute infections. In *Neonatology: Pathophysiology and Management of the Newborn,* 5th ed., Avery GB, Fletcher MA, and MacDonald MG, eds. Philadelphia: Lippincott Williams & Wilkins, 1189–1230; and Schuchat A, Zywicki SS, and Dinsmoor MJ. 2000. Risk factors and opportunities for prevention of early-onset neonatal sepsis: A multicenter case-control study. *Pediatrics* 105(1): 21–26.

Finally, infants can be infected in the nursery. Neonatal infections presenting after three to four days of age are described as late-onset, or nosocomial, infections. They occur commonly in VLBW, chronically hospitalized neonates who require invasive procedures for monitoring and support. These infections are most frequently seen in infants receiving long-term parenteral nutrition who have foreign bodies such as central lines, chest tubes, and ventriculoperitoneal shunts placed for long periods of time.

Many of these late-onset infections are caused by the same organisms seen in early-onset sepsis. In addition, numerous late-onset infections are caused by organisms that colonize the infant in the postnatal environment. Coagulase-negative Staphylococcus has emerged as the predominant neonatal pathogen causing late-onset sepsis in low birth weight infants.[8,10] Candida species, *E. coli, Klebsiella pneumoniae,* Enterococcus, and *Pseudomonas aeruginosa* are other commonly isolated pathogens.[5,7,8,11]

PREDISPOSING FACTORS FOR INFECTION

Although multiple factors have been associated with an increased risk of bacterial infections, the most important are maternal medical conditions that may predispose the fetus/infant to infection; neonatal risks factors, especially those associated with prematurity; and the nursery environment itself.

Maternal

The outcomes of fetuses and newborn infants are linked to maternal complications. Maternal fever, urinary tract infection at the time of delivery, peripartum infection, and genital bacterial colonization expose the fetus to pathogenic microorganisms and probably contribute to the initiation of preterm labor. Chorioamnionitis and prolonged and/or premature rupture of membranes (PROM) are key risk factors for neonatal sepsis.[7,12–14] The incidence of PROM is reported to be between 4 and 7 percent of all deliveries. The incidence of prolonged PROM is 1 percent of all deliveries and is associated with approximately 30 percent of all preterm births.[12,15] Maternal malnutrition, recently acquired sexually transmitted diseases, low socioeconomic status, no prenatal care, and substance abuse are also associated with prematurity and low birth weight, both of which predispose the newborn to infection.[16] Difficult or traumatic delivery and the use of invasive monitoring devices such as fetal scalp electrodes are associated with an increased frequency of neonatal infections in both term and preterm newborns.[7] Table 6-1 summarizes maternal risk factors for early-onset neonatal infections.

Neonatal

There are many neonatal risk factors for the development of infection. The most common are perinatal asphyxia, multiple births, observable congenital anomalies, and prematurity. Although no significant gender difference has

TABLE 6-2 ♦ Deficiencies in Neonatal Host Defenses That Predispose Infants to Infection

Anatomic Barriers
  Injuries during delivery (e.g., skin abrasions)
  Invasive procedures in the nursery (e.g., umbilical artery catheters, endotracheal tubes)

Phagocytic Cells
  Small polymorphonuclear leukocyte storage pool
  Decreased polymorphonuclear leukocyte adherence
  Decreased polymorphonuclear leukocyte and monocyte chemotaxis
  Decreased polymorphonuclear leukocyte intracellular killing in stressed neonates
  Decreased phagocytosis in stressed neonates

Complement
  Decreased levels of complement
  Decreased expression of complement receptors

Cellular Immunity
  Possible defects in T-cell immunoregulation

Humoral Immunity
  Decreased IgA, IgM
  Decreased IgG in premature neonates
  Impaired antibody function
  Decreased levels of fibronectin
  Decreased levels of cytokine (e.g., interferon-γ, tumor necrosis factor)

From: Bellanti JA, Zeligs BJ, and Pung Y. 1999. Immunology of the fetus and newborn. In *Neonatology: Pathophysiology and Management of the Newborn,* 5th ed., Avery GB, Fletcher MA, and MacDonald MG, eds. Philadelphia: Lippincott Williams & Wilkins, 1095. Reprinted by permission.

been documented for infections acquired *in utero,* males have a twofold higher incidence of neonatal sepsis than females. The explanation for this is not clear, but it is thought to be related to X-linked immunoregulatory genes.[7,16]

Identified abnormalities in nearly every aspect of the neonatal immune system make it anatomically competent yet inexperienced and functionally deficient. Table 6-2 summarizes deficiencies in the neonatal host defenses that may predispose newborns to infection. Other conditions predisposing neonates to acquired infection include metabolic disorders such as galactosemia; congenital or acquired immunodeficiency; loss of skin or mucosal integrity (as, for example, in epidermolysis bullosa); and neurologic impairment, which can lead to aspiration.[13,16]

Nursery Environment

Newborns can encounter microorganisms that cause nosocomial (hospital-acquired) infections in the delivery room, in the newborn nursery, or in the NICU. These microorganisms can be transmitted to infants through direct contact with an infected person (mother, visitors, hospital personnel), through indirect contact with contaminated equipment (resuscitation equipment, ventilator circuits), and through the use of contaminated products (intravenous fluids, lipid emulsions, blood). Transmission of microorganisms and yeast on the hands of hospital personnel is the most common mode of infection transmission in nurseries.[17] Colonization of an infant's skin, umbilicus, mucous membranes, and gastrointestinal tract by pathogenic microorganisms or fungi is a common prerequisite for later development of nosocomial infections. Widespread use of antibiotics in the nursery interferes with colonization by normal flora and is believed to be another contributing factor to colonization by and overgrowth of virulent organisms in the newborn.[14] The longer the hospital stay, the greater the infant's chances of acquiring a nosocomial infection as a result of invasive procedures, exposure to pathogens, and widespread antibiotic therapy.

CLINICAL PRESENTATION

Most infants with neonatal sepsis present with signs and symptoms that are subtle and nonspecific, particularly in the early stages of infection, when prompt initiation of antibiotic therapy can be most beneficial. Fetal distress (including fetal tachycardia) suggests the existence of infection contracted *in utero.* Infected newborns frequently display signs that are common to a variety of newborn disorders, making the specific diagnosis of neonatal sepsis extremely difficult. Essentially, the key to recognizing signs of sepsis is noting a change from what is "expected" or what is "normal."

The most common of the vague signs of sepsis are temperature instability, poor feeding, abdominal distention, alterations in behavior, and apnea. Table 6-3 lists symptoms that occur in the newborn with an infection. Clinical manifestations of sepsis in VLBW infants include apnea (55 percent), feeding intolerance, abdominal distention or guaiac-positive stools (43 percent), increased need for respiratory support (29 percent), as well as hypotonia (23 percent).[18] Late (and frequently more ominous) signs are those indicative of septic shock and cardiovascular dysfunction. They include tachycardia, poor perfusion, oliguria, and systemic hypotension.

Sepsis should be considered in the differential diagnosis of any neonate who is not "acting normal." A clinical diagnosis of sepsis should carry greater weight than any diagnostic laboratory test for sepsis, such as the white blood cell (WBC) count or serum C-reactive protein (CRP), because no test has 100 percent sensitivity. There is no substitute for the health care provider's clinical assessment skills because prompt recognition and treatment of sepsis are crucial in minimizing the long-term sequelae.

DIAGNOSIS

Although it is tempting to recommend a workup for sepsis in all infants with nonspecific clinical findings, this is unnecessary and in many cases impractical. The diagnosis of bacterial infection requires an integrated assessment and evaluation of the clinical signs and symptoms, trends in vital signs, laboratory information obtained from a variety of diagnostic tests, and history, including maternal history and relevant recent nursery history. When infection is suspected, a diagnostic evaluation that includes a complete blood cell (CBC) count with differential and platelet count, chest x-ray, and cultures should be conducted.[19,20] The main objective is to rule out infection in the majority of newborns and discontinue antibiotic therapy as soon as is safely possible.

Characteristics of Laboratory Tests

The ideal laboratory test should have maximum sensitivity and maximum negative predictive accuracy. See Table 6-4 for terms used to describe accuracy and reliability of laboratory

TABLE 6-3 ◆ Signs and Symptoms of Neonatal Sepsis

Clinical

General: poor feeding, irritability, lethargy, temperature instability

Respiratory: grunting, nasal flaring, intercostal retractions, tachypnea/apnea

Central nervous system: hypotonia, seizures, poor spontaneous movement

Skin: petechiae, pustulosis, sclerema, edema, jaundice

Gastrointestinal: diarrhea, hematochezia, abdominal distention, emesis, aspirates

Circulatory: bradycardia/tachycardia, hypotension, cyanosis, decreased perfusion

Laboratory

WBC count <5,000/mm^3 or >30,000/mm^3

I:T neutrophil ratio ≥0.2

Thrombocytopenia

Bacteria and leukocytes in gastric aspirate smear

Hypoglycemia

Hyponatremia

Hypocalcemia

Detection of bacterial antigen in CSF, blood, or urine (counterimmunoelectrophoresis or latex agglutination)

Changes in acute-phase reactant rates

Increase: erythrocyte sedimentation rate, C-reactive protein, haptoglobin, orosomucoid

Decrease: prealbumin, transferrin

Hyperbilirubinemia (direct)

Metabolic acidosis

Adapted from: Lott JW, and Kilb JR. 1992. The selection of antibacterial agents for treatment of neonatal sepsis, or which drug kills which bug? *Neonatal Pharmacology Quarterly* 1(1): 19–29. Reprinted by permission.

6 Clinical and Laboratory Evaluation of Neonatal Infection

TABLE 6-4 ◆ Terms Used to Describe Accuracy and Reliability of Laboratory Tests

Term	Definition
Sensitivity	The ability of a test to correctly identify those infants who truly are infected; the percentage of patients with infection who have an abnormal test
Specificity	The ability of a test to correctly identify those infants who do not have infections; the percentage of patients without infection who have a normal test
Positive predictive value (PPV)	The percentage of positive tests that are true-positive (i.e., the infant has an infection); if the test is abnormal (positive), the percentage of infants with infection
Negative predictive value (NPV)	The percentage of negative tests that are true-negative (i.e., the infant does not have sepsis); if the test is normal, the percentage of infants with no infection

Adapted from: Pincus MR. 1996. Interpreting laboratory results: Reference values and decision making. In *Clinical Diagnosis and Management by Laboratory Methods*, 19th ed., Henry JB, ed. Philadelphia: WB Saunders, 76–77; and Weinberg GA, and Powell KR. 2001. Laboratory aids for diagnosis of neonatal sepsis. In *Infectious Diseases of the Fetus and Newborn Infant*, 5th ed., Remington J, and Klein J, eds. Philadelphia: WB Saunders, 1327–1344.

tests. Health care providers want assurance that abnormal test results are reliable and accurate (high sensitivity) and that a normal test completely excludes sepsis (100 percent negative predictive value). The loss of specificity and positive predictive value is considered acceptable because the risks of unwarranted treatment with antibiotics are less than the risks of missing an infected newborn.

Evaluating diagnostic tests, or combinations of them, involves determining their validity in clinical situations. The clinical value of a test is related to its sensitivity and its specificity in the patient population being tested. Sensitivity and specificity do not change with different populations of sick and healthy patients. The predictive value of the same test can vary with age, gender, and geographic location.

Cultures

The isolation of organisms from blood or other normally sterile body fluids drawn using aseptic technique has traditionally been considered the "gold standard" for the diagnosis of sepsis or meningitis in the newborn.[3,16,21] However, systemic cultures of normally sterile body fluids are not always reliable, and the sensitivity of the culture methods is sometimes low.[3,14,22] The concentration of bacteria in the blood can be highly variable in an infected newborn infant. Therefore, the amount of blood drawn seems to be critical, with 1–2 ml of blood required for optimal results.[23,24]

Another concern regarding blood cultures is the incubation time required to detect positive culture results. Improved culture media and integration of new technology into blood culture systems could shorten the incubation time required to detect positive blood culture results. This, in turn, would change the duration of antibiotic therapy in the management of the newborn suspected of having sepsis. A recent study by Garcia-Prats and associates addressed this issue. Using a computer-assisted automated blood culture system, they obtained 455 positive blood culture results from 222 patients. Gram-positive organisms accounted for 80 percent of the positive culture results; Gram-negative organisms, for 11 percent; and yeast, for 9 percent. All cultures growing clinically significant Gram-positive and Gram-negative organisms were positive by 24 to 36 hours of incubation. Of the cultures growing yeast, 88 percent were positive by 48 hours of incubation. Prenatally administered antibiotics did not affect the time to positivity in positive blood cultures drawn on the first day of life. Although further research is needed, this study proposes the idea of reducing the duration of antibiotic therapy to 24 to 36 hours in the term, asymptomatic newborn undergoing evaluation for suspected sepsis as the result of maternal indications, rather than using the traditional 48 to 72 hours of therapy.[25]

Blood cultures from umbilical vessels have not been used extensively because of the high incidence of positive results when the outcomes of cultures of peripherally obtained cultures are negative. However, it is possible that reliable information can be elicited if the blood is drawn using fastidious technique from the umbilical artery and the infant is very young (<9 hours old) and therefore not colonized. Results of blood cultures from umbilical catheters in older infants, Broviac catheters, or peripheral central venous lines may also provide ambiguous outcomes. Ambiguities in interpretation of results can be avoided by securing blood samples for culture from both a peripheral vein and through the catheter.[6]

Performing a lumbar puncture as a routine part of a sepsis workup for early-onset sepsis has been a topic of much debate. An examination of cerebrospinal fluid (CSF) should be performed when there is a high degree of suspicion of infection based on clinical findings. Such signs include positive blood culture, hypotension, neutropenia, persistent metabolic acidosis, and neurologic signs.[3,5] (See Appendix A for more information on CSF values.) Studies have suggested that the chance of recovering an organism from the CSF of an asymptomatic infant or one presenting with respiratory distress who is being evaluated because of maternal risk factors is low.[26,27]

When sepsis presents in a newborn >72 hours of age, a urine culture should be obtained in a sterile manner by catheterization or suprapubic bladder aspiration. A bacteria count of >50,000–100,000 organisms per milliliter suggests infection.[28] Urine cultures are infrequently positive in infants <72 hours of age; the incidence of positive urine cultures in that population is as low as 1.6 percent.[3,16]

Culture and Gram's stain of surface swabs, and of nasopharyngeal and gastric aspirates, are sometimes obtained when sepsis is suspected. The isolation of pathogens from these areas indicates colonization, but is not predictive of bloodstream infection and should not influence the decision to use or not use antibiotics.[14] The sensitivity of these tests has been found to be <50 percent in predicting the organism causing sepsis; they therefore have little diagnostic value.[29] Other tests used to identify microorganisms—such as analysis of DNA, polymerase chain reaction (PCR) testing, and latex agglutination—are discussed in Chapters 1 and 3.

WBC and Differential Count Evaluation

The white blood cell count, also called the leukocyte count, and differential are frequently used in assessing neonatal sepsis. These tests are nonspecific, with both low sensitivity and low specificity for infection, but can be useful as long as their limitations are understood. There is the potential for error in interpreting the WBC evaluation. Nucleated red cells, clumps of platelets, large platelets, and unlysed red cells may all lead to false elevations in the WBC count. Because these cells are all similar in size to a WBC, they may be counted by the automated analyzer as WBCs.

The sampling site must also be taken into consideration when evaluating the WBC count. A capillary sample is the most common. When peripheral venous and arterial samples are compared to capillary, the venous samples have an 82 percent correlation, and the arterial samples have a 77 percent correlation with the capillary sample results.[30]

The differential white cell count involves the counting and categorizing of 100 WBCs based on their morphology. The results are expressed as a percentage. The WBCs are

6 CLINICAL AND LABORATORY EVALUATION OF NEONATAL INFECTION

TABLE 6-5 ◆ Reference Ranges for Neutrophil Indices in the Neonate

Index (per mm^3)	Age (hours)					
	Birth	12	24	48	72	≥120
ANC	1,800–5,400	7,800–14,400	7,200–12,600	4,200–9,000	1,800–7,000	1,800–5,400
INC	≤1,120	≤1,440	≤1,280	<800	<500	<500
I:T	<0.16	<0.16	<0.13	<0.13	<0.13	<0.12

ANC = absolute neutrophil count (mature and immature forms).
INC = immature neutrophil count (all neutrophils except segmented ones).
I:T = immature-to-total ratio (INC divided by ANC).

From: Edwards MS. 2002. Postnatal bacterial infections. In *Neonatal-Perinatal Medicine: Diseases of the Fetus and Infant*, 7th ed., Fanaroff AA, and Martin RJ, eds. Philadelphia: Mosby-Year Book, 710. Reprinted by permission. Originally adapted from: Manroe BL, et al. 1979. The neonatal blood count in health and disease. Part 1: Reference values for neutrophilic cells. *Journal of Pediatrics* 95(1): 89. Reprinted by permission.

divided into five cell types: neutrophils (divided further into mature and immature categories), lymphocytes, monocytes, eosinophils, and basophils. Manual differentials are also subject to potential errors because of interreader differences, limiting the usefulness of the leukocyte evaluation in actual clinical practice.[31]

Diagnostic decisions cannot be made solely on the findings of the WBC and differential, but the results of these evaluations should be considered in concert with the maternal history and the newborn's clinical presentation. Evaluation of the WBC count is important because the WBCs are the first cells to reach the site of infection. Although the WBC count itself is not indicative of infection, when combined with other indices, it can prove useful in predicting possible sepsis. Because of the neonate's immature immune system, the neonatal inflammatory response is not as efficient as that of the adult. This is particularly true of the WBC and neutrophil responses. The WBC and differential counts may be influenced by such factors as the newborn's age, maternal hypertension, severe asphyxia, periventricular hemorrhage, maternal fever, hemolytic disease, pneumothorax, and high altitude.[14,16,32–34]

The least helpful value is the total leukocyte count. This is normal in more than one-third of infants subsequently proved to have bacterial sepsis, particularly during the first several hours of early-onset sepsis.[22,29] Among infants whose total WBC counts are abnormal (<5,000/mm^3 or >30,000/mm^3), fewer than 50 percent are subsequently proved to be infected.[28,29] Although the total leukocyte number alone may not be helpful, a differential count that identifies the variety and number of all forms of WBCs may be helpful in evaluating for sepsis. Manroe and colleagues suggest the usefulness in calculating the absolute neutrophil count (ANC), the total immature neutrophil count (INC), and the immature-to-total (I:T) neutrophil ratio in diagnosing neonatal infections.[35] Table 6-5 presents Manroe and colleagues' reference ranges for these calculations. Also see Appendices A, B, and C for normal newborn laboratory values, normal WBC values, and neutrophil counts in newborns.

Neutrophils are the most prevalent type of WBCs in the neonate. The stages of neutrophil development from immature to mature are: myeloblast→promyelocyte→myelocyte→metamyelocyte→band→polymorphonuclear neutrophil (PMN). PMNs, also called polys or segs, are mature neutrophils and are always present in the blood of normal neonates. The bands and the metamyelocytes, less mature than the PMNs, may also be seen in the blood. The most immature neutrophils, the promyelocytes and myelocytes, reside in the bone marrow and are not normally seen in the blood. All stages of developing neutrophils exist in the marrow and are referred to as the neutrophil storage pool. Release of neutrophils from the bone marrow storage pool in response to infection usually results in an increased proportion of immature neutrophils in the blood, as well as an increased total neutrophil count. When there are more neutrophils than normal in the blood (a high total neutrophil count), neutrophilia exists. Less common in neonates than in adults, neutrophilia is also associated with asymptomatic hypoglycemia, use of oxytocin during labor, and meconium aspiration.[28]

During the first few days of life, when the neutrophil counts are normally rising, a low neutrophil count may be indicative of bacterial infection. Neutropenia, a low neutrophil concentration, may result from depletion of the neutrophil storage pool faster than it can be replenished. Neutropenia has been found to be a more accurate predictor of infection in the newborn than neutrophilia. In one study, neutropenia was seen in 77 percent of cases with confirmed or suspected sepsis and in only 23 percent of noninfected infants.[35] Asphyxia, maternal hypertension, intrauterine growth restriction, and prematurity have also been associated with persistent neutropenia after birth.[7,28,33]

During bacterial infection, increasing numbers of neutrophils from the neutrophil storage pool leave the marrow and enter the circulating blood. Initially, PMNs leave the marrow, but as the infection progresses and the demand for neutrophils increases, more immature neutrophils (bands and metamyelocytes) are released into the blood in large numbers. This "left shift" reflects the increasing concentration of immature as opposed to mature neutrophils in the blood. The I:T ratio is frequently used as an index of the left shift in neonates, although other methods of measuring this shift include the ratio of bands to segmented forms (B:S ratio), the ratio of immature to segmented (mature) neutrophils (I:M ratio), and the ratio of band forms to the total neutrophil count. The I:T ratio has a sensitivity of about 90 percent and a specificity of about 80 percent for early-onset sepsis. A number of cases of sepsis will be missed, however, if the I:T ratio is used as the only indicator of infection, and it does not seem to be as reliable an indicator for late-onset as it is for early-onset sepsis. Because most newborns will have an elevated I:T ratio at some time during an infection, repeat normal I:T ratios are reassuring. Serial CBCs have been shown to enhance the value of the WBC tests as a screen for sepsis.[36] Appendix G explains how to calculate the ratios just discussed, which can be used to evaluate the results of the WBC count.

When sepsis is present, there may also be morphologic changes in the neutrophils, such as vacuoles (visible openings), presence of toxic granules (larger-than-normal granules that stain intensely), and Dohle bodies in bacterial infections.[21,29,32] These changes are nonspecific, but have been found in 63 percent of smears from infants with confirmed sepsis and in 49 percent of smears from infants with suspected sepsis.[35]

Platelet Count

The platelet count in neonates, regardless of gestational age and birthweight, is rarely less than 100,000/mm^3 in the first ten days of life or less than 150,000/mm^3 in the next three weeks.[37] (See the chart of normal newborn values in Appendix A.) Platelet counts under 150,000/mm^3 are considered thrombocytopenic. If at any time the platelet count falls below 100,000/mm^3, the cause of the thrombocytopenia should be investigated.[13,22] Thrombocytopenia is associated with a wide variety of bacterial and viral infections. A reduction in the number of circulating platelets is an insensitive, nonspecific, and rather late indicator of serious bacterial infection. Neonates with proved bacterial sepsis or meningitis display platelet counts <100,000/mm³ in only 10–60 percent of cases.[22] Many infants with fungal infections develop low platelet counts. Therefore, fungal infections should be considered in infants who develop thrombocytopenia.[22,29] Although low platelet counts may be seen before clinical signs of sepsis are present, values may remain normal until after serious illness is present. An elevated platelet count (up to three times the normal limit) may precede or follow an infection.[22,38]

Screening Panels

Screening panels have also been used as diagnostic tools for sepsis. Rodwell and associates developed a seven-point scoring system based on white blood cell count, total and immature neutrophil counts and ratios, changes in neutrophil morphology, and thrombocytopenia to assess infants with suspected sepsis. They found that if three or more of those parameters were abnormal, their approach had 96 percent sensitivity and 99 percent negative predictive value.[39] Gerdes and Polin performed two sepsis screens 12–24 hours apart. A positive screen consisted of positive findings in two or more of the following: WBC count, I:T ratio, CRP, microerythrocyte sedimentation rate, and plasma fibronectin. This method identified all infants with sepsis and had a 100 percent sensitivity and negative predictive value.[40]

The use of a scoring system employing multiple parameters increases sensitivity at the cost of lower specificity. The shortcomings of white blood counts as indicators of sepsis (mentioned earlier) and the failure of scoring systems to identify all septic neonates leaves this approach a very useful tool, but not a definitive test for neonatal sepsis. Predicting sepsis from a panel of screening tests has been little better than relying solely on the I:T neutrophil ratio, especially in the first week of life.[37] These panels are meant to augment, not replace, health care providers' clinical assessments.

Adjunctive Tests

Because of the difficulty in differentiating infected from noninfected neonates, interest has been renewed in the use of adjunctive tests, such as acute-phase reactants and cytokines, to assist in the diagnosis of neonatal infection.

Acute-Phase Reactants: C-Reactive Protein

The acute-phase response is the body's reaction to destruction. The inflammation may be secondary to infection or trauma. There are different acute-phase reactants, one of which is C-reactive protein. The methodology for the detection of acute-phase reactants has improved with the development of new automated, quantitative specific immunoassays. Numerous studies have evaluated acute-phase reactants as predictors of neonatal sepsis. Unfortunately, it is not possible to tell whether the elevated levels of acute-phase reactants found in the presence of inflammation result from infection or another cause.

CRP is a rapid, responsive acute-phase reactant synthesized by the liver within 4–6 hours of an inflammatory stimulus, with serum CRP doubling every 8 hours thereafter. CRP peaks at approximately 36–50 hours after inflammation begins and declines rapidly with resolution of inflammation and cellular destruction.[41] CRP values do not seem to be influenced by perinatal asphyxia, hyperbilirubinemia, periventricular hemorrhage, or respiratory distress.[42] False-positive results have been seen with meconium aspiration and pneumothorax.[3]

Normal CRP reference ranges for neonates are <1.6 mg/dl on days 1–2 and <1.0 mg/dl thereafter.[21,33] The serum CRP level is elevated in 50–95 percent of infants with sepsis and necrotizing enterocolitis, but, like many tests for sepsis, the CRP level may be normal in some infants with culture-proved sepsis.[29,37] The sensitivity of CRP elevation in early detection of neonatal sepsis ranges from 47 to 100 percent, and negative predictive values are higher than positive predictive values.[37] The sensitivity of CRP is lower for early-onset (<48 hours) sepsis than for late-onset sepsis.[3] Serial CRP levels improve sensitivity significantly, however, and may be helpful in providing an index for determining the effectiveness of antibiotics and the duration of therapy in those infants with proved sepsis.[3,37,43,44] DaSilva and colleagues reviewed the use of CRP as a tool for diagnosing neonatal sepsis and concluded that it is probably the best available single diagnostic test.[45]

Cytokines

Although cytokines have not been thoroughly investigated in neonates, some researchers feel that measuring cytokines may be helpful in the early diagnosis of neonatal sepsis. Cytokines, such as interleukin-6 (IL-6), are mediators of the immune response to bacterial infections. IL-6, an inflammatory cytokine, plays a critical role in the induction of CRP in the liver. It has been hypothesized that, during bacterial infection, it may be possible to detect these molecules in the blood earlier than the acute-phase reactants. An IL-6 level higher than 100 pg/ml is 100 percent sensitive in predicting sepsis when the level is drawn in the first 12 hours of life. The sensitivity drops to 83 percent when the sample is obtained after 12 hours of age, suggesting a short half-life.[3]

Buck and associates studied IL-6 and CRP in the diagnosis of early-onset sepsis in 222 premature and term infants. Elevated IL-6 concentrations at birth were seen in 73 percent of newborns with positive blood cultures and in 87 percent with clinical sepsis but negative cultures. Seventy-eight percent of newborns without evidence of infection had normal IL-6 levels. When IL-6 and CRP levels were looked at in combination, these researchers reported 100 percent sensitivity for both culture-proved and clinical sepsis.[46]

Panero and colleagues examined IL-6 concentrations on days 1 and 2 of life. They found that, on day 1, IL-6 levels were significantly higher in infected than in healthy neonates but that the levels could not be used to distinguish between proved sepsis and clinical sepsis. IL-6 concentrations were higher in infants with late-onset infection at presentation than in the healthy control group. The levels eventually returned to normal in infants who recovered from infection.[47]

Several studies have reported that combining CRP and IL-6 measures provides more sensitivity than using either marker alone.[48,49] IL-6 is a very early marker of infection, but levels can become normal even if infection continues. The simultaneous determination of CRP can help because the rise in CRP levels occurs 12–48 hours after the onset of infection, at a time when IL-6 levels would have fallen.[22] One study noted that a combined parameter of IL-6 at ≥50 pg/ml and CRP at ≥1.0 mg/dl yielded a sensitivity of 96 percent, a specificity of 74 percent, a positive predictive value of 49 percent, and a negative predictive value of 99 percent.[49] Although more information is needed to determine the role of these tests in diagnosis of early-onset sepsis, when these two markers are combined, the sensitivity becomes 100 percent for infected infants at any postnatal age.[50]

SUMMARY

Accurate diagnosis of neonatal sepsis is difficult because of the imperfect diagnostic sensitivity of independent laboratory tests. Even blood cultures have an unacceptably low sensitivity. In order to treat all newborns who have sepsis while minimizing the unnecessary use of antibiotics in those without infection, neonatal health care providers must consider predisposing factors to infection, history, clinical presentation of the newborn, and laboratory data. Recognition and management of neonatal sepsis require a multidimensional approach for optimal results.

REFERENCES

1. Stoll BJ, et al. 1996. Early-onset sepsis in very low birthweight neonates: A report from the National Institute of Child Health and Human Development Neonatal Research Network. *Journal of Pediatrics* 129(1): 72–80.
2. Msall ME, et al. 1991. Risk factors for major neurodevelopmental impairments and need for special education resources in extremely premature infants. *Journal of Pediatrics* 119(4): 606–614.
3. Kaftan H, and Kinney JS. 1998. Early onset neonatal bacterial infections. *Seminars in Perinatology* 22(1): 15–23.
4. Philip AG. 1994. The changing face of neonatal infection: Experience at a regional medical center. *Pediatric Infectious Disease Journal* 13(12): 1098–1102.
5. Thilo EH, and Rosenberg AA. 1999. The newborn infant. In *Current Pediatric Diagnosis and Treatment*, 14th ed., Hay WW, et al., eds. Stamford, Connecticut: Appleton & Lange, 61–70.
6. Klein JO. 2001. Bacterial sepsis. In *Infectious Diseases of the Fetus and Newborn Infant*, 5th ed., Remington JS, and Klein JO, eds. Philadelphia: WB Saunders, 943–998.
7. Stoll BJ. 2004. Infections of the neonatal infant. In *Nelson Textbook of Pediatrics*, 17th ed., Behrman RE, Kliegman RM, and Jenson HB, eds. Philadelphia: WB Saunders, 623–640.
8. Stoll BJ, et al. 2002. Late-onset sepsis in very low birth weight neonates: The experience of the NICHD Neonatal Research Network. *Pediatrics* 110(2): 285–291.
9. Stoll BJ, et al. 2002. Changes in pathogens causing early-onset sepsis in very-low-birth-weight infants. *New England Journal of Medicine* 347(4): 240–247.
10. Patrick CC. 1990. Coagulase-negative staphylococci: Pathogens with increasing clinical significance. *Journal of Pediatrics* 116(4): 497–507.
11. Baltimore RS. 1998. Neonatal nosocomial infections. *Seminars in Perinatology* 22(1): 25–32.
12. Belady PH, Farkouh LJ, and Gibbs RS. 1997. Intra-amniotic infection and premature rupture of membranes. *Clinics in Perinatology* 24(1): 43–57.
13. Philip AG. 1996. Neonatal infection. In *Neonatology: A Practical Guide*, 4th ed., Philip AG, ed. Philadelphia: WB Saunders, 182–203.
14. Freij BJ, and McCracken GH. 1999. Acute infections. In *Neonatology: Pathophysiology and Management of the Newborn*, 5th ed., Avery GB, Fletcher MA, and MacDonald MG, eds. Philadelphia: Lippincott Williams & Wilkins, 1189–1230.
15. Watts D, et al. 1992. The association of occult amniotic fluid infection with gestational age and neonatal outcome among women in premature labor. *Obstetrics and Gynecology* 79(3): 351–357.
16. Edwards MS. 2002. Postnatal bacterial infections. In *Neonatal-Perinatal Medicine: Diseases of the Fetus and Infant*, 7th ed., Fanaroff AA, and Martin RJ, eds. Philadelphia: Mosby-Year Book, 706–718.
17. Harris JS, and Goldmann DA. 2001. Infections acquired in the nursery: Epidemiology and control. In *Infectious Diseases of the Fetus and Newborn Infant*, 5th ed., Remington JS, and Klein JO, eds. Philadelphia: WB Saunders, 1371–1418.
18. Fanaroff AA, et al. 1998. Incidence, presenting features, risk factors, and significance of late onset septicemia in very low birth weight infants. *Pediatric Infectious Disease Journal* 17(7): 593–598.
19. Lott JW, and Kilb JR. 1992. The selection of antibacterial agents for treatment of neonatal sepsis, or which drug kills which bug? *Neonatal Pharmacology Quarterly* 1(1): 19–29.
20. McCourt M. 1994. At risk for infection: The very-low-birth-weight infant. *Journal of Perinatal and Neonatal Nursing* 7(4): 52–64.
21. Gerdes JS. 1991. Clinicopathologic approach to the diagnosis of neonatal sepsis. *Clinics in Perinatology* 18(2): 361–381.
22. Papoff P. 2000. The use of hematologic data to evaluate infections in neonates. In *Hematologic Problems of the Neonate*, Christensen RD, ed. Philadelphia: WB Saunders, 389–404.
23. Schelonka RL, et al. 1996. Volume of blood required to detect common neonatal pathogens. *Journal of Pediatrics* 129(2): 275–278.
24. Kellogg JA, et al. 1997. Frequency of low level bacteremia in infants from birth to two months of age. *Pediatric Infectious Disease Journal* 16(4): 381–385.
25. Garcia-Prats JA, et al. 2000. Rapid detection of microorganisms in blood cultures of newborn infants utilizing an automated blood culture system. *Pediatrics* 105(3): 523–527.
26. Wiswell TE, et al. 1995. No lumbar puncture in the evaluation for early neonatal sepsis: Will meningitis be missed? *Pediatrics* 95(6): 803–806.
27. Schwersenski J, McIntyre L, and Bauer CR. 1991. Lumbar puncture frequency and cerebrospinal fluid analysis in the neonate. *American Journal of Diseases of Children* 145(1): 54–58.
28. Paxton J. 1999. Neonatal infections. In *Core Curriculum for Neonatal Intensive Care Nursing*, 2nd ed., Deacon J, and O'Neill P, eds. Philadelphia: WB Saunders, 413–441.
29. Isaacs D, and Moxon ER. 1999. *Handbook of Neonatal Infections: A Practical Guide*. London: WB Saunders, 53–75.
30. Shaw N. 2003. Assessment and management of the hematologic system. In *Comprehensive Neonatal Nursing: A Physiologic Approach*, 3rd ed., Kenner C, and Lott J, eds. Philadelphia: WB Saunders, 580–623.
31. Schelonka RL, et al. 1995. Differentiation of segmented and band neutrophils during the early newborn period. *Journal of Pediatrics* 127(2): 298–300.
32. Walters MC, and Abelson HT. 1996. Interpretation of the complete blood count. *Pediatric Clinics of North America* 43(3): 599–622.
33. Horns KM. 2000. Neoteric, physiologic, and immunologic methods for assessing early-onset neonatal sepsis. *Journal of Neonatal and Perinatal Nursing* 13(4): 50–66.
34. Polinski C. 1996. The value of the white blood cell count and differential in the prediction of neonatal sepsis. *Neonatal Network* 15(7): 13–23.
35. Manroe BL, et al. 1979. The neonatal blood count in health and disease. Part 1: Reference values for neutrophilic cells. *Journal of Pediatrics* 95(1): 89–98.
36. Greenberg DN, and Yoder BA. 1990. Changes in the differential white blood cell count in screening for Group B streptococcal sepsis. *Pediatric Infectious Disease Journal* 9(12): 886–889.
37. Weinberg GA, and Powell KR. 2001. Laboratory aids for diagnosis of neonatal sepsis. In *Infectious Diseases of the Fetus and Newborn Infant*, 5th ed., Remington J, and Klein J, eds. Philadelphia: WB Saunders, 1327–1344.
38. Vora AJ, and Lilleyman JS. 1993. Secondary thrombocytosis. *Archives of Disease in Childhood* 68(1): 88–90.
39. Rodwell RL, et al. 1993. Hematologic scoring system in early diagnosis of sepsis in neutropenic newborns. *Pediatric Infectious Disease Journal* 12(5): 372–376.
40. Gerdes JS, and Polin RA. 1987. Sepsis screen in neonates with evaluation of plasma fibronectin. *Pediatric Infectious Disease Journal* 6(5): 443–446.
41. Jaye DL, and Waites KB. 1997. Clinical applications of C-reactive protein in pediatrics. *Pediatric Infectious Disease Journal* 16(8): 735–747.
42. Schouten-Van Meeteren NYN, et al. 1992. Influence of perinatal conditions on C-reactive protein production. *Journal of Pediatrics* 120(4 part 1): 621–624.
43. Ehl S, et al. 1997. C-reactive protein is a useful marker for guiding duration of antibiotic therapy in suspected neonatal bacterial infection. *Pediatrics* 99(2): 216–221.

44. Benitz WE, et al. 1998. Serial serum C-reactive protein levels in the diagnosis of neonatal infection. *Pediatrics* 102(4): e41.
45. DaSilva O, Ohlsson A, and Kenyon C. 1995. Accuracy of leukocyte indices and C-reactive protein for diagnosis of neonatal sepsis: A critical review. *Pediatric Infectious Disease Journal* 14(5): 362–366.
46. Buck C, et al. 1994. Interleukin-6: A sensitive parameter for the early diagnosis of neonatal bacterial infection. *Pediatrics* 93(1): 54–58.
47. Panero A, et al. 1997. Interleukin-6 in neonates with early and late onset infection. *Pediatric Infectious Disease Journal* 16(4): 370–375.
48. Onal EE, et al. 1999. Interleukin-6 concentration in neonatal sepsis. *Lancet* 353(9148): 239–240.
49. Doellner H, et al. 1998. Interleukin-6 concentrations in neonates evaluated for sepsis. *Journal of Pediatrics* 132(2): 295–299.
50. Messer J, et al. 1996. Evaluation of interleukin-6 and soluble receptors of tumor necrosis factor for early diagnosis of neonatal infection. *Journal of Pediatrics* 129(4): 574–580.

NOTES

NOTES

CHAPTER 7

Management of Neonatal Infection, Sepsis, and Complications

CATHERINE WITT, RNC, MS, NNP

The primary principle in management of infections in the newborn is removing or killing the invading microorganism, primarily through antimicrobial therapy. However, management of neonatal infection must also address its effects on the infant and any complications that arise. Collateral care includes respiratory support, correction of acidosis and other metabolic abnormalities, treatment of cardiogenic shock, and perhaps the use of nitric oxide or extracorporeal membrane oxygenation to improve oxygen delivery to the tissues. Each infant's individual signs, symptoms, laboratory findings, and general condition determine the course of treatment.

EVALUATION

Treatment of neonatal infection begins with evaluation of the infant, including risk factors, physical presentation, and laboratory findings. Because newborns present with a narrow range of symptoms for a variety of problems, it can be difficult to determine the cause. For example, respiratory distress has several etiologies, including prematurity, retained lung fluid, air leaks, and pneumonia. The clinician must determine which of the infants showing respiratory distress should be evaluated for infection and placed on antimicrobials. Knowledge of risk factors for infection, the signs and symptoms of sepsis, and experience in caring for newborns allow the practitioner to make appropriate clinical judgments. Because the consequences of untreated sepsis in the newborn are severe, most practitioners agree that it is preferable to err on the side of caution, even if some infants are treated unnecessarily.

When an infant is demonstrating signs and symptoms of infection, a workup for it and the initiation of antimicrobial therapy must be considered. Although it is prudent for clinicians to avoid indiscriminate use of antibiotics that may lead to further development of resistant organisms, the infant who is exhibiting signs and symptoms of infection must be treated promptly. If the blood cultures and/or cerebrospinal fluid (CSF) do not indicate an infection after 48–72 hours, the antimicrobials can be discontinued. When the mother has received antimicrobial agents prior to delivery, they may interfere with the infant's cultures, causing a false-negative culture in an infant who really is infected. Thus, if the mother was

7 MANAGEMENT OF NEONATAL INFECTION, SEPSIS, AND COMPLICATIONS

FIGURE 7-1 ♦ Management of the neonate whose mother received intrapartum antimicrobial prophylaxis (IAP) for prevention of early-onset Group B streptococcal (GBS) disease.

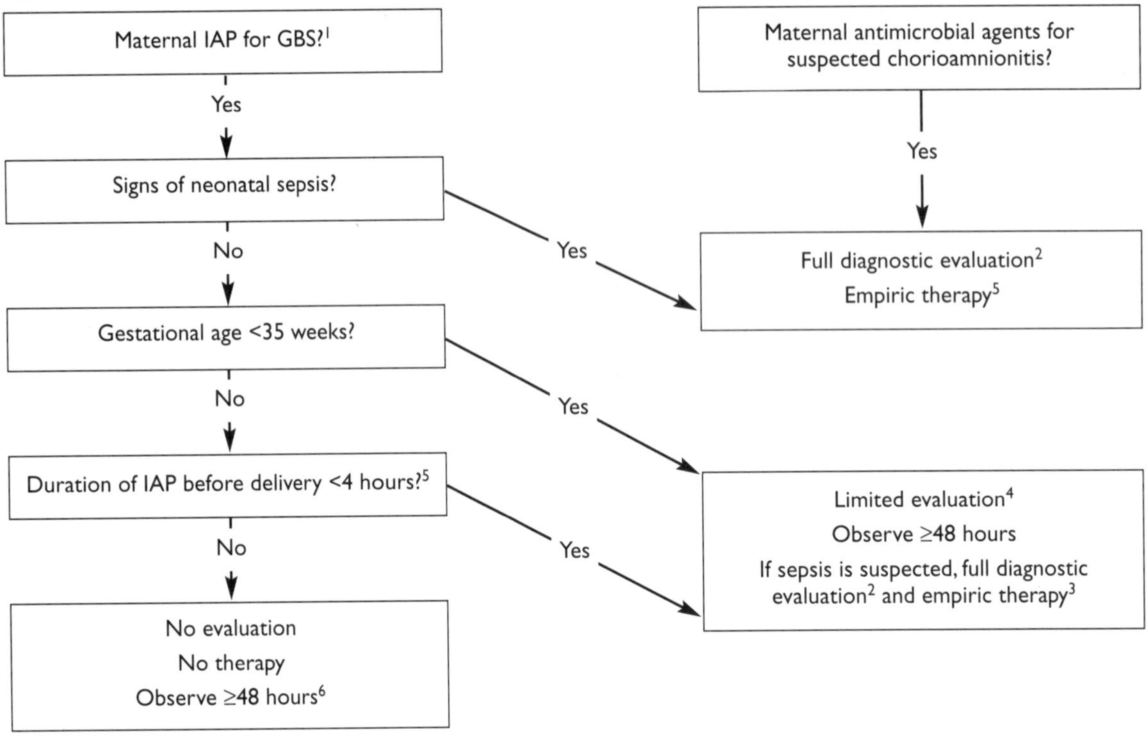

```
Maternal IAP for GBS?[1]                    Maternal antimicrobial agents for
         │                                   suspected chorioamnionitis?
        Yes                                              │
         ▼                                              Yes
Signs of neonatal sepsis? ─────Yes──────┐                │
         │                              ▼                ▼
        No                     Full diagnostic evaluation[2]
         ▼                           Empiric therapy[5]
Gestational age <35 weeks?────Yes──────┐
         │
        No
         ▼
Duration of IAP before delivery <4 hours?[5]            Limited evaluation[4]
         │                                               Observe ≥48 hours
        No                  ────Yes──────▶  If sepsis is suspected, full diagnostic
         ▼                                   evaluation[2] and empiric therapy[3]
    No evaluation
    No therapy
    Observe ≥48 hours[6]
```

[1] If no maternal IAP for GBS was administered despite an indication being present, data are insufficient on which to recommend a single management strategy.

[2] Includes CBC count with differential, blood culture, and chest radiograph if respiratory abnormalities are present. When sighs of sepsis are present, a lumbar puncture, if feasible, should be performed.

[3] Duration of therapy varies depending on results of blood culture, cerebrospinal fluid findings (if obtained), and the clinical course of the infant. If laboratory results and clinical course do not indicate bacterial infection, duration may be as short as 48 hours.

[4] CBC including WBC count with differential and blood culture.

[5] Applies only to penicillin, ampicillin, or cefazolin and assumes recommended dosing regimens.

[6] A healthy-appearing infant who was ≥38 weeks gestation at delivery and whose mother received ≥4 hours of IAP before delivery may be discharged home after 24 hours *if* other discharge criteria have been met and a person able to comply fully with instructions for home observation will be present. If any one of these conditions is not met, the infant should be observed in the hospital for at least 48 hours and until criteria for discharge are achieved.

From: American Academy of Pediatrics. 2003. *Red Book: Report of the Committee on Infectious Diseases,* 26th ed. Elk Grove Village, Illinois: American Academy of Pediatrics, 590. Reprinted by permission.

treated for infection during labor, the newborn's antimicrobial course may need to be extended, despite negative cultures.[1] The decision to treat an asymptomatic infant is more difficult. The likelihood of an asymptomatic infant being infected depends on a variety of risk factors. These include maternal colonization with Group B Streptococcus (GBS), premature or prolonged rupture of membranes, chorioamnionitis, maternal urinary tract infection, maternal temperature elevation, fetal tachycardia, low Apgar score at five minutes, meconium-stained fluid, and preterm delivery. The more risk factors, the higher is the possibility for infection in the newborn.

If the mother was colonized with GBS and was treated with antimicrobial prophylaxis during labor, the infant is greater than 38 weeks, and there are no other risk factors, the American Academy of Pediatrics recommends observation of the infant for 24 hours, with no further workup if the baby remains asymptomatic. The infant may be discharged at 24 hours of age, provided his caretakers understand how to observe for signs and symptoms of infection and are able to communicate any concerns to health care professionals. If the mother was not treated during labor or received fewer than two doses of antimicrobials, the infant should be observed for at least 48 hours in the hospital. When sepsis is suspected, especially in the presence of other risk factors, or when the baby is less than 35 weeks, he should have a full workup and be started on antibiotics.[2] The decision about duration of therapy can be made when laboratory test results are received. Figure 7-1 provides guidelines for evaluating and managing suspected infection in the infant whose mother is colonized with Group B Streptococcus.

TYPES OF INFECTIONS

Respiratory Tract Infections

Pneumonia is often a presentation of neonatal infection, occurring in as many as 10 percent of NICU patients, and is a common cause of mortality in perinatally acquired infections.[3] Group B Streptococcus is usually the cause of perinatally acquired pneumonia. *Escherichia coli*, *Haemophilus influenzae*, Klebsiella, and Enterobacter are also likely causative organisms. Infants in the NICU are at risk for nosocomially or late-onset acquired respiratory infections caused by *Staphylococcus aureus*, Pseudomonas, Klebsiella, or *Serratia marcescens*.[4,5]

Infants are at increased risk for pneumonia for a variety of reasons, including immaturity of the lungs and the immune system, as well as hospitalization. Absence of secretory immunoglobulin A (IgA) during the first few days after birth means that the ability of the mucosa of the respiratory tract to prevent the adherence or entry of bacteria is reduced. Alveolar macrophage activity also appears to be reduced in the neonate because preterm infants and term infants have a decreased number of lung macrophages until 48–72 hours after delivery.[6,7]

Congenital pneumonia is acquired *in utero* or during labor and delivery. It can be acquired transplacentally when bacteria crossing the placenta invade the fetal lungs or as an ascending infection, with bacteria from the vaginal flora contaminating the amniotic fluid or membranes. Fetal asphyxia causing gasping of amniotic fluid introduces the bacteria into the lung.

Aspiration of vaginal bacteria during delivery or colonization of the infant's skin and mucosal surfaces followed by aspiration of oropharyngeal secretions may also lead to pneumonia in the newborn. Onset of infection in these infants may be delayed by several hours or days.

Nosocomial pneumonia is a particular problem for preterm and low birth weight infants, those requiring prolonged hospitalization, and babies requiring mechanical ventilation. Invasive procedures (particularly intubation), poor handwashing by health care personnel, and colonization with atypical flora increase the risk of hospital-acquired pneumonia.[8]

Pathology

Pneumonia is characterized by inflammation of the bronchioli and adjacent alveoli. Vascular congestion, edema, leukocyte infiltration, epithelial damage, and exudate of plasma proteins cause atelectasis and formation of hyaline membranes. Areas of necrosis and multiple small abscesses may be seen in the lungs of infants with pneumonia caused by staphylococci species. In addition, pneumonia is thought to be associated with alterations in surfactant

FIGURE 7-2 ♦ Chest x-ray of infant with pneumonia.

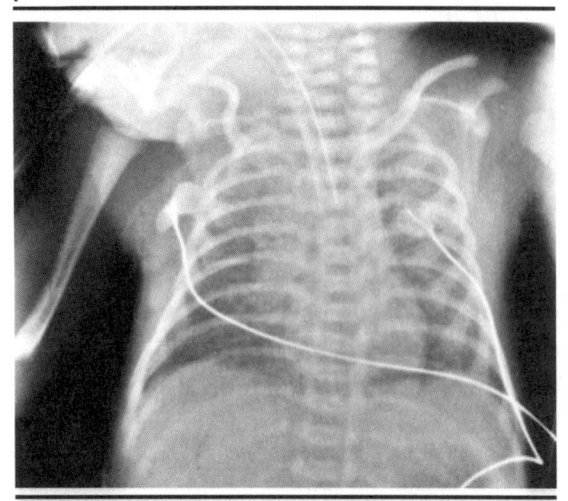

From: Trotter C, and Carey BE. 2000. Radiology basics: Overview and concepts. *Neonatal Network* 19(2): 36. Reprinted by permission.

production and function. Accompanying cardiogenic shock may result in damage to Type II pneumocytes, further decreasing surfactant production.[9] Increased vascular permeability resulting from damage to capillary endothelium leads to interstitial and alveolar edema and hemorrhage. These changes result in a decrease in functional residual capacity and lung compliance, leading to hypoxemia, respiratory acidosis, and, frequently, pulmonary hypertension and pulmonary hemorrhage.

Clinical Manifestations

The presentation of pneumonia is often nonspecific. Infants with early-onset (less than 48 hours after birth) pneumonia frequently have a history of fetal tachycardia, fetal distress, low Apgar scores, and need for resuscitation.[8] Most present with respiratory distress and cyanosis either immediately after birth or within the first few hours following delivery. Apnea and bradycardia in the term infant should alert the practitioner to the possibility of infection, and the infant should be treated accordingly until sepsis is ruled out. Temperature instability, poor perfusion, irritability, lethargy, and poor feeding or feeding intolerance may also be signs of infection. Infants in the NICU with nosocomial pneumonia may present with increased oxygen requirements and need for ventilator support, apnea, bradycardia, temperature instability, and feeding intolerance.

Diagnosis

Chest radiography may be significant for diffuse, homogeneous atelectasis, often similar to what is seen in hyaline membrane disease. Pleural effusions, increased perihilar streaking, or lobular consolidation may also be present (Figure 7-2). Other disease processes, such as hyaline membrane disease, may complicate the practitioner's ability to interpret the findings. A blood culture and complete blood count (CBC) with differential may be helpful in identifying the neonate with pneumonia. A culture and Gram's stain of pulmonary secretions obtained from an endotracheal tube can aid in the identification of pathogens, although initial cultures are frequently negative, even in the presence of clinical disease.[8] Amniotic fluid cultures and placental pathology indicate the presence or absence of chorioamnionitis and may provide clues for possible organisms, but cannot diagnose the presence or absence of the organism in the neonatal lung. Because microbial colonization occurs rapidly after insertion of the tube, cultures not obtained immediately may reflect colonization rather than infection and are difficult to interpret.

Management

In addition to treating the infant with antimicrobials, caregivers need to make ongoing assessments of the infant's need for oxygen and mechanical ventilation, with monitoring of oxygen saturation and arterial blood gases. Disruption of surfactant function and atelectasis interferes with lung expansion, leading to hypoxia and hypercarbia. In addition, increased vascular permeability leads to interstitial edema and further inhibits gas exchange. Keeping the infant well oxygenated and providing appropriate respiratory support are essential to avoid additional complications.

Pulmonary hypertension can occur in response to hypoxia and acidosis. In addition, many infants with congenital pneumonia are depressed at birth, requiring resuscitation and this also places them at higher risk for pulmonary hypertension.[8] Persistent pulmonary hypertension of the newborn (PPHN) is treated primarily with oxygen and mechanical ventilation, with the goal being to increase pulmonary blood flow and decrease right-to-left shunting. Correction of acidosis and maintenance of systemic blood pressure are also critical. Minimizing stimulation and eliminating agitation may prevent transient episodes of hypoxia, which contribute to pulmonary vascular resistance, and sedation and paralysis may be necessary to prevent agitation. Some infants with pulmonary hypertension may respond to respiratory or metabolic alkalosis, which can be induced by hyperventilation or sodium bicarbonate infusion. However, the risks of compromising cerebral blood flow from hyperoxemia and hypocarbia make this approach controversial, and it should be used with caution.

Inhaled nitric oxide has been shown to dilate pulmonary vasculature specifically and has been used with success in some infants with pulmonary hypertension due to pneumonia or other causes.[10-13] Surfactant replacement has also been shown to have some success in limited studies, for treatment of both respiratory distress caused by bacterial pneumonia and pulmonary hemorrhage.[14-18] Extracorporeal membrane oxygenation may be used in infants >34 weeks gestation who do not respond to other means of medical support.[19,20]

Meningitis

Meningitis is an acute inflammation of the membranes lining the brain and spinal column. It is caused by bacterial or viral microorganisms as well as fungi. The incidence of bacterial meningitis is 0.4–1 per 1,000 live births.[4,21] Predisposing factors for meningitis include prematurity, low birth weight, perinatal and intrauterine infections, and prolonged rupture of the membranes. Male infants have a statistically higher risk for infection and meningitis than do females.[22] Neonates may acquire meningitis either transplacentally or by aspiration or inhalation of the microorganisms that cause it. Development of bacteremia gives the microorganisms access to the CSF. Of infants with positive blood cultures, about 25 percent develop meningitis, with a higher incidence in late-onset infections.[4] The most common causative organisms for neonatal meningitis are Group B β-hemolytic Streptococcus, *E. coli*, and *Listeria monocytogenes*.[23,24]

Pathology

Meningitis causes multiple pathologic changes in the neonate, regardless of the causative organism. Most characteristic is a purulent exudate that covers the meninges and the ependymal surfaces of the ventricles. Perivascular inflammation and inflammation of the intracranial vessels can be seen, as can thrombophlebitis, leading to occlusion of veins in the subependymal zone. Inflammation of the ventricles of the brain is also present in about 75 percent of infants with meningitis. Hydrocephalus and noninfectious encephalopathy occur in almost 50 percent of meningitis cases.[25] Subdural effusions are rare in neonates, but occur in 10–20 percent of infants who develop meningitis between 3 and 12 months of age.[25,26]

Clinical Manifestations

Initially, the infant with meningitis presents with signs and symptoms similar to those of any generalized infection. These may include lethargy, poor feeding or feeding intolerance, temperature instability, respiratory distress, and apnea. Greater irritability and signs and symptoms of increased intracranial pressure (bulging fontanel, hypertension, tremors or twitching); seizure activity; persistent, severe vomiting; alterations in consciousness; and diminished muscle tone may be apparent. Seizures occur in 20–50 percent of infants with meningitis and may be more common with Gram-negative bacterial disease.[24]

Diagnosis

The diagnosis of meningitis is based on the presence of clinical signs and symptoms of the disease and confirmed by analysis of CSF, which is difficult in newborns because they tend to have higher limits of normal than do children or adults. Premature infants may have persistent elevated white blood cell (WBC) counts without infection. Abnormal CSF findings include:

- A CSF leukocyte count of ≥32/mm^3, with 60 percent polymorphonucleocytes
- CSF glucose <50–75 percent of serum glucose level
- Protein >100–180 mg/dl[4]
- Presence of microorganisms on Gram's stain smears
- Positive culture

The presence of one or more of these findings may be sufficient to make the diagnosis, although a positive culture is considered the definitive finding.[24,27]

Management

Infants with suspected or confirmed meningitis require aggressive management with antimicrobials, as well as supportive therapy. The selection of appropriate antimicrobial therapy is based on the sensitivity of the causative microorganism to various drugs and on the ability of the drug to achieve adequate CSF levels in relation to serum levels. Ampicillin and an aminoglycoside are recommended for initial therapy of neonatal meningitis, until the specific microorganism is identified. A third-generation cephalosporin may also be considered; they are the drug of choice for Gram-negative bacterial meningitis because their high concentrations in the serum allow achievement of adequate CSF concentrations without dose-related toxicity.[4,24] CSF studies should be repeated 24–48 hours after initiation of therapy; the CSF should be sterile by at least 72 hours. Therapy is usually continued for at least two weeks after a negative culture for Gram-positive microorganisms and for three weeks for Gram-negative microorganisms. Fungal infections may require treatment for as long as six weeks.[26]

In addition to antimicrobial therapy, multisystem supportive therapy is required for the newborn with meningitis. Mechanical ventilation, seizure control, fluid management, cardiopulmonary monitoring, and blood pressure support are frequently needed. Acute observation and monitoring of the infant are essential because infants who become critically ill with meningitis can deteriorate quickly and need rapid interventions. Placement of a percutaneous central venous catheter for parenteral nutrition and extended antimicrobial therapy may be indicated. Families need educational and emotional support during the long-term hospitalizations involved with this infection, particularly if complications develop. Use of corticosteroids to decrease long-term neurologic sequelae has been studied in older infants with some success, but the utility of this therapy in neonates is uncertain.[24,28]

Prognosis

The mortality rate for neonatal meningitis is high, ranging from 10 to 30 percent, depending on the microorganism, the general health of the infant, and the supportive care required.[26] Although the infant may appear healthy at discharge, the morbidity associated with meningitis is significant. Careful developmental follow-up of these patients is essential. Destruction of brain tissue, hemorrhages, and infarcts causing necrosis to vital brain cells may cause extensive brain damage, leading to death or poor neurologic outcomes. Long-term complications of meningitis include perceptual difficulties, reading problems, hearing loss, and mental retardation. It is estimated that 15–50 percent of survivors have some degree of neurologic abnormality.[24,29,30]

Urinary Tract Infections

Neonatal urinary tract infections (UTIs) have an incidence rate of approximately 1 percent in term infants and up to 3 percent in preterm infants.[31] UTIs are more common in male than in female infants during the newborn period (the reverse is true after the newborn period) and in infants born to mothers with UTIs. Bacteriuria may occur as an isolated UTI, or it may be associated with generalized sepsis.

UTIs are most commonly caused by *E. coli*, with other Gram-negative organisms, such as Klebsiella, seen occasionally. Infection with Gram-positive microorganisms, with the exception of enterococci and occasionally GBS, is rare. Because *E. coli* and GBS are both normal bacterial flora in the female genital tract, the neonate is exposed to these potential pathogens during birth. UTIs can be the result of a congenital anomaly that obstructs urine flow, causing urinary stasis and bacterial growth. Vesicoureteral reflux, which provides easy access for bacteria to the kidneys, is an important risk factor. In addition, some studies have suggested that uncircumcised male infants are at slightly higher risk for UTIs than are circumcised males.[32–34] All infants with positive urine cultures should have radiologic evaluation of the urinary tract. A renal ultrasound can be used to rule out congenital anomalies, followed by a voiding cystourethrogram (VCUG) at least two weeks after antimicrobial therapy has been completed.[35]

UTIs may also be caused by iatrogenic factors, such as bacterial invasion secondary to an invasive procedure like a suprapubic bladder tap or a urethral catheter. Iatrogenic complications can be minimized by using good handwashing practices, careful skin preparation, and aseptic technique during invasive procedures.

Neural tube defects like spina bifida and myelomeningocele are often accompanied by a neurogenic bladder. Little or no nerve enervation to the bladder makes it difficult for the organ to move urine into the urinary tract. Urinary flow is impeded, and bacterial growth occurs unchecked, resulting in a UTI.

Clinical Manifestations

Most neonates with UTIs are asymptomatic. When clinical symptoms are seen, they tend to be nonspecific findings, such as temperature instability, failure to thrive or poor weight gain, abdominal distention, hepatomegaly, direct hyperbilirubinemia, intermittent cyanosis, thrombocytopenia purpura, and sometimes proteinuria and hematuria.[25]

Diagnosis

Diagnosis of a UTI is made by examination, Gram's stain, and culture of a urine specimen obtained under sterile conditions. Suprapubic bladder aspiration or sterile bladder catheterization may be used for specimen collection. A culture should not be collected by a urine bag because of the potential for contamination by bacteria on the perineum. The presence of more than 50,000 colony-forming units in a specimen obtained by bladder catheterization confirms a diagnosis. If the urine is obtained by suprapubic bladder tap, any number of bacteria should be considered significant.[36] A Gram's stain of the unspun urine will often provide the identity of the bacteria. If a UTI is suspected, a blood culture should be drawn to determine if neonatal septicemia is also present.

Management

Antimicrobial therapy is started as soon as the presumptive diagnosis of a UTI is made. Initial treatment should include intravenous antimicrobials because septicemia is found in 15–30 percent of UTIs.[26] Oral antimicrobials may be used if intravenous (IV) access becomes a problem during the course of the therapy and there is no accompanying septicemia. A repeat urine culture should be obtained 48–72 hours after initiation of therapy. The repeat culture should be sterile or should show a significant decrease in the amount of bacteria.[25,37]

Broad-spectrum antibiotics, such as ampicillin and gentamicin, may be used pending identification of the organism and sensitivity testing.

Otitis Media

Otitis media, inflammation of the middle ear, is probably a more frequent complication in newborns than diagnosis would indicate. The difficulty of viewing the tympanic membrane in neonates means that its inspection is not a routine part of the newborn exam. Consequently, the incidence of otitis media in the neonate is uncertain. It is estimated to occur in up to 34 percent of term newborns from birth to eight weeks of age.[38] Autopsy reports on infants from NICUs suggest that the incidence of otitis media is significantly higher than that estimate in preterm infants and in those requiring intubation, mechanical ventilation, and continuous positive airway pressure.[26]

Symptoms of otitis media are nonspecific and include irritability, lethargy, fever, cough, diarrhea, vomiting, tachypnea, and anorexia. Associated conjunctivitis is seen in about 50 percent of patients.[26]

Diagnosis of otitis media is made by otoscopic examination of the eardrum. The eardrum appears red and may be bulging. If perforation has occurred, serous drainage may be present. Tympanometry is unreliable because the tympanic membrane tends to appear thicker in the neonate than in older infants and children.

Treatment of otitis media includes the administration of broad-spectrum antibiotics. If the infant does not respond to treatment, tympanocentesis should be considered for culture and sensitivity so that specific antimicrobials can be selected.

Osteomyelitis and Septic Arthritis

Infection of the long bone is referred to as osteomyelitis; infection of the membrane lining the joint (the synovium) is called septic arthritis. These infections may occur separately or in conjunction with one another in the newborn period. The incidence is not known, but both conditions are uncommon, occurring in 1–3 per 1,000 neonates in the NICU.[26]

During the first 12 months after birth, capillaries cross the epiphysial plate of long bones, providing a direct communication between the metaphysis and the joint space. This allows for rapid growth of bone and conversion from cartilage to bone. Consequently, infection from the blood can easily spread to the bone, and infection at one site can readily spread to another. These capillaries disappear at approximately one year of age.

Organisms responsible for osteomyelitis and/or septic arthritis most commonly include GBS, *S. aureus*, and Gram-negative organisms such as Klebsiella and *E. coli*. Pseudomonas, *H. influenzae*, and *Candida albicans* are also associated with these conditions. *S. aureus* is one of the most common organisms because it has collagen-binding receptors that allow it to attach to the cartilage. In addition, it is frequently resistant to common antibiotics such as penicillin.

Infection frequently occurs following a traumatic injury, such as a cephalhematoma, or from invasive procedures, such as heelsticks, venipunctures, umbilical catheterization, and attachment of fetal-monitoring scalp electrodes. Extensions of soft tissue, ear, and sinus infections have also been reported.[39] Premature infants and sick full-term infants are more vulnerable and may have systemic illness, but these infections may occur in older infants, most commonly between two and four weeks of age.[40]

FIGURE 7-3 ◆ X-ray showing soft-tissue edema in 5-week-old, 1,690 gm neonate with osteomyelitis.

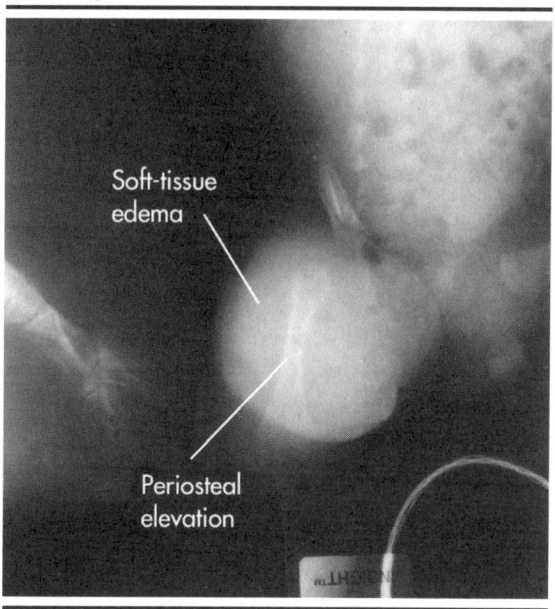

From: McPherson DM. 2002. Osteomyelitis in the neonate. *Neonatal Network* 21(1): 15. Reprinted by permission.

FIGURE 7-4 ◆ Femur x-ray of same infant, now 7 weeks old with bony destruction.

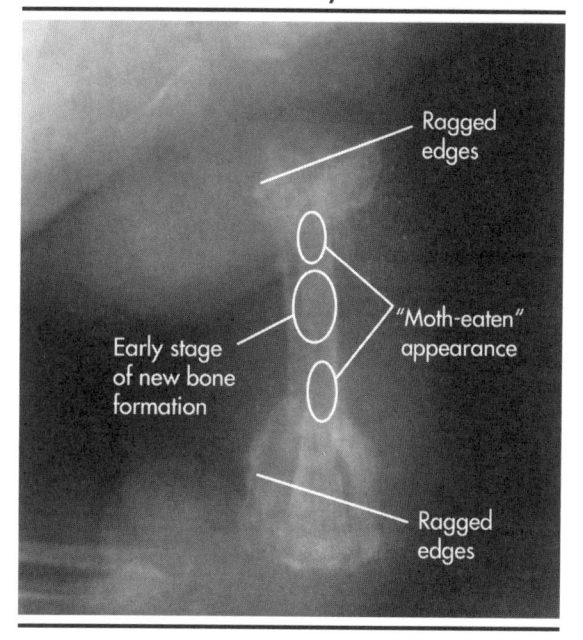

From: McPherson DM. 2002. Osteomyelitis in the neonate. *Neonatal Network* 21(1): 15. Reprinted by permission.

Diagnosis

Early diagnosis and treatment are important to prevent complications such as effects on the growth plate and loss of motion or degenerative arthritis. The infant may initially present with nonspecific symptoms of infection, such as fever, lethargy, and poor feeding. These are followed by swelling, pain, erythema, and decreased movement of the affected limb. A complete blood count may show increased leukocytes, especially immature cells. Older infants and children may have higher erythrocyte sedimentation rates, but there is little information on this in the neonate.

Blood cultures should be obtained from infants who are suspected of having osteomyelitis or septic arthritis. Needle aspirations of fluid or pus in the involved bone or joint should be obtained for Gram's stain and culture. Initial radiographs may be normal or show nonspecific soft tissue swelling or widening of the articular space (Figure 7-3). These alterations are followed by destruction and necrosis of the bone, illustrated on x-ray by irregular areas of decreased density (Figure 7-4). Subluxation and destruction of the joint and lifting of periosteum from the bone may also be seen.

Management

Treatment of osteomyelitis and septic arthritis includes long-term antibiotic therapy, continuing for three to four weeks after resolution of symptoms. Antimicrobial selection is based on results of the Gram's stain and culture of any aspirated fluid. Vancomycin is usually used for Gram-positive infections, and cefotaxime or gentamicin for Gram-negative organisms. If no fluid is available or the organism is not identified, an antistaphylococcal drug and an aminoglycoside are used.[26]

Draining the joint space or bone by needle aspiration or surgery relieves pressure on the

FIGURE 7-5 ◆ Scalded skin syndrome secondary to staphylococcal infection.

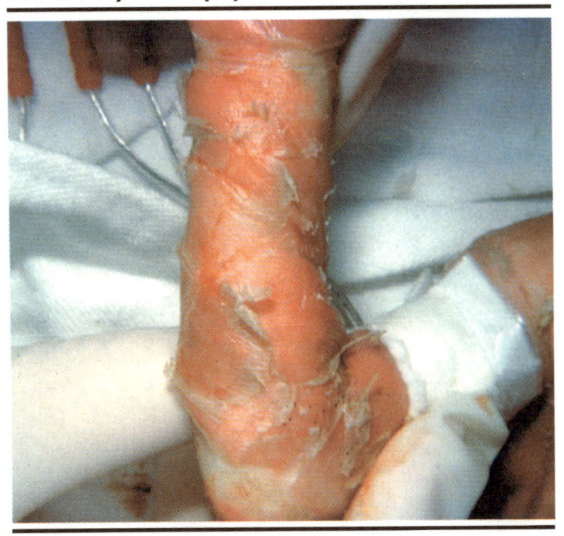

Courtesy of Dr. David A. Clark, Albany Medical Center, Albany, New York. Reprinted by permission.

joint and prevents vascular compromise. This may also be necessary to rid the area of pockets of bacteria. Physical therapy should be instituted after the initial swelling and pain have subsided. Full range of motion may take several months to return.

Prognosis

Death from osteomyelitis and septic arthritis is rare when these conditions are accurately diagnosed and appropriately treated. However, bone deformations, damage to the growth plate, contractures, and muscle weakness can lead to disability of the infected limb.

Cutaneous Infections

Most cutaneous infections in the neonate are caused by *S. aureus* or by Group A or B streptococci. Cutaneous infections can have several clinical presentations, with pustular lesions being the most common. Pustules may present as solitary lesions or in clusters. They are most commonly seen in the diaper area or periumbilically, but they may spread to other parts of the body. A Gram's stain and culture of a smear from an intact lesion can identify the microorganism causing the lesion. In the absence of systemic signs and symptoms of illness or extensive involvement, the pustules can usually be treated with a mild cleansing or antiseptic agent. If more extensive or systemic involvement is suspected, such as cellulites or fever, parenteral antibiotics may be indicated.[41]

Omphalitis

Omphalitis is usually caused by Staphylococcus or Streptococcus. It is characterized by erythema around the umbilicus and a wet, malodorous stump. Invasion of the bloodstream or peritoneal cavity by microorganisms occurs via the umbilical vessels. Parenteral antibiotics are necessary to treat the infant.

Staphylococcal Scalded Skin Syndrome

Staphylococcal scalded skin syndrome presents as a generalized erythema, followed by eruption of large blisters and peeling of the epidermis, often in large sections. It is associated with bullous impetigo, toxic epidermal necrolysis, Ritter's disease, and nonstreptococcal scarlatina. The most common cause is phage Group II staphylococci. The pathogenesis of these diseases appears to be the release of an exotoxin that damages epidermal cell walls. Presentation begins with a generalized erythema, edema, and tenderness, followed by bullous eruption, desquamation, and peeling of the epidermis, often in large sheets. The usual sites of infection include the conjunctiva, neck, and umbilicus.

Treatment should not be initiated until blood, eye, nasopharynx, and other cultures are obtained. This infection may be treated with nafcillin or oxycillin; vancomycin may be used if the Staphylococcus is resistant to nafcillin. Figure 7-5 shows a baby with scalded skin syndrome.

Necrotizing Fasciitis

Necrotizing fasciitis is an infection of the deep fascia with secondary necrosis of the subcutaneous tissue. It is usually caused by Staphylococcus species (most commonly, *S. aureus*), *E. coli,* Klebsiella, or anaerobic bacteria. It is uncommon in the newborn, but may be associated with infection following surgical procedures, birth trauma, or other cutaneous infections. Subcutaneous tissues, including muscle layers, are invaded, and the microorganisms spread along the fascial planes. Skin and tissue may feel "woody," with indistinct borders to the lesion.

Treatment involves antibiotic coverage (usually nafcillin), extensive surgical excision, and resection of the destroyed tissue. Hyperbaric oxygen therapy has been used with some success in older infants and children, but there is limited experience with its use in infants. Hyperbaric oxygen uses oxygen under pressure to increase oxygen tissue levels higher than what can be achieved with 100 percent inhaled O_2. The increased oxygen improves blood flow to the tissues and acts directly on anaerobic bacteria as well as enhancing leukocyte and macrophage activity.

Neonatal Ophthalmia

Infections of the eye may be caused by a number of organisms in the newborn, with Chlamydia being the most common. Staphylococci, streptococci, *Neisseria gonorrhoeae*, and Haemophilus species are also seen. Bacterial infections usually present with redness and edema of the eyelid, with purulent discharge. Although a culture and Gram's stain of the discharge may be helpful in selecting the proper antimicrobial agent, identified bacteria may not be the cause of the conjunctivitis. Normal skin floras are often seen in the sample. Frequently, the causative agent of the conjunctivitis is not determined.

Common organisms such as staphylococci or streptococci can be treated with topical antibiotic ointment such as erythromycin, sulfacetamide sodium, or gentamycin ointment. Gram-negative rods such as *Pseudomonas aeruginosa* can cause a virulent infection with complications such as septicemia, meningitis, and brain abscess.[42] Prompt diagnosis and treatment, including a blood culture and parenteral antimicrobial therapy, are essential. Parenteral antimicrobial therapy should also be used for infections caused by *N. gonorrhoeae*.

Chlamydia eye infections may begin in the first few days of life, but symptoms may not be seen until two to three weeks after delivery. It is most often acquired from the maternal vaginal canal during delivery. Intense swelling and redness of the eyelids and copious purulent discharge are common with chlamydial infections. Oral erythromycin is more effective than topical therapy in treating Chlamydia and should be initiated as soon as the infection is suspected.[26]

Viral conjunctivitis is frequently associated with upper respiratory infections. Infants with viral conjunctivitis generally have watery or mucopurulent, but rarely purulent, discharge. Antibiotic ointments will not be effective in treating viral conjunctivitis, but because cultures often identify common skin bacteria as well, antibiotic ointment is sometimes used if the cause of conjunctivitis is unclear.

COMPLICATIONS OF INFECTION

Septic Shock

Cardiogenic shock is a frequent complication of neonatal sepsis. Hypoxemia and inadequate tissue perfusion make it impossible for the infant's system to provide adequate oxygen and nutrients to the tissues and to remove metabolic waste products. Shock is an unstable state. If untreated, it can cause progressive tissue damage and death.[43,44]

The events of septic shock are caused by the infant's response to the release of toxins by the microorganisms responsible for infection. That response involves hemodynamic, metabolic, and clinical changes. The released toxins may be of bacterial, viral, fungal, or protozoal origin.

The most common etiologic agent in septic shock is endotoxin, a complex lipopolysaccharide released by Gram-negative bacteria.[45]

Gram-negative bacteria are the most common organisms responsible for septic shock.

However, Gram-positive organisms also produce toxins, such as the exotoxin produced by *S. aureus*, Clostridia species, and species of Streptococcus. These toxins are released from the microorganism during phagocytosis, or disintegration of the organism, and are normally cleared by the reticuloendothelial system (RES). If the RES is able to clear the toxin effectively, septic shock will not develop. When the RES is not functioning well, however, or there is an overwhelming production of toxins, the infant's system will be unable to clear the toxins efficiently, and they will accumulate.

The symptoms seen in septic shock result from compensatory mechanisms triggered by the infant's defense system and from the direct effects of the toxins. Endotoxin release produces an immune response that leads to alterations in vascular tone and permeability. These changes can be vasodilation, increased vascular permeability leading to third-spacing of fluid, and hypotension.[43,46] The polysaccharide component of endotoxin produces a complement-consuming, anaphylaxis-like reaction in the infant, with release of histamine and serotonin. The release of these chemicals causes further vasodilation, hypotension, decreased oxygen delivery at the cellular level, and cellular injury and/or death.[47] Although less is known about the effects of the exotoxins produced by Gram-positive organisms, they appear to have similar results, producing profound hypotension and multiorgan failure.[48]

The hypotension associated with septic shock impairs normal blood flow and oxygen delivery to the tissues, interfering with normal cell function.[47] The decreased availability of oxygen at the cellular level interferes with electron transport and glucose metabolism, resulting in the production of lactic acid and subsequent metabolic acidosis. If the changes leading to metabolic acidosis are not reversed rapidly, the cycle can become progressively worse and eventually lead to cell death. In addition, endotoxins affect the metabolism of essential substrates, such as glucose, fat, and protein, further impairing cellular functioning.

Cellular energy is derived from the conversion of oxygen and nutrients to adenosine triphosphate (ATP) within the cell. There are two mechanisms, or pathways, for ATP production: aerobic and anaerobic. During normal, aerobic metabolism, protein, carbohydrates, and fats are metabolized through the Krebs cycle in the mitochondria of the cell. Glucose is converted to pyruvate; and ATP, water, and carbon dioxide are released. The aerobic pathway is efficient, yielding 36 units of ATP per molecule of glucose. During anaerobic metabolism, lack of sufficient oxygen causes pyruvate to be converted to lactic acid and only 2 units of ATP are produced per molecule of glucose. Therefore, anaerobic metabolism is a very inefficient pathway for energy production. The anaerobic pathway occurs in the cytoplasm of the cell, and lactic acid easily diffuses into the extracellular fluid. Figure 7-6 shows the aerobic Krebs cycle and Figure 7-7, the anaerobic glycolytic pathway.

Release of catecholamine and glucagon is stimulated during sepsis, increasing lipolysis, which leads to free fatty acid (FFA) elevation. Transport of FFAs across the mitochondrial membrane is impaired, so the FFAs accumulate in the bloodstream, inhibiting pyruvate dehydrogenase and blocking glucose metabolism and further reducing available energy.

This lack of oxygen and energy affects the metabolism in all cells in the body, leading to significant cellular damage, including decreased mitochondrial function, decreased cell wall integrity and failure of the potassium-sodium pump, and rupture of lysosomes, releasing digestive enzymes within the cell. Within a short time,

FIGURE 7-6 ♦ Aerobic metabolism: The Krebs cycle.

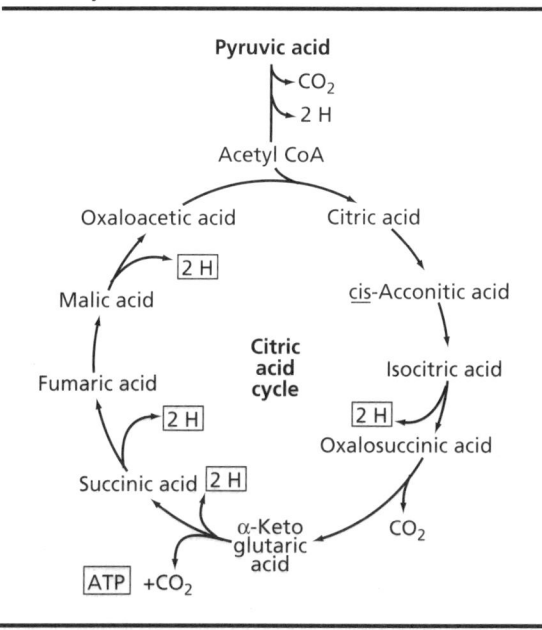

From: Porth CM. 2003. Cell and tissue characteristics. In *Pathophysiology: Concepts of Altered Health States*, 6th ed. Philadelphia: Lippincott Williams & Wilkins, 76. Reprinted by permission.

FIGURE 7-7 ♦ Anaerobic metabolism: The glycolytic pathway.

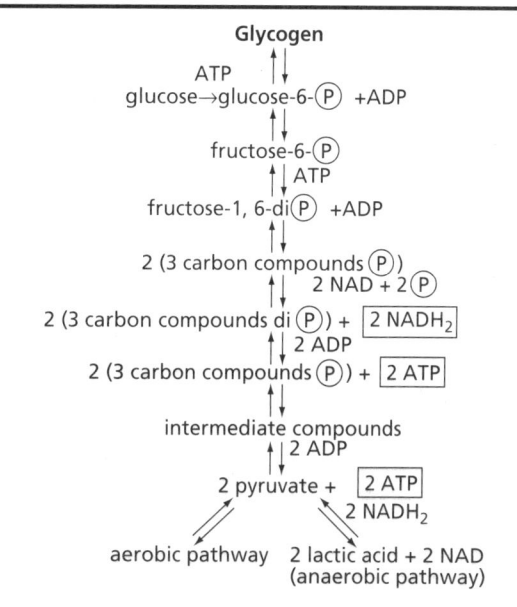

From: Porth CM. 2003. Cell and tissue characteristics. In *Pathophysiology: Concepts of Altered Health States*, 6th ed. Philadelphia: Lippincott Williams & Wilkins, 76. Reprinted by permission.

sufficient tissue damage can occur to make the process irreversible.[47]

The effects of septic shock are essentially the same as those of general shock. In the face of decreased central and peripheral venous pressure, blood flow is redistributed, with reduction of flow to the skin, gut, and kidney and preservation of flow to the heart, lung, and adrenal glands. This is controlled by both local and systemic responses to hypotension and hypoperfusion.

Local Responses

At the local level, the brain, kidney, and heart respond to decreased perfusion by reducing resistance to flow through vasodilation of arterioles. The exact mechanism of the stimulus for this autoregulation is not known, but it may be modulated at the tissue level by local metabolic feedback secondary to acidosis, hypoxia, and hypercarbia. All organs are capable of microcirculatory changes that enhance oxygen extraction locally when blood flow is reduced. Changes include opening of previously closed capillaries, adjustments in hemoglobin-oxygen affinity secondary to local pH reduction, and secretion of procoagulant and antithrombotic substances.[49] These changes allow for increased blood flow and oxygen delivery to the tissues and slower passage of blood through the affected area, allowing more time for diffusion of oxygen.

In septic shock, these compensatory mechanisms may be impaired because of microembolism (if disseminated intravascular coagulopathy is present) or altered vascular autoregulation. Histamine and prostacyclin release may decrease vascular tone and increase capillary permeability, leading to third-spacing of fluid and decreased intravascular volume.

Systemic Responses

Vascular resistance and blood flow to an organ depend on the interplay between local autoregulation and the response to the effects of sympathetic nervous system (SNS) stimulation and humoral stimulation. At the systemic level, control of regional vascular beds by the autonomic nervous system (ANS) and circulating hormones helps maintain blood pressure and organ perfusion pressure and distributes available cardiac output to organs with high metabolic demands (brain, heart). Also, systemic responses enhance compromised organ function and perfusion by restoring pH and improving blood volume and cardiac output.[47]

Arterial tone may vary significantly from one organ to another in response to a low cardiac output caused by differences in autoregulation and in the degree of sympathetic enervation. When cardiac output decreases, the ANS is stimulated, causing an increased discharge of sympathetic adrenergic nerve fibers and the local release of norepinephrine. The afferent input for this response is from cardiopulmonary receptors in the atria and arterial baroreceptors. Sympathetic stimulation causes peripheral vasoconstriction, increased heart rate, and increased cardiac contractility. The degree of vasoconstriction depends on the adrenergic enervation of each organ. The splanchnic, renal, integumentary, and skeletal-muscle vascular beds are most responsive to sympathetic vasoconstriction; the coronary and cerebral circulations have a lower response. The net result is a redistribution of blood flow away from the gut, kidney, skin, and muscle and preservation of blood flow to the heart and brain.

The underlying process causing the shock may also affect blood flow distribution. For adequate function, some organs require more blood flow than that needed for metabolism. The kidneys require high blood flow for proper filtration and excretion of wastes; skin blood flow determines heat transfer and, thus, regulation of temperature. These organs have very low resting oxygen extraction because of the high levels of blood flow to them and can tolerate large decreases in blood flow without hypoxia. However, reductions in blood flow diminish the functional ability of these organs. Redistribution of blood flow helps match a limited systemic oxygen supply to organ oxygen demands. An increase in total systemic vascular resistance helps maintain diastolic blood pressure and myocardial perfusion. In septic shock, however, these mechanisms are not effective in maintaining the blood pressure and myocardial perfusion for very long.[47]

Because the venous system is also richly enervated with sympathetic fibers, there may be venoconstriction with sympathetic stimulation during shock, causing a decrease in the volume of blood remaining in the veins and improving systemic venous return. When cardiac output is decreased, sympathetic stimulation of the adrenal medulla releases epinephrine and norepinephrine into the circulation, and stimulation of the kidney indirectly promotes the release of renin. Circulating adrenergic hormones enhance the local sympathetic responses and cause vasoconstriction and increased myocardial contractility. Epinephrine also causes an increase in heart rate. Renin, released from the kidney in response to decreased perfusion of the macula densa, catalyzes conversion of angiotensinogen to angiotensin I, which is then converted to angiotensin II as it passes through the pulmonary vascular bed (Figure 7-8).

Angiotensin II stimulates the release of aldosterone from the adrenal gland and can cross the blood-brain barrier to promote the release of arginine vasopressin from the pituitary gland. Vasopressin release is also stimulated by a decreased atrial or aortic pressure. Angiotensin II, aldosterone, and vasopressin each causes vasoconstriction, thus potentiating the effects of the SNS in low-perfusion states. Aldosterone and vasopressin also increase salt and water retention, to help increase blood volume and restore perfusion.

INFECTION IN THE NEONATE

Local Metabolic Effects

Stimulation of the sympathoadrenal system and the release of vasoactive peptides during shock cause vasoconstriction that can override local autoregulatory effects. Tissue with low metabolic activity, such as skin or muscle, may experience intense vasoconstriction with only a moderate reduction in cardiac output. Metabolism in these tissues can be sustained only by increases in the fractional extraction of oxygen and other nutrients. When these increases are inadequate to maintain metabolism, there will be a decrease in oxygen tension and a resultant desaturation of venous blood, with an increase in lactic acid and other metabolic by-products. This change to anaerobic metabolism, with decreased energy and heat production and increased accumulation of waste products, rapidly depletes cellular energy stores and, eventually, causes irreversible tissue injury. With sustained tissue ischemia, cell metabolism is depressed and cell membrane function is disrupted, resulting in intracellular edema and loss of cellular integrity. Direct injury to the vascular endothelium increases vascular permeability, causing interstitial edema.

The edema and tissue injury may not manifest until local blood flow is restored. Following ischemia and reperfusion, the availability of oxygen may influence the degree of injury. Several endogenous substances, including amines, peptides, fatty acids, purines, calcium, and free oxygen radicals, have been implicated in the damage that occurs during ischemia or reperfusion. Circulating neutrophils and platelets may contribute to local vascular injury.[51]

Effects on Specific Organs

Septic shock has important effects on many organs. They include the heart, lungs, kidneys, liver, and the stomach and intestines.

FIGURE 7-8 ♦ The renin-angiotensin feedback system.

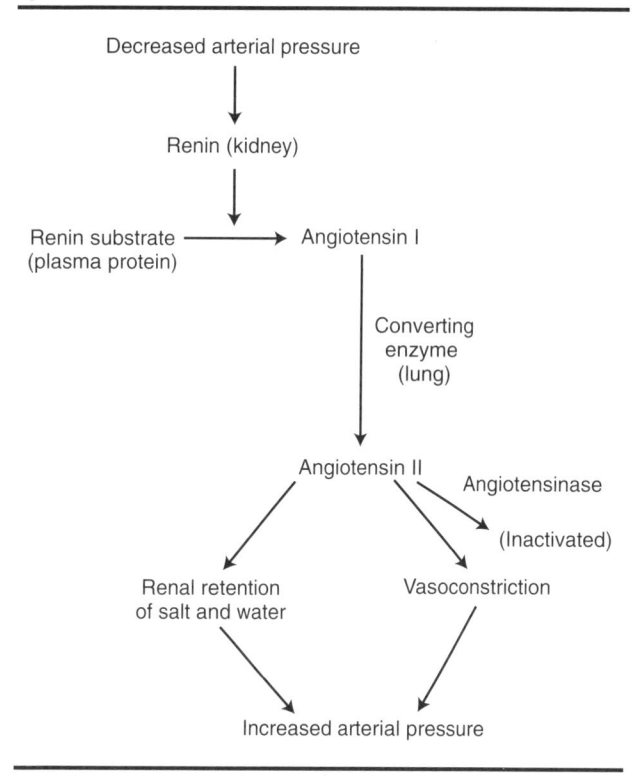

From: Guyton AC, and Hall JE. 2000. Dominant role of the kidney in long-term regulation of arterial pressure and in hypertension: The integrated system of pressure control. In *Textbook of Medical Physiology*, 10th ed., Guyton AC, and Hall JE, eds. Philadelphia: WB Saunders, 201. Reprinted by permission.

Heart. The initial expansion in pulmonary and peripheral resistance increases the preload, or venous return, to the heart. It also augments the afterload, or resistance the heart must work against with each contraction, thus increasing the workload and oxygen requirements of the myocardium.[52]

As the pH and oxygen levels fall, the myocardium must rely on stored glycogen for energy. As these energy stores are depleted, myocardial function decreases, and blood flow to vital organs, including the heart, begins to fail. The resulting hypoxemia and ischemia lead to myocardial dysfunction, poor contractility, and bradycardia.

7 MANAGEMENT OF NEONATAL INFECTION, SEPSIS, AND COMPLICATIONS

Lungs. Changes in pulmonary function include alterations in capillary permeability and gas exchange. Acidosis and hypoxia may increase pulmonary vascular resistance, with right-to-left shunting through the foramen ovale and the ductus arteriosus. Hypoxia may also damage Type II alveolar cells, leading to decreased surfactant production.

Left-sided heart failure resulting from ischemia may produce pulmonary edema, causing a decrease in functional residual capacity and lung compliance, alveolar collapse, and increased small-airway resistance. The ventilation-perfusion mismatch impairs gas exchange; there may be sequestration of platelets and neutrophils in the pulmonary capillaries, with release of proteases. Perivascular leakage, potentiated by histamine and bradykinin, increases the extravascular lung water produced by greater capillary permeability. Advanced shock states are marked by extensive loss of capillary endothelial integrity, with interstitial and intra-alveolar hemorrhage.[53]

Kidneys. Renal blood flow normally makes up 25 percent of cardiac output, but it may be reduced to as low as 10 percent in shock.[54] In shock, renal blood flow is redistributed, with decreased flow to the cortex. Low perfusion of the kidney leads to impaired clearance of waste products and damage to the kidney itself. Renal tubular injury may progress to cellular necrosis, with accumulation of proteinaceous and cellular debris. Initially, decreased blood flow results in increased sodium and water reabsorption, caused by the secretion of aldosterone and antidiuretic hormone. This mechanism fails with continued low perfusion of the kidney; the kidney is then unable to clear hydrogen and potassium ions, toxic substances, and drugs or to excrete water. End results are a decreased glomerular filtration rate, decreased urinary output, renal tubular acidosis and/or necrosis, electrolyte abnormalities, and renal hypertension.

Liver. Decreased hepatic blood flow and hypoxemia produce cellular injury and decreased metabolic activity. Elevated liver enzymes and indirect and direct hyperbilirubinemia may be seen. Coagulation derangements may result from inadequate regeneration of clotting factors. Lactic acid, normally cleared by the liver, is produced by it. Cytoplasmic lysosomal enzymes and RES function decrease. Diminished protein and carbohydrate metabolism impairs the liver's detoxification abilities.

Stomach and intestines. Decreased blood flow to the stomach and intestines causes reduced motility, decreased absorption of nutrients, and increased production of lactic acid. Prolonged hypoxia and ischemia may result in damage and infarction to the bowel, raising the risk of invasion of the bowel wall by bacteria. Damage to the mucosal lining of the gastrointestinal (GI) tract may contribute to intravascular volume depletion by allowing third-spacing of fluid.

Clinical Manifestations

The infant with septic shock may present with fulminant disease that takes a rapid course, but frequently the signs and symptoms of septic shock are subtle, vague, or misleading. Early signs of septic shock include poor perfusion, pallor, tachycardia, hypotension, apnea, and respiratory distress. Lethargy or irritability, decreased tone, temperature instability, and feeding intolerance may also be seen. Infants in the initial stages of cardiogenic shock may display signs of increased cardiac output; vasodilatation; warm, flushed, and dry skin; and respiratory alkalosis. As the infant's condition worsens, decreased cardiac output with cold, cyanotic extremities, decreased central venous pressure, and metabolic acidosis develop.[55]

Diagnosis

The diagnosis of septic shock depends on identifying the signs and symptoms of shock and is confirmed by a positive blood culture.

Knowledge of risk factors and presentation is essential. The clinician must also understand the general course of and treatment protocols for septic shock because untreated septic shock leads to irreversible injury and death.

Management

If septic shock is suspected, aggressive therapy must be instituted promptly. Cultures of blood and urine should be obtained, and appropriate antimicrobial and supportive therapy must be instituted. Initial measures for managing septic shock are aimed at all three of these goals:

1. Improving cardiac output and tissue perfusion by interventions that compensate for the primary pathophysiologic disturbances
2. Treating the underlying cause
3. Reducing excessive demands for blood flow to make the best use of available cardiac output

Of course, identification and treatment of the specific cause of the sepsis are critical. A sepsis workup and initiation of antimicrobials should be done immediately. Broad-spectrum antimicrobials, with coverage for Gram-negative rods, are used initially.[26,56]

Ventilatory status should be assessed and appropriate respiratory support provided to optimize oxygen delivery. Intubation and mechanical ventilation are indicated to reduce the work of breathing. Decreased perfusion stimulates the ventilatory drive, increasing the metabolic demands of the respiratory muscles. In severe shock with decreased cardiac output, 20 percent of the cardiac output may be directed to the respiratory muscles. Interstitial or alveolar pulmonary edema increases the work of breathing even more by decreasing compliance and increasing airway resistance.[26,56]

Tissue perfusion can be expanded by improving cardiac output. Four variables affect cardiac output: heart rate, filling volume, contractility, and afterload. Under normal conditions, neonates and infants have a fast heart rate. This means that their ability to sustain cardiac output through an increase in heart rate is limited. Although initially effective, the higher rate has a high energy cost and cannot be maintained. Filling volume is influenced by blood volume and heart rate—the amount of time between contractions allowed for filling of the ventricles. Contractility depends in part on the health of the cardiac muscle as well as the amount of stretch achieved with ventricular filling. Afterload refers to the pressure the left ventricle must pump against to send blood to the rest of the body.

Restoring adequate circulating volume is an immediate goal, with infusion of normal saline, ringer's lactate solution, or blood products. The object of therapy is prompt restoration of vascular volume to support adequate tissue perfusion and prevent the cumulative effects of prolonged underperfusion of tissues. Prolonged underperfusion leads to harmful secondary effects, including increased capillary permeability and pulmonary disease, which complicate therapy. Transfusion of packed red blood cells may also be needed to maintain a normal hemoglobin concentration and to increase oxygen availability to the tissues; blood transfusion is appropriate only if anemia is present.

Excessive speed in volume replacement is dangerous. Some vascular beds (brain) dilate maximally in response to systemic hypotension. If systemic pressure is raised abruptly, there is no time for the vasculature to constrict partially, and the higher pressure is transmitted to the capillaries, where it can cause capillary injury, edema, or hemorrhage. Effects on the circulation should be evaluated after each infusion. If expansion of intravascular volume and tachycardia cannot maintain perfusion, inotropic support may be useful to help improve cardiac contractility and function.[7,56]

Inadequate tissue perfusion leads to metabolic acidosis, which decreases myocardial function even further, progressively lessening perfusion. Inotropic drugs are not effective in severe acidosis because the circulation is unresponsive to sympathomimetic amines in that state. A recurrence of acidosis after the initial acidosis is corrected suggests continuing underperfusion. Sodium bicarbonate administration is a temporary measure to restore acid-base balance, but it cannot prevent the effects of accumulated wastes and lactic acid. Repeated administration of sodium bicarbonate causes hypernatremia and hyperosmolarity and cannot neutralize the ongoing lactic acidosis associated with inadequate tissue perfusion. Tromethamine (THAM) can be used in lieu of bicarbonate if hypernatremia is present, but THAM should not be used for longer than 24 hours. Hyperkalemia may occur, especially with decreased renal perfusion.

Hypocalcemia may occur in neonatal sepsis as a result of the parathyroid gland's impaired ability to control calcium balance. Because the ionized fraction of calcium is metabolically active, hypocalcemic effects may occur even with normal total serum calcium levels. Hypocalcemia depresses cardiac contractility and may lead to cardiac arrhythmias.[55]

Monitoring

Septic shock is an acute, life-threatening medical emergency. The neonate's response to therapy must be monitored constantly. Components of monitoring include blood pressure, heart rate, electrocardiogram (ECG) (rate and rhythm), arterial blood gases, pulse oximetry (oxygenation), end tidal PCO_2 (ventilation), respiratory rate and pattern, and systemic perfusion. Systemic perfusion can be observed or assessed by warmth of extremities, temperature, capillary filling time, peripheral pulses, urinary output, and central venous pressure.

DISSEMINATED INTRAVASCULAR COAGULOPATHY

Disseminated intravascular coagulopathy (DIC) is another potential complication of maternal or neonatal infection. Venous stasis (with clot formation) or injury or insult to endothelial tissue activates the clotting mechanism inappropriately, leading to production of thrombin and proteolytic enzymes. Thrombin initiates the formation of intravascular fibrin, the deposition of platelets, and the formation of intravascular thrombi.[57] The body attempts to maintain homeostasis through fibrinolysis, or breakdown of the clot. As plasma acts to dissolve the clot, fibrin degradation products are formed. Naturally occurring factors (anticoagulation factors, heparin, and intrinsic factors V, VIII, and XII) are used in the fibrinolysis process. When these factors are depleted, clot formation continues unchecked. The result is widespread formation of small, ineffective clots throughout the vascular system, consumption of clotting factors, and hemorrhage.

Many of the homeostasis factors used in the fibrinolysis are either produced by or filtered in the liver. The immaturity of the neonate's liver—even in the healthy term newborn—puts neonates at greater risk than adults for depletion of the fibrinolysis components and subsequent development of DIC. Another risk factor for the development of DIC in neonates is a low level of vitamin K, which assists in clotting and clot formation. In addition, the immaturity of the immune system adversely affects the infant's ability to achieve a balance between compensatory mechanisms to sustain function and persistent alterations that result in further injury.

SUMMARY

Treatment of infection requires careful assessment of the underlying causative organism and its effects on each individual body system. The causative organism must be identified as soon as possible and appropriate antibiotic therapy initiated. Careful attention must be paid to the function of each organ system and supportive care provided.

REFERENCES

1. Baker CJ. 1997. Group B streptococcal infections. *Clinics in Perinatology* 24(1): 59–70.
2. American Academy of Pediatrics. 2003. *Red Book: Report of the Committee on Infectious Diseases*, 26th ed. Elk Grove Village, Illinois: American Academy of Pediatrics, 584–591.
3. Gaynes RP, et al. 1998. Nosocomial infections among neonates in high risk nurseries in the United States. *Pediatrics* 98(3): 357–361.
4. Klein JO. 2001. Bacterial sepsis and meningitis. In *Infectious Diseases of the Fetus and Newborn Infant*, 5th ed., Remington JS, and Klein JO, eds. Philadelphia: WB Saunders, 943–998.
5. Whitsett JA, et al. 1999. Acute respiratory disorders. In *Neonatology: Pathophysiology and Management of the Newborn*, 5th ed., Avery GB, Fletcher MA, and MacDonald MG, eds. Philadelphia: Lippincott Williams & Wilkins, 485–508.
6. Alenghat E, and Esterly JR. 1984. Alveolar macrophages in perinatal infants. *Pediatrics* 74(2): 221–223.
7. Perez EM, and Weisman LE. 1997. Novel approaches to the prevention and therapy of neonatal bacterial sepsis. *Clinics in Perinatology* 24(1): 213–229.
8. Barnett ED, and Klein JO. 2001. Bacterial infections in the neonate. In *Infectious Diseases of the Fetus and Newborn Infant*, 5th ed., Remington JS, and Klein JO, eds. Philadelphia: WB Saunders, 999–1018.
9. LeVine AM, et al. 1996. Surfactant content in children with inflammatory lung disease. *Critical Care Medicine* 24(6): 1062–1067.
10. Abman SH, and Kinsella JP. 1995. Inhaled NO for persistent pulmonary hypertension of the newborn: The physiology matters! *Pediatrics* 96(6): 1153–1155.
11. Kinsella JP, et al. 1997. Randomized, multicenter trial of inhaled nitric oxide and high frequency ventilation in severe persistent pulmonary hypertension of the newborn. *Journal of Pediatrics* 131(1): 55–62.
12. Kinsella JP, and Abman SH. 1998. Controversies in the use of inhaled nitric oxide therapy in the newborn. *Clinics in Perinatology* 25(2): 203–218.
13. Kinsella JP, and Abman SH. 1995. Recent developments in the pathophysiology and treatment of persistent pulmonary hypertension of the newborn. *Journal of Pediatrics* 126(6): 853–864.
14. Pandit PB, Dunn MS, and Colucci EA. 1995. Surfactant therapy in neonates with respiratory deterioration due to pulmonary hemorrhage. *Pediatrics* 95(1): 32–36.
15. Fetter WPF, et al. 1995. Surfactant replacement therapy in neonates with respiratory failure due to bacterial sepsis. *Acta Paediatrica* 84(1): 14–16.
16. Kinsella JP, and Shaul PW. 2004. Physiology of nitric oxide in the developing lung. In *Fetal and Neonatal Physiology*, 3rd ed., Polin RA, Fox WW, and Abman SH, eds. Philadelphia: WB Saunders, 733–743.
17. Dekowski SA, and Holtzman RB. 1998. Surfactant replacement therapy: An update on applications. *Pediatric Clinics of North America* 45(3): 549–572.
18. Lotze A, et al. 1998. Multicenter study of surfactant (beractant) use in the treatment of term infants with severe respiratory failure. *Journal of Pediatrics* 132(1): 40–47.
19. Cornish JD, et al. 1993. Efficacy of venovenous extracorporeal membrane oxygenation for neonates with respiratory and circulatory compromise. *Journal of Pediatrics* 122(1): 105–109.
20. Klein MD, and Whittlesey GC. 1994. Extracorporeal membrane oxygenation. *Pediatric Clinics of North America* 41(2): 365–384.
21. Bell AH, et al. 1989. Meningitis in the newborn: A 14 year review. *Archives of Disease in Childhood* 64(6): 873–874.
22. Washburn TC, Medearis DN Jr, and Childs B. 1965. Sex differences in susceptibility to infections. *Pediatrics* 35(1): 57–61.
23. Edwards MS. 2002. Postnatal bacterial infections. In *Neonatal-Perinatal Medicine: Diseases of the Fetus and Newborn*, 7th ed., Fanaroff AA, and Martin RJ, eds. St. Louis: Mosby-Year Book, 706-745.
24. Pong A, and Bradley JS. 1999. Bacterial meningitis and the newborn infant. *Infectious Disease Clinics of North America* 13(3): 711–733.
25. Cole FS. 1998. Bacterial infections of the newborn. In *Avery's Diseases of the Newborn*, 7th ed., Taeusch HW, and Ballard RA, eds. Philadelphia: WB Saunders, 490–512.
26. Freij BJ, and McCracken GH Jr. 1999. Acute infections. In *Neonatology: Pathophysiology and Management of the Newborn*, 5th ed., Avery GB, Fletcher MA, and McDonald MG, eds. Philadelphia: Lippincott Williams & Wilkins, 1189–1230.
27. Ahmed A, et al. 1996. Cerebral spinal fluid values in the term neonate. *Pediatric Infectious Disease Journal* 15(4): 298–303.
28. Wald ER, et al. 1995. Dexamethasone therapy for children with bacterial meningitis. *Pediatrics* 95(1): 21–28.
29. Wald ER, et al. 1986. Long-term outcome of Group B streptococcal meningitis. *Pediatrics* 77(2): 217–221.
30. Unhanand M, et al. 1993. Gram-negative enteric bacillary meningitis: A twenty-one year experience. *Journal of Pediatrics* 122(1): 15–21.
31. Verma RP, and Pizzica A. 1998. Early neonatal urinary tract infection: A case report and review. *Journal of Perinatology* 18(6 part 1): 480–484.
32. Wiswell TE, and Roscelli JD. 1986. Corroborative evidence for the decreased incidence of urinary tract infections in circumcised male infants. *Pediatrics* 78(1): 96–99.
33. To T, et al. 1998. Cohort study on circumcision of newborn boys and subsequent risk of urinary tract infection. *Lancet* 352(9143): 1813–1816.
34. Herzog LW. 1989. Urinary tract infections and circumcision: A case controlled study. *American Journal of Diseases of Children* 143(3): 348–350.
35. Dick PT, and Feldman W. 1996. Routine diagnostic imaging for childhood urinary tract infections: A systematic overview. *Journal of Pediatrics* 128(1): 15–22.
36. Barkemeyer BM. 1993. Suprapubic aspiration of urine in very low birth weight infants. *Pediatrics* 92(3): 457–459.
37. Thomas KS. 2003. Assessment and management of genitourinary dysfunction. In *Comprehensive Neonatal Nursing: A Physiologic Perspective*, 3rd ed., Kenner C, and Lott JW, eds. Philadelphia: WB Saunders, 673–699.
38. Marchant CD, et al. 1984. Course and outcome of otitis media in early infancy: A prospective study. *Journal of Pediatrics* 104(6): 826–831.
39. Ogden JA. 1998. Pathophysiology of neonatal osteomyelitis and septic arthritis. In *Fetal and Neonatal Physiology*, 2nd ed., Polin RA, and Fox WM, eds. Philadelphia: WB Saunders, 2382–2387.
40. McPherson DM. 2002. Osteomyelitis in the neonate. *Neonatal Network* 21(1): 9–22.
41. Darmstadt GL, and Dinulos JG. 2001. Bacterial infections. In *Textbook of Neonatal Dermatology*, Eichenfield LF, Frieden IJ, and Esterly NB, eds. Philadelphia: WB Saunders, 179–200.
42. Shah SS, et al. 1999. Bacteremia, meningitis, and brain abscesses in a hospitalized infant: Complications of *Pseudomonas aeruginosa* conjunctivitis. *Journal of Perinatology* 19(6): 462–465.
43. Anderson M, and Blumer JL. 1997. Advances in the therapy for sepsis in children. *Pediatric Clinics of North America* 44(1): 179–205.
44. Wiessner WH, Casey LC, and Zbilut JP. 1995. Treatment of sepsis and septic shock: A review. *Heart & Lung* 24(5): 380–392.
45. Morrison DC, et al. 1999. Structure-function relationships of bacterial endotoxins: Contribution to microbial sepsis. *Infectious Disease Clinics of North America* 13(2): 313–340.

46. Gilstrap LC, and Faro S. 1997. Pregnancy and septic shock. In *Infections in Pregnancy*, 2nd ed., Gilstrap LC, and Faro S, eds. New York: Wiley, 113–134.
47. Guyton AC, and Hall JE. 2001. Circulatory shock and physiology of its treatment. In *Textbook of Medical Physiology*, 10th ed., Guyton AC, and Hall JE, eds. Philadelphia: WB Saunders, 253–363.
48. Sriskandan S, and Cohen J. 1999. Gram-positive sepsis: Mechanisms and differences from Gram-negative sepsis. *Infectious Disease Clinics of North America* 13(2): 397–412.
49. Symeonides S, and Balk RA. 1999. Nitric oxide in the pathogenesis of sepsis. *Infectious Disease Clinics of North America* 13(2): 449–463.
50. New MI, and Rapaport R. 1997. The adrenal cortex. In *Pediatric Endocrinology*, Sperling MA, ed. Philadelphia: WB Saunders, 281–315.
51. Hazinski MF. 1992. Cardiovascular disorders. In *Nursing Care of the Critically Ill Child*, 2nd ed., Hazinski MF, ed. St. Louis: Mosby-Year Book, 117–394.
52. Walther FJ, et al. 1985. Cardiac output in newborn infants with transient myocardial dysfunction. *Journal of Pediatrics* 107(5): 781–785.
53. Schwarz RH. 1993. Septic shock. In *Obstetric and Perinatal Infections*, Charles D, ed. St. Louis: Mosby-Year Book, 95–103.
54. Brion LP, Satlin LM, and Edelmann CM Jr. 1999. Renal disease. In *Neonatology: Pathophysiology and Management of the Newborn*, 5th ed., Avery GB, Fletcher MA, and MacDonald MG, eds. Philadelphia: Lippincott Williams & Wilkins, 887–973.
55. Witek-Janusek L, and Cusack C. 1994. Neonatal sepsis: Confronting the challenge. *Critical Care Nursing Clinics of North America* 6(2): 405–419.
56. Dellinger RP. 1999. Current therapy for sepsis. *Infectious Disease Clinics of North America* 13(2): 495–508.
57. Pugh M. 1997. DIC screening in the newborn. *Neonatal Network* 16(7): 57–60.

NOTES

CHAPTER 8

Pharmacologic Management of Neonatal Infection

Debra Sansoucie, EdD, RNC, NNP

Despite improvements in antimicrobial therapy, advances in neonatal life support measures, and timely recognition of perinatal risk factors for infection, sepsis continues to be a major cause of morbidity and mortality in the newborn infant. Preterm and low birth weight neonates are particularly susceptible to vertically and nosocomially acquired infections.[1] Because of the often insidious presentation and rapid progression of neonatal infection, early detection and timely management are imperative. Thus, antimicrobial treatment is often initiated even when indications are minimal and the diagnosis of infection is presumptive.

In addition to prompt antimicrobial management and optimal supportive therapy, adjunctive therapies designed to augment deficits in the neonate's own host defenses are being investigated.[1-4] These therapies appear quite promising as supplements to conventional treatments; however, these approaches warrant further study to prove their safety and efficacy before they can be recommended for routine use in the management of neonatal infection. This chapter reviews the principles that guide use of both conventional pharmacologic and adjunctive therapies in treating infection in neonates.

Pharmacotherapeutic Agents

An antimicrobial agent is any chemical used to treat infectious disease by inhibiting or killing pathogens. An antibiotic is defined as any antimicrobial substance that is derived from a living organism, such as molds, bacteria, and some plants. The term *antibiotic* was intended to distinguish between chemical therapeutic agents, such as sulfonamide drugs, and those extracted from the secretions of living organisms, such as penicillin; however, many of these drugs and their derivatives are now synthesized or manufactured in the laboratory. Thus, the term *antibiotic* is currently used to describe a substance produced in whole or in part by chemical synthesis that in small amounts kills or inhibits the growth of other microorganisms.[5]

The ideal antimicrobial agent has several important properties:
- **It inhibits or destroys the pathogen without damaging the host.** The agent does this by disrupting the pathogen's metabolism without

at the same time harming normal human metabolism, usually by targeting some aspect of the pathogen's metabolic process that differs from the host's. This is known as selective toxicity.

- **It is bactericidal rather than bacteriostatic in its action.** Bacteriostatic agents are inhibitory. This means that they act to prevent the growth of pathogens but do not destroy their ability to reproduce. Final destruction of the organism is dependent on the host's defense mechanisms. Bactericidal agents actually kill the organisms against which they are used. This difference becomes exceptionally significant when the host is comparatively immunocompromised, as is the newborn.
- **It has the capacity to kill pathogens before they mutate and become resistant to it.** The agent should be the least likely to induce development of antibiotic resistance in mutant microbes.

Other important factors include the ability to rapidly reach bactericidal levels in the body and to sustain them for extended periods; the lack of production of an allergic response or harmful side effects when administered for a prolonged period; effectiveness against a broad range of microbes commonly encountered in the intensive care nursery; and the ability to remain active in the presence of plasma, body fluids, and exudates.[5]

Finally, the fact that approximately one-fourth of infected neonates will concurrently have bacterial meningitis demonstrates the importance of the ideal antimicrobial agent's ability to attain therapeutic concentrations in the cerebrospinal fluid (CSF).[6]

Basic Mechanisms of Antibiotic Action

Antimicrobial agents target microbes at various sites within the cell, where they act to inhibit essential biochemical events. These agents may work to inhibit cell wall synthesis, cell membrane function, cellular protein synthesis, or cellular nucleic acid synthesis.[5,7,8]

Inhibition of Cell Wall Synthesis

The most common mechanism of antibiotic activity involves disruption of the bacterial cell wall. The cell wall of a bacterium consists of a rigid outer layer. It maintains the shape of the bacterium and protects the inner cell membrane from osmotic or mechanical trauma. Because the internal osmotic pressure of the bacterial cell is several times higher than that of the surrounding environment, any substance that destroys the wall or prevents its synthesis in growing cells leads to lysis of the cell.[5,7]

The major structural component of the bacterial cell wall is the peptidoglycan layer. This layer is synthesized in stages, each of which occurs at a different site in the cell. Cell wall rigidity is attained by cross-linking of peptide chains as a result of transpeptidation reactions in which a peptide bond produced inside of the cell is traded for a peptide bond outside the cell. This reaction is catalyzed by the enzymes D-alanine and D-alanine transpeptidase-carboxypeptidases. These penicillin-binding proteins (PBPs) are the target of β-lactam antibiotics. When growing bacteria are exposed to these antibiotics, the antibiotic binds to the PBPs, inhibiting synthesis and causing cell death. The peptidoglycan layer is much thicker in the cell wall of Gram-positive than of Gram-negative bacteria.[5,7,8]

Cell wall inhibitors have a remarkable lack of toxicity to human host cells and are used extensively in the care of neonates. This lack of toxicity is attributed to the absence of a bacterial-type cell wall, with its peptidoglycan component, in human cells. Examples of the classes of antibiotics that inhibit cell wall synthesis include the β-lactam drugs (penicillins and cephalosporins) and glycopeptides (vancomycin).[5,7,8]

Inhibition of Cell Membrane Function

The cytoplasmic membrane binds the cytoplasm of all living cells. This membrane plays a vital role in the cell by serving as a selective permeability barrier and carrying out active transport functions, thereby controlling the internal composition of the cell. If the functional integrity of the cytoplasmic membrane is disrupted, cell damage or death results.

Antibiotics whose primary target is the cell membrane do not discriminate as effectively between microorganisms and host tissues as do those that interfere with cell wall synthesis. Because of their relative lack of selective toxicity, few of these antibiotics are used clinically. Examples of those currently employed in neonatal care include amphotericin and fluconazole.[5,7]

Inhibition of Protein Synthesis

Protein synthesis is the end result of transcription, in which DNA-dependent ribonucleic acid is synthesized, and translation, in which RNA-dependent protein is synthesized. Antibiotics that interfere with either of these processes prevent the manufacture of protein and thus affect cell viability. The precise mechanisms of action of drugs that inhibit protein synthesis in bacteria are not fully established. Drugs from this class that are commonly used in neonates include clindamycin and aminoglycosides.[5]

Inhibition of Nucleic Acid Synthesis

Any agent that interrupts the structure of the DNA molecule may have deleterious effects on cell division and metabolism. Processes that antimicrobial agents may inhibit include DNA precursor synthesis, DNA replication, and RNA polymerase formation.

Although several known antimicrobial agents disrupt the structure and function of DNA, few are utilized clinically because they lack selective toxicity.[5,7] There has been some recent use of these agents in neonates, but data regarding their safety and efficacy in this population are limited.[9] Examples of drugs from this class include sulfonamides, flucytosine, acyclovir, and zidovudine.[5]

Resistance to Antibiotics

Despite the success achieved in the struggle against infectious disease since the discovery of antibiotics, the ability of pathogens to develop resistance to various antibiotics is a serious threat to the continued efficacy of these agents.

Microorganisms exhibit resistance to drugs through several different mechanisms. Some bacteria produce enzymes that destroy the active drug. Others alter their structure to change or eliminate the drug's target or modify their metabolic pathway to effectively bypass the reaction inhibited by the drug. Still others develop an altered enzyme that can still perform its cellular function but that is less affected by the drug than the original enzyme was. Finally, the microorganism may alter its cellular permeability to the drug.[5,7]

Drug resistance may develop via random spontaneous mutation that results in an altered susceptibility to the drug. Once the mutation has taken place, exposure to the drug serves only to allow the growth of resistant organisms over sensitive organisms. A second way in which drug resistance may develop is when a resistance trait is genetically transmitted from a resistant cell to a sensitive one. Environmental exposure of host cells to antibiotics may favor the growth of drug-resistant pathogens that may then transfer their genetic resistance to previously sensitive pathogens. Infectious drug blockage of this kind is significant because it may result in resistance to multiple drugs. Multiple-drug resistance is now seen globally, making successful treatment of many bacterial infections difficult if not impossible.[5,7] Each nursery must study resistance patterns and restrict unnecessary use of broad-spectrum antibiotics to ensure appropriate use of antimicrobial therapy.

Principles of Antibiotic Pharmacology in the Neonate

Antibiotics administered to a newborn are distributed according to the drugs' own chemical and physical properties into the various compartments of the body, which are composed of water, fat, and protein. The rapidly shifting physiologic processes during the first few weeks of life dramatically affect the pharmacokinetic properties of these agents in newborns. Disease states and gestational age may also influence absorption, distribution, metabolism, and excretion of a drug. Therefore, the unique physiology of the term and preterm infant must be considered when establishing standards of safety and efficacy for antimicrobial products.[6]

Absorption

Absorption refers to the movement of a drug from its site of administration into the bloodstream. Absorption influences the time to achievement of peak plasma concentrations and their duration. Multiple unique characteristics may affect the newborn's oral absorption of antibiotics. These include, but are not limited to, alkaline gastric pH, prolonged gastric emptying and intestinal transit time, and decreased pancreatic enzyme activity.[6,10] The net effect of these features on the neonate's oral absorption is to make it quite variable—and therefore difficult to predict—compared with that of older infants and children. In addition, infant formula or milk products in the gastrointestinal (GI) tract may further increase gastric pH and delay absorption of acidic drugs. Diarrhea, caused by bacterial or viral infections, can further decrease drug absorption.[11] Diseases that limit available gastrointestinal surface area, such as short bowel syndrome, have the greatest negative impact on oral drug absorption.[10]

To bypass these absorptive barriers and decrease the time to achievement of therapeutic serum levels, the parenteral route of drug administration is recommended for treating neonatal sepsis. Intravenous (IV) drug delivery is preferred over intramuscular (IM) injection, which can be affected by vasomotor instability, decreased muscle tone, and oxygenation. In addition, the neonate's low ratio of skeletal muscle mass to body mass may adversely affect rate and extent of absorption of a drug delivered IM.[10,11]

Distribution

After a drug has been absorbed into the bloodstream, it is distributed into various body compartments, tissues, and cells. Several factors, including extracellular fluid volume, body composition, and plasma proteins, are important determinants of drug dosage and interval of administration in the neonate.

Extracellular fluid volume influences both the concentration and the effect of water-soluble drugs because the majority of these agents must pass through extracellular fluid to reach their receptors. Extracellular fluid volume decreases from 65 percent of body weight early in the third trimester to 40 percent at term, with a corresponding increase in intracellular water. Thus, for infants born prematurely, extracellular fluid volume is increased relative to total body water. For example, an infant born at 32 weeks gestation will have an extracellular fluid volume of approximately 53 percent compared to a total body water of 83 percent. The physiologic loss of approximately 10 percent of body weight during the first week after delivery reflects mobilization of both extracellular and intracellular fluid, with preterm neonates experiencing a more rapid and pronounced loss of total body water (10–15 percent). These shifts may have important implications for the use of antibiotics in newborns, particularly for drugs that are distributed primarily in the extracellular fluid. A premature neonate treated with an aminoglycoside, for example, would require a higher relative dose to achieve a desired serum concentration than would a term neonate.[9,11]

Body composition also affects the distribution of fat-soluble drugs. While body water decreases, body fat correspondingly increases. Adipose tissue is responsible for about 4 percent of the body weight of a preterm infant weighing 1,500 gm. Body fat to total body mass increases to approximately 13 percent at term. As the percentage of fat increases, so does the volume of distribution of lipophilic compounds. Therefore, distribution of these drugs is more limited in preterm than in term neonates.[9]

Because only free, unbound drug can act in the body, the extent to which a drug binds to plasma proteins alters both its action and effect. Levels of albumin and other plasma proteins are lower in infants than in older children and adults and are proportionately lower in preterm neonates. Moreover, neonatal proteins have less affinity for many drugs. As a result of reduced protein binding, drugs may reach higher than expected unbound serum levels. This may affect amounts of ampicillin, nafcillin, ceftriaxone, and chloramphenicol, to name a few, potentially intensifying both their therapeutic and their toxic effects.[9]

Drugs that bind to plasma proteins may also compete for binding sites with endogenous compounds, such as bilirubin, resulting in higher levels of free bilirubin in the serum. However, the extent of protein binding by an antibiotic does not always correlate with this potentially adverse reaction.[9] Once bilirubin is bound to protein, most antibiotic agents are unable to displace it because they have less binding affinity for albumin. Only sulfonamides, moxalactam, cefoperazone, and ceftriaxone have been shown to significantly displace bilirubin from albumin-binding sites.[6]

Metabolism

Many antibiotics undergo biotransformation before they are eliminated from the body. Biotransformation provides for more rapid clearance of the drug by converting it to a more polar, less lipid-soluble molecule. Although the chief organ for drug metabolism is the liver, the kidneys, intestine, lungs, and skin are also capable of biotransformation.

Neonates, whose liver represents 40 percent of their total body mass (compared with 2 percent in adults), have a much greater surface area for drug metabolism. At the same time, the relative immaturity of the neonatal liver and hepatic enzyme system inhibits drug metabolism. Furthermore, glucuronidation, which renders drugs more water soluble to assist in renal excretion, is decreased in newborns compared with older neonates and infants. Chloramphenicol-induced "gray baby syndrome" results from the neonate's reduced rate of glucuronide conjugation, leading to toxic accumulation of the drug and, ultimately, cardiovascular collapse. Newborns being treated with chloramphenicol must be given decreased dosages, and serum levels must be followed carefully.[10,11]

Despite the foregoing observations, the influences of gestational age, birth weight, illness, and other factors on drug metabolism in the neonate are not yet clearly defined.[10]

Excretion

Excretion refers to the movement of a drug or its metabolites from the tissues back into the circulation and finally into organs of elimination to be removed from the body. The chief pathway for elimination of antibiotics from the body is by renal excretion. This represents the net effect of glomerular filtration, tubular secretion, and tubular reabsorption.

A neonate's kidneys differ from an adult's in that they receive less cardiac output, have decreased renal plasma flow, have diminished tubular function, and also have a low glomerular filtration rate (GFR). The GFR of term infants is one-fourth that of adults, and the rate is lower than that of premature neonates. In infants ≥34 weeks gestation, GFR appears to increase in relation to postnatal age; whereas, in infants ≤34 weeks gestation, GFR increases with postconceptional age. Thus, both postconceptional and postnatal age must be considered when establishing guidelines for dose and frequency of administration of antibiotics in preterm infants.[9–11]

There is a significant increase in renal function during the first two weeks of life. This change may have a profound impact on antibiotic pharmacokinetics. Neonates, especially preterm infants, may experience sustained serum concentrations and prolonged half-life values of many drugs in the first days and weeks of life. For example, the half-life of β-lactam antibiotics is two times higher in a two-week-old infant than in an adult.[6] Because renal function changes continuously during the first month of life, determinations of drug dosage and frequency must take each infant's specific timetable into account.

Renal development, renal diseases, or coexisting illnesses that further decrease renal blood flow may also profoundly affect dosing requirements.[10] Dosage and frequency must be scrupulously defined when administering antibiotic agents to newborn infants.

SELECTION OF ANTIMICROBIAL AGENTS

In any infant in whom sepsis is suspected, antimicrobial therapy should be initiated as soon as the diagnostic evaluation has been completed. Disease progression in the neonatal population is far too swift to await confirmation from blood or other cultures. The choice of antimicrobial agents should be based on a variety of factors. These include timing and setting of the disease, prevalent organisms and their patterns of antimicrobial susceptibility, site of the suspected infection, penetration of the specific antibiotic to that site, and safety of the antibiotic.[3,9]

For early-onset disease, initial therapy should provide coverage for Gram-positive cocci and Gram-negative enteric bacilli, particularly Group B Streptococcus (GBS) and *Escherichia coli*, as well as *Listeria monocytogenes*. Treatment for late-onset disease (acquired after day 4 of life) must include coverage for nosocomially acquired microbes. These include *Staphylococcus aureus*, *Staphylococcus epidermidis*, and Gram-negative enteric bacilli such as Pseudomonas species.[1,3] In certain clinical circumstances, addition of other antibiotics may be considered. For example, coverage for anaerobic organisms may be warranted if bowel perforation or peritonitis is suspected.[12]

It is important to verify the susceptibility of microorganisms isolated from culture and to adjust coverage as necessary. Most commonly, the duration of therapy is a minimum of 7–10 days for bacterial sepsis and 21 days for meningitis caused by GBS or Gram-negative enteric bacilli. In the absence of positive cultures at 72 hours, a clinical decision is usually made whether to continue treatment for neonatal sepsis.[1]

The most common antimicrobial agents used to treat neonatal infection and sepsis are discussed in this section. Appendix D provides additional information on antibiotic agents, including doses.

Antibiotics Used in Neonatal Infection

Aminoglycosides

The aminoglycosides have been used extensively for therapy of neonatal sepsis and meningitis because of their broad-spectrum antibacterial activity against Gram-negative enteric pathogens. Aminoglycosides are bactericidal agents that act by disrupting normal protein synthesis in the bacterial cell. However, because of their low therapeutic index and the emergence of aminoglycoside-resistant strains among Gram-negative enteric bacilli, many neonatal units have limited their use.[3,9]

Among aminoglycosides, gentamicin and tobramycin are the drugs of choice in most nurseries. Amikacin is also suitable for use in the neonatal population, but it is frequently reserved for

FIGURE 8-1 ♦ The structure of penicillin.

The common portion of all penicillins is 6-APA. This molecule occurs naturally (R_1 = penicillin G) or may be modified at "R" to produce a variety of "synthetic" penicillins, such as R_2 = methicillin, R_3 = ampicillin.

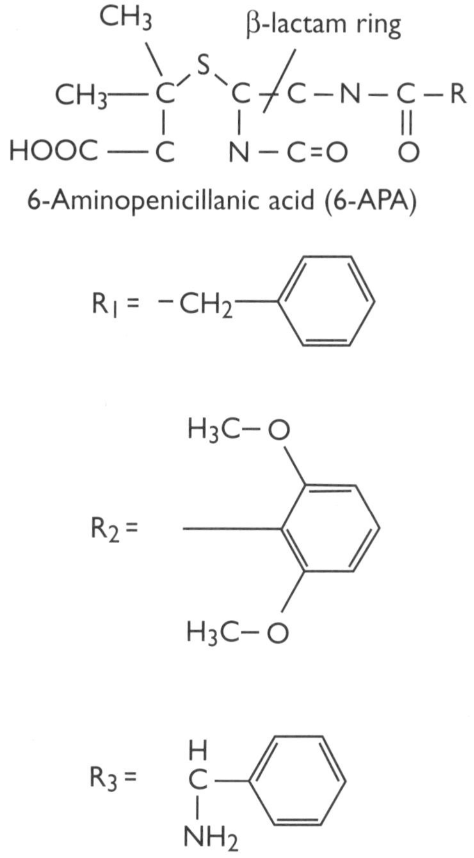

6-Aminopenicillanic acid (6-APA)

From: Burton GRW. 2000. *Microbiology for the Health Sciences*, 6th ed. Philadelphia: Lippincott Williams & Wilkins, 127. Reprinted by permission.

treatment of infections caused by multiply-resistant organisms because it is less likely to be degraded by the bacterial enzymes that inactivate gentamicin and tobramycin.[3,9] In nurseries that have experienced a heightened resistance to gentamicin, amikacin may be used as a primary drug for treatment of virulent Gram-negative infections. There is no consistent evidence that exclusive use of amikacin increases the emergence of resistant bacterial strains.[3,9]

When combined with penicillins, aminoglycosides provide synergistic bacterial activity *in vitro* against enterococci, GBS, *L. monocytogenes*, *S. aureus*, and some Gram-negative enteric rods.[6] Serum levels should be observed after five half-lives or after three to five doses have been administered and thereafter to document adjustments to maintain appropriate levels.[9] Although aminoglycosides have been implicated as contributing to ototoxicity in neonates, the risk of toxicity has been proved to be minimal when these agents are administered in the proper dosage and when serum concentrations are closely monitored and maintained within the recommended therapeutic range.[3,9]

β-*Lactam Antibiotics*

The unique β-lactam ring contained in their chemical structure defines the antibiotics in the β-lactam group, which includes the penicillins and the cephalosporins (Figure 8-1). The β-lactams exert their bactericidal effects by binding to specific targets on the cytoplasmic membrane. These targets are bacterial enzymes involved in cell wall synthesis and are known as penicillin-binding proteins (PBPs). Because PBPs catalyze the final cross-linking of the cell wall structure, inhibition of this process leads to a loss of cell wall integrity, and cell lysis ultimately ensues.[5]

Resistance to β-lactam antibiotics may be attributed to a variety of mechanisms, including inactivation of the drug, alteration of the target site, and blockage of the drug's transport into the cell. β-lactamases, enzymes that split the β-lactam ring of the penicillins and cephalosporins to form inactive compounds, constitute the primary mode of bacterial resistance. β-lactamases are responsible for many resistant strains of Gram-positive and Gram-negative bacteria, including most staphylococci and enteric Gram-negative bacilli as well as many *Neisseria gonorrhoeae* strains. In fact, semisynthetic penicillins and cephalosporins were developed in an effort to find compounds that β-lactamase could not counteract.[5,10]

Resistance may also be mediated by alteration in the PBPs, as in penicillin resistance in *Streptococcus pneumoniae* and *N. gonorrhoeae*. Finally, the antibiotic must pass through the cell wall to reach the susceptible PBPs located on the cytoplasmic membrane. Although the cell wall of Gram-positive bacteria does not present a major barrier to drug entry, the complex outer membrane of Gram-negative bacteria may retard or restrict access.[5,10] In a phenomenon known as tolerance, some GBS organisms are inhibited but not killed by penicillin.[3]

Penicillin and semisynthetic penicillins. Penicillin is one of the oldest and most widely used drugs for treatment of neonatal bacterial infection. It is a safe and effective choice for treatment against streptococci, susceptible pneumococci, meningococci, susceptible gonococci, and *Treponema pallidum*.[6,9] Ampicillin is the penicillin usually administered (in combination with an aminoglycoside) as initial empiric therapy for neonatal sepsis and meningitis because of its safety and broad antimicrobial coverage. Ampicillin is more effective than penicillin against most strains of enterococci and *L. monocytogenes*, as well as some Gram-negative pathogens. However, it is less efficacious against Groups A and B streptococci or susceptible strains of staphylococci and pneumococci. Ampicillin and gentamicin have demonstrated synergistic activity against enterococci, *L. monocytogenes*, and GBS.[5,6,9]

Anti-staphylococcal penicillins are useful for infections caused by susceptible *S. aureus* or *S. epidermidis*. This class of drugs includes nafcillin and oxacillin. Also known as penicillinase-resistant penicillins, these antistaphylococcal penicillins block inactivation by most staphylococcal β-lactamases as the result of a substituted side chain in the β-lactam ring that hinders the enzyme's attachment.[5,6]

Anti-pseudomonas penicillins, which include the carboxypenicillins and the acylampicillins, are semisynthetic penicillins with increased activity against *Pseudomonas aeruginosa*. The carboxypenicillins, including ticarcillin, are also more active against strains of Enterobacter, Serratia, and certain strains of Proteus that are not susceptible to the earlier penicillins.[5] Ticarcillin demonstrates increased activity against *P. aeruginosa* when compared with carbenicillin.[6] Its primary use in the newborn is in treating serious Gram-negative infections, including those caused by *P. aeruginosa*, in combination with an aminoglycoside. Clavulinic acid, a powerful inhibitor of several bacterial β-lactamases, substantially enhances the activity of ticarcillin against Gram-negative enteric organisms, anaerobes, and methicillin-susceptible *S. aureus*. Limited clinical use suggests that the administration of ticarcillin-clavulanate, usually in combination with an aminoglycoside, may provide safe and efficacious treatment against serious nosocomially acquired Gram-negative infection, making it potentially very useful in the neonatal population.[5,6,9]

The acylampicillins, another class of antipseudomonas penicillins, include mezlocillin, azlocillin, and piperacillin. These drugs display activity against a wide range of Gram-positive and Gram-negative bacteria. Their most important feature is activity against *P. aeruginosa*, and of the three, piperacillin is the most effective against this organism. These drugs are useful against enterococci and many anaerobes, including *Bacteroides fragilis*. When used in combination with an aminoglycoside, they provide valuable treatment for multiresistant Gram-negative enteric organisms such as Enterobacter and *Serratia marcescens*.[5,6,9]

Renal function should be monitored routinely when penicillins are administered parenterally because elimination occurs primarily via the kidneys. Because reversible bone-marrow suppression may be associated with high-dose therapy, white blood cell (WBC) counts should be observed once or twice weekly during the course of treatment.[6,9]

Cephalosporins. The cephalosporins are widely used β-lactam antibiotics that are similar to the penicillins in structure and mode of action. They are classified into generations based on the general features of their antimicrobial activity rather than their time of introduction into clinical use. The role of first- and second-generation cephalosporins is limited in neonates. However, the third-generation cephalosporins, which include cefotaxime, ceftriaxone, and ceftazidime, have proved to be efficacious in the treatment of neonatal infections because of their notably enhanced activity against enteric Gram-negative bacilli. Although they have excellent activity against Enterobacteriaceae, they are not suitable as monotherapy for empiric treatment of presumed sepsis because of their limited activity against staphylococci and other Gram-positive organisms. In addition, none of the third-generation cephalosporins is active against *L. monocytogenes* or enterococci.[5,6,9]

The third-generation cephalosporins are effective when used alone or in combination with an aminoglycoside for the treatment of serious infections, including meningitis caused by Gram-negative organisms. The appropriateness of using a third-generation cephalosporin in combination with ampicillin as routine initial coverage for suspected sepsis has been challenged because of the potential for rapidly developing resistance in the presence of a large reservoir of organisms. Exposure of some Gram-negative bacteria, such as *P. aeruginosa* or *Enterobacter cloacae*, to these agents can result in a uniform resistance to all third-generation cephalosporins via production of chromosomally mediated, highly powerful β-lactamases.[6,9]

The third-generation cephalosporins are primarily excreted by the kidneys. Serum creatinine and WBC count with differential should be monitored in infants receiving parenteral therapy because of the potential for renal or bone marrow toxicity.[6,9]

Carbapenems. Imipenem is a member of a comparatively new class of β-lactam antibiotics, the carbapenems. These agents have a remarkably wide spectrum of activity against Gram-positive and Gram-negative bacteria, including anaerobes.[6,9] *Stenotrophomonas maltophilia* (formerly referred to as *Pseudomonas maltophilia*), *Enterococcus faecium*, and *Pseudomonas cepacia* are the only three antimicrobial species that have demonstrated resistance against the carbapenems.[9]

Imipenem is generally well tolerated; however, a high incidence of seizure activity noted after its use for treatment of bacterial meningitis in infants has resulted in its judicious use in infants and children. Carbapenems should be used only when the infectious agent has demonstrated resistance to other classes of antibiotics.[6,9,13]

Clindamycin

The primary role of clindamycin in antibacterial therapy for the neonate is in the treatment of infections caused by anaerobes, including *B. fragilis*. Clindamycin is a bacteriostatic agent and is generally used with other antimicrobials. For example, empiric therapy for necrotizing enterocolitis often consists of a regimen including ampicillin or vancomycin, an aminoglycoside, and clindamycin. Indications for use include treatment of bacteremia, pulmonary and other deep-tissue infections, and peritonitis.[9,12]

The drug's serum half-life is prolonged in preterm neonates less than four weeks of age, but term infants demonstrate half-life values comparable to those published for adults. Elimination is by hepatic inactivation and renal excretion; therefore, liver function should be monitored. Adverse effects are rare.[9]

Vancomycin

Vancomycin is a narrow-spectrum, bactericidal antibiotic active against staphylococci, streptococci, enterococci, and other Gram-positive bacteria. Vancomycin is a complex glycopeptide that interferes with bacterial cell wall synthesis, alters plasma membrane function, and inhibits RNA synthesis. It is used extensively to treat nosocomial infections caused by methicillin-resistant staphylococci and is the drug of choice for documented infections caused by *S. epidermidis* and other coagulase-negative staphylococci.[5,6,9] Vancomycin has customarily been used along with a third-generation cephalosporin for initial empiric therapy of suspected nosocomial late-onset sepsis in the neonate. Recently, however, the striking rise in vancomycin-resistant enterococci and global concern that vancomycin resistance may extend to include other Gram-positive organisms such as staphylococci, should discourage its use for empiric therapy of neonatal sepsis and antimicrobial prophylaxis of very low birth weight infants.[6]

Although initial experience with vancomycin suggested a moderate incidence of ototoxicity and nephrotoxicity, more recent evidence indicates that the drug is well tolerated and safe when administered intravenously, particularly in neonates. The drug is not metabolized by the body and is eliminated unchanged in the urine.[5,6,9]

Serum levels should be observed after the fifth half-life or third to fifth dose, and renal function should be monitored.[6,9]

Antifungal-Agent Therapy

Because of the increasing complexity of neonatal care, disseminated candidiasis is occurring with increasing frequency, especially in preterm infants. Growing use of corticosteroids, broad-spectrum antibiotics, and central venous catheters in the treatment of very low birth weight infants has been associated with escalating systemic fungal infection.[14] Early recognition and treatment of these infections are of the utmost importance in ameliorating morbidity and mortality in this patient population.

Antifungal drugs may be divided into three basic categories: amphotericin B, flucytosine, and the imidazole derivatives fluconazole and itraconazole. Itraconazole has not been used extensively in children. Although amphotericin B is the broadest spectrum of these drugs, it is also the most toxic. Flucytosine has a narrow spectrum of activity and is usually used in combination with amphotericin B.[15]

Amphotericin B

Despite its toxicity, amphotericin B is the antimicrobial agent of choice for severe fungal infections. It binds with ergosterol and other sterols in the fungal cell membrane and disrupts cellular integrity, ultimately resulting in lysis of the cell. Drug resistance develops slowly, perhaps as a result of a decreased concentration of ergosterol in the cell membrane.[15]

Amphotericin B has a wide spectrum of activity and is effective for many varieties of cutaneous, mucocutaneous, deep-tissue, and disseminated fungal infections. Because it is not absorbed well from the gastrointestinal tract, it is used intravenously to treat systemic fungal infections and severe superficial mycoses.

Amphotericin B is not well distributed into the CSF following intravenous administration. Therefore, infants with fungal meningitis may require intrathecal administration of the drug.[15,16]

Dosing guidelines have been established based largely on data from studies of older children and adults; there has been little research in neonates or infants. Because the pharmacokinetics of amphotericin B are predictable, it is not suggested that serum levels be obtained as a guide to therapy.[16]

There have been few studies on the toxicity of amphotericin B in infants and children; however, available data suggest that toxicity is probably similar to that in adults, who frequently experience nausea, vomiting, headache, chills, and fever during infusion of the drug.[16] Additionally, potential adverse effects include decreased renal blood flow and glomerular filtration rate; damage to tubular epithelium, with resultant urinary loss of potassium; decreased reabsorption of sodium; renal tubular acidosis; and nephrocalcinosis. Seizures or cardiac arrhythmias may occur if the drug is administered too rapidly or if the dose is too concentrated. Pretreatment with an analgesic prior to infusion is recommended. Other reported adverse effects include bone marrow suppression, eosinophilia, GI bleeding, skin rash, liver failure, flushing, and anaphylaxis. Renal and hepatic function, blood counts, and serum electrolytes should be monitored carefully for the duration of the therapy.[11,16]

Liposomal Amphotericin B

There are three lipid formulations of amphotericin B currently available in the U.S. These include amphotericin B lipid complex, amphotericin B colloidal dispersion, and liposomal amphotericin B. Although the lipid formulations are significantly more expensive than conventional amphotericin B, they have been reported to reduce toxicity and to increase efficacy and clinical tolerance.[17,18]

Liposomal amphotericin B consists of amphotericin B within a bilayer liposomal drug delivery system and may be used for treatment of systemic fungal infections resistant to conventional amphotericin B or for patients with renal or hepatic dysfunction.[15] Its uptake by macrophages and transport to infected areas appear to play major parts in increasing efficacy and reducing toxicity.[13,19,20]

In one study, researchers found that liposomal amphotericin B was not associated with fever, chills, or phlebitis. Hematologic parameters remained within normal limits. Sixteen of 40 infants did experience hypokalemia.[19] The initial dose of liposomal amphotericin B is 1 mg/kg; the dose is increased by 1 mg/kg each day to a maximum dose of 5 mg/kg every 24 hours. The infusion is administered over 2 hours. The higher doses are used in treating meningitis and osteoarthritis. Despite reports of minimal side effects, serum electrolytes, creatinine, blood urea nitrogen (BUN), and complete blood count (CBC) should be monitored.[13]

Amphotericin B lipid complex and amphotericin B colloidal dispersion may also be used as alternative therapy for fungal infections when amphotericin B is contraindicated because of impaired renal function or concomitant use of other nephrotoxic agents and in cases of treatment failure.[17,21] These formulations have been found to be safe and well tolerated in preterm infants with invasive fungal infections and renal dysfunction.[17,21]

Flucytosine

Flucytosine (5-fluorocytosine) is a fluorine analog of cytosine, a normal body constituent. Its mechanisms of action include interference with DNA synthesis and cell growth. Flucytosine has a narrow spectrum of activity but is active against many fungi, including Candida and Cryptococcus. There are data that suggest synergism with amphotericin B, resulting in an augmented antifungal effect.[15,16]

Flucytosine is well absorbed from the GI tract; levels in the CSF range from 60 to 90 percent of the serum values.[15,16] Flucytosine has been used extensively in infants, usually in conjunction with amphotericin B. It is recommended as an adjunctive therapy to amphotericin B for treatment of cryptococcal meningitis, and some have suggested this combination for patients with Candida meningitis or neonatal candidiasis.

Toxicity includes transient neutropenia and hepatocellular damage. Other adverse effects include severe diarrhea and rash. However, few untoward side effects have been noted, even with prolonged use. Because the drug is excreted by the kidneys, dosages must be monitored and reduced in infants with renal impairment.[15,16] Renal and hepatic function and WBC counts should be monitored periodically during treatment.[11]

Fluconazole

The imidazole-derived antifungal agent fluconazole may be administered either orally or intravenously. It acts by inhibition of fungal ergosterol synthesis. Fluconazole has been shown to penetrate well into body tissues, including CSF and skin. It is effective in the treatment of systemic infections, meningitis, and severe superficial mycoses caused by Candida species. It has also been shown to be effective against Coccidioides and dermatophytes.[16]

Adverse reactions may include headache, nausea, vomiting, diarrhea, elevated liver enzyme levels, rash, and anaphylaxis.[11] Because the drug is excreted primarily by the kidneys, dosages must be monitored and reduced in infants with renal impairment.[15,16] Renal and hepatic function should be monitored periodically during treatment.[11]

Antiviral Agent Therapy

The past decade has seen remarkable progress in the treatment of viral diseases in adults. Unfortunately, the development of antiviral medications for children, especially neonates, has lagged seriously. Antiviral drugs target the steps of viral replication that are regulated by virus-specific enzymes and that are independent of host cell substrates. Because viruses utilize host cell machinery and closely mimic host cell replication, many antiviral agents tend to have a low therapeutic index and high levels of toxicity.

Although the newborn can suffer from numerous viral infections for which therapies currently exist, this discussion focuses on four drugs used in the treatment of herpes simplex virus (HSV), varicella-zoster virus (VZV), cytomegalovirus (CMV), and human immunodeficiency virus (HIV). These drugs are all purine nucleoside analogs that act by incorporating themselves into the nucleic acids of viral DNA or RNA, where they cause abnormal transcription and translation, leading to loss of viral infectivity. They also act by phosphorylation to triphosphates that inhibit DNA and RNA polymerases.[22]

Acyclovir

Acyclovir, an acyclic analog of guanosine, has demonstrated significant *in vitro* antiviral activity against herpesviruses, especially HSV and VZV.[23] Acyclovir is available in three forms: intravenous, oral, and topical. It is excreted primarily unchanged by glomerular filtration, with the remainder being excreted by tubular secretion.[11]

Because acyclovir is taken up selectively by virus-infected cells, it has a very low toxicity for normal host cells. It therefore has an excellent safety profile and is well tolerated. The primary adverse effect of acyclovir is alteration of renal function. Dehydration, preexisting renal insufficiency, and high doses of acyclovir are risk factors for renal toxicity. Adequate hydration of the infant during treatment may decrease the potential for this adverse effect. In infants with renal insufficiency, dosage adjustments are required.[11,22,23]

Although there have been reports of central nervous system (CNS) toxicity after IV administration of acyclovir, this has not been documented in the newborn. However, oral administration has been associated with neutropenia in the neonatal population. Other reported toxicities, although rare, include bone marrow suppression, serum transaminase elevation, and allergic reactions. Phlebitis at the IV site has also been observed.[11,22,23]

Vidarabine

When phosphorylated to its active form, vidarabine blocks viral DNA synthesis by inhibiting viral DNA polymerase. This drug has established clinical efficacy against infections with HSV-1, HSV-2, and VZV and has been utilized intravenously to treat neonatal HSV infections and herpes simplex encephalitis. IV administration of vidarabine requires dilution in large volumes of fluid and infusion over 12–18 hours. The large fluid volumes needed for dilution prevent its intramuscular use. It cannot be administered orally because intestinal absorption causes the drug to be deaminated. Because there are no significant differences in outcomes between acyclovir and vidarabine in the treatment of neonatal HSV infection, the safety and ease of administration of acyclovir support its recommendation as the treatment of choice.[23]

Topical preparations of vidarabine are available for ophthalmic use and are effective for the treatment of the acute keratoconjunctivitis that frequently accompanies HSV infection in the newborn. Potential adverse reactions include temporary burning, mild irritation, pain, conjunctival injection, punctal occlusion, superficial punctate keratitis, and photophobia.[11]

Ganciclovir

Ganciclovir is a derivative of acyclovir that contains an additional hydroxymethyl group on its side chain. It competitively inhibits viral DNA polymerase and may be incorporated within viral DNA to cause early termination of DNA replication. This drug is active against CMV, HSV, and VZV. Although acyclovir remains the drug of choice for treatment of congenital HSV and VZV, ganciclovir is the only medication under evaluation for the treatment of congenital CMV.[23] Because cellular kinases convert the drug to ganciclovir triphosphate, it preferentially concentrates in CMV-infected cells. The drug must be given intravenously because it is poorly absorbed after oral administration. The primary route of drug elimination is via the kidneys, and it is excreted 90 percent unchanged.[11,22]

Ganciclovir has been shown to cause clinically significant neutropenia and thrombocytopenia in clinical trials; and, unlike acyclovir, it is mutagenic, teratogenic, and carcinogenic. Other adverse reactions include nausea, vomiting, hepatitis, and CNS dysfunction with disorientation and psychosis. Allergic reactions with skin rash and eosinophilia have also been reported. Phlebitis and local pain with severe tissue reaction have been observed after extravasation of IV-administered ganciclovir. Because of its toxicity profile, it should be used only for newborns with severe symptomatic infection. A CBC must be closely monitored for the duration of therapy.[11,22,23]

Zidovudine

Zidovudine is a nucleoside analog that inhibits HIV replication by interfering with viral reverse transcriptase, an enzyme essential for retroviral DNA synthesis. Zidovudine is converted inside the cell to an active triphosphate compound, metabolized via hepatic glucuronidation, and renally excreted. It is available as an oral syrup, which is well absorbed but only 65 percent bioavailable as a result of significant first-pass metabolism. The intravenous form of the drug must be diluted to a concentration not exceeding 4 mg/ml prior to administration. Adverse effects include anemia and neutropenia, which occur frequently during therapy and must be carefully monitored. Headaches, nausea, myalgia, and insomnia are also common.[11,22,23]

Zidovudine was the first drug licensed for the treatment of HIV/AIDS. The seminal antiviral trial, PACTG 076, indicated that zidovudine reduced the incidence of HIV transmission from 25 percent to 8 percent when pregnant women were treated beginning at 20 weeks gestation, as well as intravenously during delivery, and the newborn was treated during the first six weeks of life. Although these data are encouraging, the potential for long-term toxicities in the mother and the newborn is under investigation.[23]

ADJUNCTIVE THERAPIES FOR NEONATAL SEPSIS

Neonates face multiple challenges from potentially infectious pathogens both during and after birth. This is complicated by compromised immunity in the term newborn, with preterm infants being even more susceptible to serious infection. Because the newborn's innate mechanisms for combating infection are not fully developed, early and effective therapy for preventing and treating sepsis is imperative. Several adjunctive therapies targeted at augmenting host defenses are being investigated for use in conjunction with conventional management to improve the outcome of neonatal sepsis. This section briefly describes the most promising of these therapies.

Intravenous Immunoglobulin

Of the immunoglobulins (IgG, IgA, IgM, IgD, and IgE), IgG is the only one that is actively transported across the placenta to the fetus. This process begins after 32 weeks gestation; therefore, infants born before that time have significantly diminished serum IgG levels. Because endogenous synthesis does not commence until about 24 weeks after birth, serum levels continue to decrease in the infant as maternally derived antibodies are utilized postnatally. Moreover, transplacentally acquired antibodies are limited in function to the specific organisms to which the mother has been exposed. Immunoglobulins are an important constituent of the immune response to infections involving encapsulated organisms, such as GBS and *E. coli*, and the mother may lack these antibodies.[2,24]

These immunologic deficiencies have prompted investigators to study the efficacy of intravenous immune globulin (IGIV) for the prevention and treatment of neonatal infections. The commercially available IGIV preparation used in the majority of studies is a plasma-derived, concentrated form of IgG antibodies pooled from a donor population. There are substantial functional differences between immunoglobulin preparations from different manufacturers, as well as between lots from the same manufacturer. Thus, various IGIV products may have significantly different antibody titers to specific pathogens, especially to GBS infection. Furthermore, differences in populations of infants, predominant pathogens, study design, and IGIV dosage and schedule make the conflicting findings of these studies difficult to assess.[2,24]

Hyperimmune and human monoclonal antibody preparations have been developed to decrease the variability of pathogen-specific antibody among different lots and products of IGIV.[24] These preparations target five serotypes of GBS. In an animal model comparing these type-specific GBS antibody compounds against standard IGIV for GBS sepsis, the type-specific preparations showed higher protective activities against serotypes Ia, II, and III than did standard IGIV. These protective activities were sustained even when lower doses of the monoclonal and hyperimmune globulins were compared with higher doses of standard IGIV.[25]

When used as prophylaxis or adjunctive therapy for infection in the neonate, IGIV has been shown to be safe, with minimal short-term adverse effects. However, animal data indicate that IGIV may suppress the immune response when given in high doses.[26,27] In addition, an outbreak of hepatitis C associated with administration of IGIV caused manufacturers to more closely supervise virucidal processing of their product.[28] Large, prospective, randomized, placebo-controlled trials must be completed to rule out potential complications and long-term problems with this therapy.

Review of currently available data suggests that IGIV cannot be recommended for routine treatment or prevention of neonatal bacterial infection. Certain clinical situations, such as sick preterm infants with overwhelming infection or preterm infants with low IgG levels and recurrent infection, may warrant its consideration.[2,24]

As noted previously, IGIV products that are pathogen-specific must be developed and tested carefully in large trials. A randomized trial of 510 children with bronchopulmonary dysplasia and/or prematurity who received monthly prophylaxis with respiratory syncytial virus immune globulin (RSV-IGIV) demonstrated promising results. RSV-IGIV was shown to be safe and well tolerated, and it reduced hospitalizations by 41 percent in children receiving the treatment.[29] As a result, RSV-IGIV has been approved by the U.S. Food and Drug Administration for prevention of severe RSV infections in infants <24 months with bronchopulmonary dysplasia and/or prematurity.[30]

Granulocyte Transfusions

Septic neonates are often neutropenic because of decreased bone marrow neutrophil reserves and circulating-pool depletion. In addition to this quantitative deficiency, qualitative deficiencies include decreased chemotaxis, impaired opsonization, decreased phagocytosis, and diminished bactericidal activity.[24] Granulocyte transfusions have been investigated in an attempt to decrease the high mortality rate among neutropenic septic neonates.

The results of numerous investigations of granulocyte transfusion for neonates with sepsis have been inconsistent.[31–35] Most of these studies have been uncontrolled and have differed in the patient populations, the choice of granulocyte preparation, and the timing and frequency of granulocyte transfusions, making them difficult to compare. In a pilot study, Cairo and colleagues established that granulocyte transfusions were more efficacious than IGIV in the adjuvant treatment of infants with neutropenia and overwhelming bacterial sepsis. This report also noted, however, that granulocyte transfusions have several potentially life-threatening complications, such as fluid overload, transmission of infectious agents, pulmonary insufficiency, alloimmunization, and graft-versus-host disease.[36] Because of these concerns, as well as the high costs of obtaining purified granulocytes, this treatment cannot currently be recommended as a standard of care.[2,24]

Colony-Stimulating Factors G-CSF and GM-CSF

Colony-stimulating factors (CSFs) are glycoprotein hormones that regulate the proliferation and differentiation of myeloid progenitor cells and the function of mature blood cells. They stimulate the reproduction of myeloid colonies and the release of neutrophils from storage pools. It has also been demonstrated that these factors augment chemotaxis and the phagocytic killing function of mature cells.[2,24] Initially described in the 1960s, these proteins have been cloned in bacteria and cell lines and are being investigated for prophylaxis and treatment of neonatal sepsis.[24] These factors include granulocyte colony-stimulating factor (G-CSF) and granulocyte-monocyte colony-stimulating factor (GM-CSF).

G-CSF has been utilized in newborn infants with presumed sepsis because of its potential to ameliorate the neutropenia associated with sepsis and to improve neutrophil function. The results of a randomized, placebo-controlled trial of 42 infants <72 hours of age with suspected sepsis revealed that G-CSF induced a significant dose-dependent increase in peripheral blood and bone marrow absolute neutrophil concentration and in functional activation of neutrophils (C3bi expression) with no acute toxicity.[37] At two-year follow-up, no long-term adverse effects were noted.[38]

Use of GM-CSF for seven days in 20 very low birth weight neonates at 72 hours of age was investigated in a randomized, placebo-controlled trial. Results showed increased absolute neutrophil count, absolute monocyte count, platelet count, C3bi expression, and bone-marrow neutrophil-storage pool.[39] Prophylactic administration of GM-CSF in preterm infants <1,000 gm is being studied to determine if it reduces the incidence of nosocomial infection in this high-risk population.[24]

Based on current evidence, G-CSF and GM-CSF may be appropriate agents for adjuvant treatment in neonatal sepsis.[24] Large, prospective, randomized, placebo-controlled trials are needed to replicate the results of earlier studies before these therapies can be recommended for routine use.

SUMMARY

Neonatal sepsis continues to be associated with high morbidity and mortality, especially in ill and preterm neonates. Developmental changes that occur during the newborn period affect the cause of bacterial infections, an infant's response to infection, the agents used for treatment, and the pharmacologic properties of antimicrobial agents. These factors make early identification and effective pharmacologic management of infection one of the greatest challenges in neonatal care.

Designing an optimal therapeutic regimen requires a thorough understanding of the pharmacology of the drug being considered as well as the unique physiology of the neonate being treated. Adjunctive therapies, targeted at augmenting defenses of the immunocompromised neonate, also offer potential strategies for treatment and prevention of infection. As continued research affords a greater understanding of the complexities of neonatal infection and sepsis, an increasingly effective array of treatment strategies will improve morbidity and mortality.

REFERENCES

1. Klein JO, and Marcy SM. 2001. Bacterial sepsis and meningitis. In *Infectious Diseases of the Fetus and Newborn Infant*, 5th ed., Remington JS, and Klein JO, eds. Philadelphia: WB Saunders, 943–998.
2. Bellanti J, Ziligs B, and Pung YH. 1999. Immunology of the fetus and newborn. In *Neonatology: Pathophysiology and Management of the Newborn*, 5th ed., Avery G, Fletcher MA, and MacDonald M, eds. Philadelphia: Lippincott Williams & Wilkins, 1093–1121.
3. Hickey SM, and McCracken G. 2002. Postnatal bacterial infections. In *Neonatal-Perinatal Medicine: Diseases of the Fetus and Infant*, 7th ed., Fanaroff AA, and Martin RJ, eds. St. Louis: Mosby-Year Book, 706–745.
4. Coles FS. 1998. Immunology. In *Avery's Diseases of the Newborn*, 7th ed., Taeusch HW, and Ballard RA, eds. Philadelphia: WB Saunders, 435–452.
5. Willett HP. 1992. Antimicrobial agents. In *Zinsser Microbiology*, 20th ed., Joklik WD, et al., eds. Norwalk, Connecticut: Appleton & Lange, 153–187.
6. Saez-Llorens X, and McCracken GH. 2001. Clinical pharmacology of antibacterial agents. In *Infectious Diseases of the Fetus and Newborn Infant*, 5th ed., Remington JS, and Klein JO, eds. Philadelphia: WB Saunders, 1419–1466.
7. Murray PR, et al. 2002. *Medical Microbiology*, 4th ed. St. Louis: Mosby-Year Book, 11–24, 186, 215.
8. Burton GRW. 2000. *Microbiology for the Health Sciences*, 6th ed. Philadelphia: Lippincott Williams & Wilkins, 123–139.
9. Edwards MS. 1997. Antibacterial therapy in pregnancy and neonates. In *Clinics in Perinatology: Infections in Perinatology*, Stoll BJ, and Weisman LE, eds. Philadelphia: WB Saunders, 251–266.
10. Blumer JL, and Reed MD. 1992. Principles of neonatal pharmacology. In *Pediatric Pharmacology: Therapeutic Principles in Practice*, 3rd ed., Yaffe SJ, and Aranda JV, eds. Philadelphia: WB Saunders, 164–177.
11. Chestnut DH. 2000. *Handbook of Pediatric Drug Therapy*, 2nd ed. Springhouse, Pennsylvania: Springhouse, 1–4, 325–327.
12. Cavaliere T. 1995. Pharmacological treatment of neonatal sepsis: Antimicrobial agents and immunotherapy. *Journal of Obstetric, Gynecologic, and Neonatal Nursing* 24(7): 647–658.
13. Taketomo C, Hodding J, and Kraus D. 2003. *Pediatric Dosage Handbook*., 10th ed., Hudson, Ohio: Lexi-Comp, 98–103, 595–597.
14. Edwards MS. 2002. Fungal and protozoal infections. In *Neonatal-Perinatal Medicine: Diseases of the Fetus and Infant*, 7th ed., Fanaroff AA, and Martin RJ, eds. St. Louis: Mosby-Year Book, 745–754.
15. Lebel MH, Lebel P, and Mills EL. 1992. Antifungal agents for systemic mycotic infections. In *Pediatric Pharmacology: Therapeutic Principles in Practice*, 3rd ed., Yaffe SJ, and Aranda JV, eds. Philadelphia: WB Saunders, 261–275.
16. Miller MJ. 2001. Fungal infections. In *Infectious Diseases of the Fetus and Newborn Infant*, 5th ed., Remington JS, and Klein JO, eds. Philadelphia: WB Saunders, 813–853.
17. Robinson RF, and Nahata MC. 1999. A comparative review of conventional and lipid formulations of amphotericin B. *Journal of Clinical Pharmacy and Therapeutics* 24(4): 249–257.
18. Koren G, et al. 1988. Pharmacokinetics and adverse effects of amphotericin B in infants and children. *Journal of Pediatrics* 113(3): 559–563.
19. Scarella A, et al. 1998. Liposomal amphotericin B treatment for neonatal fungal infections. *Pediatric Infectious Disease Journal* 17(2): 146–148.
20. Hiemenz JW, and Walsh TJ. 1996. Lipid formulations of amphotericin B: Recent progress and future directions. *Clinical Infectious Diseases* 22(supplement 2): S133–S144.
21. Linder N, et al. 2003. Treatment of candidaemia in premature infants: Comparison of three amphotericin B preparations. *Journal of Antimicrobial Chemotherapy* 52(4): 663–667.
22. Patel JA, and Ogra PL. 1992. Antiviral chemotherapy. In *Pediatric Pharmacology: Therapeutic Principles in Practice*, 3rd ed., Yaffe SJ, and Aranda JV, eds. Philadelphia: WB Saunders, 365–389.
23. Whitley RJ, and Kimberlin DW. 1997. Treatment of viral infections during pregnancy and the neonatal period. In *Clinics in Perinatology: Infections in Perinatology*, Stoll BJ, and Weisman LE, eds. Philadelphia: WB Saunders, 267–283.

24. Perez EM, and Weisman LE. 1997. Novel approaches to the prevention and therapy of neonatal bacterial sepsis. In *Clinics in Perinatology: Infections in Perinatology*, Stoll BJ, and Weisman LE, eds. Philadelphia: WB Saunders, 213–230.
25. Hill HR, et al. 1991. Comparative protective activity of human monoclonal and hyperimmune polyclonal antibody against Group B streptococci. *Journal of Infectious Diseases* 163(4): 792–798.
26. Kim KS. 1987. Efficacy of human immunoglobulin and penicillin G in treatment of experimental Group B streptococcal infection. *Pediatric Research* 21(3): 289–292.
27. Weisman LE, and Lorenzetti P.M. 1988. High dose human intravenous immunoglobulin (IVIG) appears to suppress the enhancing effect of subinhibitory levels of penicillin on the opsonophagocytosis of Group B streptococcal sepsis: A current assessment. *Pediatric Research* 23: 47A.
28. Flora K, et al. 1996. An outbreak of acute hepatitis C among recipients of intravenous immunoglobulin. *Annals of Allergy and Asthma Immunology* 76(2): 160–162.
29. The PREVENT Study Group. 1997. Reduction of respiratory syncytial virus hospitalization among premature infants and infants with bronchopulmonary dysplasia using respiratory syncytial virus immune globulin prophylaxis. *Pediatrics* 99(1): 93–99.
30. American Academy of Pediatrics, Committee on Infectious Disease, Committee on Fetus and Newborn. 1997. Respiratory syncytial virus immune globulin intravenous: Indications for use. *Pediatrics* 99(4): 645–650.
31. Baley JE, et al. 1987. Buffy coat transfusions in neutropenic neonates with presumed sepsis: A prospective, randomized trial. *Pediatrics* 80(5): 712–720.
32. Cairo MS, et al. 1984. Improved survival of newborns receiving leukocyte transfusions for sepsis. *Pediatrics* 74(5): 887–892.
33. Cairo MS, et al. 1987. Role of circulating complement and polymorphonuclear leukocyte transfusion in treatment and outcome in critically ill neonates with sepsis. *Journal of Pediatrics* 110(6): 935–941.
34. Laurenti F, et al. 1981. Polymorphonuclear leukocyte transfusion for the treatment of sepsis in the newborn infant. *Journal of Pediatrics* 98(1): 118–123.
35. Wheeler JG, et al. 1987. Buffy coat transfusions in neonates with sepsis and neutrophil storage pool depletion. *Pediatrics* 79(3): 422–425.
36. Cairo MS, et al. 1992. Randomized trial of granulocyte transfusions versus intravenous immune globulin therapy for neonatal neutropenia and sepsis. *Journal of Pediatrics* 120(2 part 1): 281–285.
37. Gillian E, et al. 1994. A randomized, placebo controlled trial of recombinant human granulocyte colony-stimulating factor administration in newborn infants with presumed sepsis: Significant induction of peripheral and bone marrow neutrophilia. *Blood* 84(5): 1427–1433.
38. Rosenthal J, et al. 1996. A two-year follow-up of neonates with presumed sepsis treated with recombinant human granulocyte colony-stimulating factor during the first week of life. *Journal of Pediatrics* 128(1): 135–137.
39. Cairo M, et al. 1995. Results of a phase I/II trial of recombinant human granulocyte-macrophage colony-stimulating factor in very low birth-weight neonates: Significant induction of circulatory neutrophils, monocytes, platelets, and bone marrow neutrophils. *Blood* 86(7): 2509–2515.

NOTES

Notes

APPENDIX A

Normal Laboratory Values for Evaluation of Infection and CSF Findings in Term and Premature Infants

A-1 ◆ Normal Laboratory Values for Evaluation of Infection

Value	Gestational Age (wk) 28	Gestational Age (wk) 34	Full-Term Cord Blood	Day 1	Day 3	Day 7	Day 14
Hb (g/dl)	14.5	15.0	16.8	18.4	17.8	17.0	16.8
Hematocrit (%)	45	47	53	58	55	54	52
Red cells (mm^3)	4.0	4.4	5.25	5.8	5.6	5.2	5.1
MCV (µ^3)	120	118	107	108	99	98	96
MCH (pg)	40	38	34	35	33	32.5	31.5
MCHC (%)	31	32	31.7	32.5	33	33	33
Reticulocytes (%)	5–10	3–10	3–7	3–7	1–3	0–1	0–1
Platelets (1,000s/mm^3)			290	192	213	248	252

MCV = mean corpuscular volume; MCH = mean corpuscular hemoglobin; MCHC = mean corpuscular hemoglobin concentration.

From: Klaus MH, and Fanaroff AA, eds. 2001. *Care of the High-Risk Neonate,* 5th ed. Philadelphia: WB Saunders, 574. Reprinted by permission.

APPENDIX A

CSF Findings in Term and Premature Infants

A-2 ◆ Cerebrospinal Fluid Values in High-Risk Neonates Without Meningitis

Value	Term	Preterm
WBC count (cells/mm^3)		
No. of infants	87	30
Mean	8.2	9.0
Median	5	6
SD	7.1	8.2
Range	0–32	0–29
± 2 SD	0–22.4	0–25.4
Percentage PMN	61.3%	57.2%
Protein (mg/dl)		
No. of Infants	35	17
Mean	90	115
Range	20–170	65–150
Glucose (mg/dl)		
No. of infants	51	23
Mean	52	50
Range	34–119	24–63
CSF/blood glucose(%)		
No. of infants	51	23
Mean	81	74
Range	44–248	55–105

PMN = polymorphonuclear cells; CSF = cerebrospinal fluid.

From: Klaus MH, and Fanaroff AA, eds. 2001. *Care of the High-Risk Neonate,* 5th ed. Philadelphia: WB Saunders, 580. (Adapted from: Sarff L, Platt L, and McCracken G. 1976. Cerebrospinal fluid evaluation in neonates: Comparison of high risk infants with and without meningitis. *Journal of Pediatrics* 88[3]: 473–477.) Reprinted by permission

A-3 ◆ Cerebrospinal Fluid Values in First 24 Hours of Life in 135 Full-Term Infants

Value	Range	Mean	2 SD
Red blood cells	0–1,070	9	0–884
Polymorphs	0–70	3	0–27
Lymphocytes	0–20	2	0–24
Protein	32–240	63	27–144
Sugar	32–78	51	35–64
Chloride	680–760	720	660–780

From: Naidoo T. 1968. The cerebrospinal fluid in the healthy newborn infant. *South African Medical Journal* 42(35): 933–935. Reprinted by permission

A-4 ◆ Cerebrospinal Fluid Values on First and Seventh Days in Full-Term Infants

	Day 1 (n = 135)		Day 7 (n = 20)	
Value	Range	Mean	Range	Mean
Red blood cells	0–620	32	0–48	3
Polymorphs	0–26	7	0–5	2
Lymphocytes	0–16	5	0–4	1
Protein	40–148	73	27–65	47
Sugar	38–64	48	48–62	55
Chloride	680–760	720	720–760	720

From: Naidoo T. 1968. The cerebrospinal fluid in the healthy newborn infant. *South African Medical Journal* 42(35): 933–935. Reprinted by permission

A-5 ♦ Cerebrospinal Fluid Values of Healthy Term Newborns

Value	0–24 Hours	1 Day	7 Days	>7 Days
Color	Clear of xanthochromic	Clear of xanthochromic	Clear of xanthochromic	
Red blood cells/mm³	9 (0–1,070)	23 (6–630)	3 (0–48)	
Polymorphonuclear leukocytes/mm³	3 (0–70)	7 (0–26)	2 (0–5)	
Lymphocytes	2 (0–20)	5 (0–16)	1 (0–4)	
Protein (mg/dl)	63 (32–240)	73 (40–148)	47 (27–65)	
Blucose (mg/dl)	51 (32–78)	48 (38–64)	55 (48–62)	
Lactate dehydrogenase (IU/liter)	22–73	22–73	22–73	0–40

From: Klaus MH, and Fanaroff AA, eds. 2001. *Care of the High-Risk Neonate,* 5th ed. Philadelphia: WB Saunders, 581. (Modified from: Naidoo T. 1968. The cerebrospinal fluid in the healthy newborn infant. *South African Medical Journal* 42[35]: 933–935; and Neches W, and Platt M. 1968. Cerebrospinal fluid LDH in 287 children, including 53 cases of meningitis of bacterial and non-bacterial etiology. *Pediatrics* 41[6]: 1097–1103.) Reprinted by permission.

A-6 ♦ Cerebrospinal Fluid Values in Very Low Birth Weight Infants on Basis of Birth Weight

	≤1,000 gm		1,001–1,500 gm	
Value	Mean ± SD	Range	Mean ± SD	Range
Birth weight (gm)	763 ± 115	550–980	1,278 ± 152	1,020–1,500
Gestational age (wk)	26 ± 1.3	24–28	29 ± 1.4	27–33
Leukocytes/mm³	4 ± 3	0–14	6 ± 9	0–44
Erythrocytes/mm³	1,027 ± 3,270	0–19,050	786 ± 1,879	0–9,750
PMN leukocytes (%)	6 ± 15	0–66	9 ± 17	0–60
MN leukocytes (%)	86 ± 30	34–100	85 ± 28	13–100
Glucose (mg/dl)	61 ± 34	29–217	59 ± 21	31–109
Protein (mg/dl)	150 ± 56	95–370	132 ± 43	45–227

PMN = polymorphonuclear; MN = mononuclear.

From: Klaus MH, and Fanaroff AA, eds. 2001. *Care of the High-Risk Neonate,* 5th ed. Philadelphia: WB Saunders, 581. (Modified from: Rodriguez AF, Kaplan SL, and Mason EO. 1990. Cerebrospinal fluid values in the very low birth weight infant. *Journal of Pediatrics* 116[6]: 971–974.) Reprinted by permission.

APPENDIX B

White Cell and Differential Counts in Premature Infants

White Cell and Differential Counts in Premature Infants

Birth Weight	<1,500 gm			1,500–2,500 gm		
Age in Weeks	1	2	4	1	2	4
Total count ($\times 10^3/mm^3$)						
Mean	16.8	15.4	12.1	13.0	10.0	8.4
Range	6.1–32.8	10.4–21.3	8.7–17.2	6.7–14.7	7.0–14.1	5.8–12.4
Percent of Total						
Polymorphs						
Segmented	54	45	40	55	43	41
Unsegmented	7	6	5	8	8	6
Eosinophils	2	3	3	2	3	3
Basophils	1	1	1	1	1	1
Monocytes	6	10	10	5	9	11
Lymphocytes	30	35	41	9	36	38

From: Klaus MH, and Fanaroff AA, eds. 2001. *Care of the High-Risk Neonate,* 5th ed. Philadelphia: WB Saunders, 576. Reprinted by permission.

APPENDIX C

Leukocyte Values and Neutrophil Counts in Term and Premature Infants

C-1 ◆ Leukocyte Values in Term and Premature Infants (10³ cells/µl)

Age (hours)	Total White Cell Count	Neutrophils	Bands/Metas	Lymphocytes	Monocytes	Eosinophils
Term Infants						
0	10.0–26.0	5.0–13.0	0.4–1.8	3.5–8.5	0.7–1.5	0.2–2.0
12	13.5–31.0	9.0–18.0	0.4–2.0	3.0–7.0	1.0–2.0	0.2–2.0
72	5.0–14.5	2.0–7.0	0.2–0.4	2.0–5.0	0.5–1.0	0.2–1.0
144	6.0–14.5	2.0–6.0	0.2–0.5	3.0–6.0	0.7–1.2	0.2–0.8
Premature Infants						
0	5.0–19.0	2.0–9.0	0.2–2.4	2.5–6.0	0.3–1.0	0.1–0.7
12	5.0–21.0	3.0–11.0	0.2–2.4	1.5–5.0	0.3–1.3	0.1–1.1
72	5.0–14.0	3.0–7.0	0.2–0.6	1.5–4.0	0.3–1.2	0.2–1.1
144	5.5–17.5	2.0–7.0	0.2–0.5	2.5–7.5	0.5–1.5	0.3–1.2

From: Klaus MH, and Fanaroff AA. 2001. *Care of the High-Risk Neonate*, 5th ed. Philadelphia: WB Saunders, 577. (Originally from: Oski F, and Naiman J. 1982. *Hematologic Problems in the Newborn*. Philadelphia: WB Saunders.) Reprinted by permission.

C-2 ◆ Total Neutrophil Count Reference Range in the First 60 Hours of Life

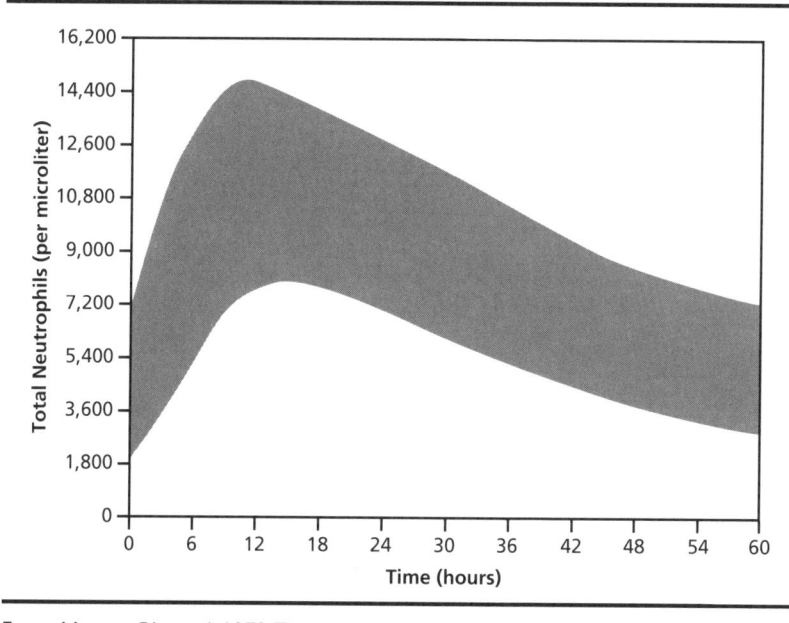

From: Manroe BL, et al. 1979. The neonatal blood count in health and disease. Part 1: Reference values for neutrophilic cells. *Journal of Pediatrics* 95(1): 91. Reprinted by permission.

Appendix C

APPENDIX D

Antibacterial Agents Used to Treat Neonatal Infection

APPENDIX D

Antibiotic Route	Susceptible Microorganisms	Dose — Infants 0–4 weeks of age BW <1,200 gm	Dose — Infants <1 week of age BW 1,200–2,000 gm	Dose — Infants <1 week of age BW >2,000 gm	Dose — Infants ≥1 week of age BW 1,200–2,000 gm	Dose — Infants ≥1 week of age BW >2,000 gm	Comments
Amikacin[1,2] IV (preferred): Infuse over 30 minutes.	*Escherichia coli* Enterobacter Proteus Serratia Pseudomonas	7.5 mg/kg/dose every 18–24 hours	7.5 mg/kg/dose every 12 hours	7.5–10 mg/kg/dose every 12 hours	7.5–10 mg/kg/dose every 8–12 hours	10 mg/kg/dose every 8 hours	Follow peak and trough levels: Peak: 20–30 µg/ml Trough: 5–10 µg/ml Use for microorganisms resistant to gentamicin. Assess renal function.
Ampicillin[3] IV (preferred): Infuse no faster than 100 mg/minute. Give over at least 3–5 minutes; may give over 10–30 minutes.	*Escherichia coli* Group B β-hemolytic streptococci *Haemophilus influenzae,* *Listeria monocytogenes* *Neisseria gonorrhoeae* *Proteus mirabilis,* *Shigella,* *Salmonella*	25–50 mg/kg/dose every 12 hours	25–50 mg/kg/dose every 12 hours	25–50 mg/kg/dose every 8 hours	25–50 mg/kg/dose every 8 hours	25–50 mg/kg/dose every 6 hours	Serum levels not necessary. Renal excretion. Rare CNS excitation and seizure activity.
Cefotaxime IV: Over 30 minutes preferred; over 5 minutes minimum.	*Neisseria* *Haemophilus influenzae*	50 mg/kg/dose every 12 hours	50 mg/kg/dose every 12 hours	50 mg/kg/dose every 8–12 hours	50 mg/kg/dose every 8 hours	50 mg/kg/dose every 6–8 hours	Adverse effects are rare, but may include: rash, diarrhea, alteration in bowel flora, leukopenia, granulocytopenia, eosinophilia.

(continued on next page)

INFECTION IN THE NEONATE

Antibiotic Route	Susceptible Microorganisms	Dose — Infants 0–4 weeks of age BW <1,200 gm	Dose — Infants <1 week of age BW 1,200–2,000 gm	Dose — Infants <1 week of age BW >2,000 gm	Dose — Infants ≥1 week of age BW 1,200–2,000 gm	Dose — Infants ≥1 week of age BW >2,000 gm	Comments
Ceftazidime IV (preferred): Infusion over 30 minutes preferred; over 5 minutes, minimum.	Serratia Acinetobacter Pseudomonas aeruginosa	50 mg/kg/dose every 12 hours	50 mg/kg/dose every 12 hours	50 mg/kg/dose every 8–12 hours	50 mg/kg/dose every 8 hours	50 mg/kg/dose every 8 hours	Adverse effects are infrequent, but may include: rash, diarrhea, slightly elevated hepatic enzymes, eosinophilia.
Ceftriaxone[4] IV: Infusion over 30 minutes preferred, over at least 4 minutes minimum. IM: (only if IV access is unavailable)	Neisseria gonorrhoeae N. meningitidis E. coli Haemophilus influenzae Gram-positive cocii S. pneumoniae S. aureus Klebsiella P. mirabilis Serratia Enterobacter	50 mg/kg/dose every 24 hours	50 mg/kg/dose every 24–36 hours	50 mg/kg/dose every 24 hours	50 mg/kg/dose every 24 hours	50–75 mg/kg/dose every 24 hours	***Not recommended for use in neonates with hyperbilirubinemia.*** Rash, sludging in gall bladder, diarrhea, eosinophilia, thrombocytosis, leukopenia, increased BUN and serum creatinine, slightly elevated hepatic enzymes, hypersensitivity reactions.
Clindamycin IV (preferred): Infuse over 30–60 minutes.	Staphylococcus aureus Streptococcus pneumoniae, Anaerobic bacteria, such as Bacteroides fragilis	5 mg/kg/dose every 12 hours	5 mg/kg/dose every 12 hours	5 mg/kg/dose every 8 hours	5 mg/kg/dose every 8 hours	5–7.5 mg/kg/dose every 6 hours	***Should not be used to treat meningitis.*** Monitor liver and GI functions. Pseudomembranous colitis. Poor CSF penetration.

(continued on next page)

191

Dose

Antibiotic Route	Susceptible Microorganisms	Infants 0–4 weeks of age BW <1,200 gm	Infants <1 week of age BW 1,200–2,000 gm	Infants <1 week of age BW >2,000 gm	Infants ≥1 week of age BW 1,200–2,000 gm	Infants ≥1 week of age BW >2,000 gm	Comments
Erythromycin IV: Infuse slowly over 60 minutes.	*Chlamydia trachomatis, Ureaplasma urealyticum,* Staphylococcus, Streptococcus, *Listeria monocytogenes.*	10 mg/kg/dose every 12 hours	10 mg/kg/dose every 12 hours	10 mg/kg/dose every 12 hours	10 mg/kg/dose every 8 hours	10 mg/kg/dose every 8 hours	
Gentamicin[1,2] IV (preferred): Infuse over 30 minutes.	*E. coli,* Enterobacter, Proteus, Serratia, Pseudomonas Synergistic antibacterial activity with penicillins against Group B Streptococcus and *S. aureus.*	2.5 mg/kg/dose every 18–24 hours	2.5 mg/kg/dose every 12 hours	2.5 mg/kg/dose every 12 hours	2.5 mg/kg/dose every 8–12 hours	2.5 mg/kg/dose every 8 hours	Ototoxicity. Nephrotoxicity. Monitor therapeutic levels: *Peak:* 4–10 µg/ml *Trough:* 0.5–2 µg/ml Patients with PDA may need higher dose. Half-life prolonged in preterm and asphyxiated neonates. Poor CSF penetration. Neuromuscular blockade.

(continued on next page)

INFECTION IN THE NEONATE

Antibiotic Route	Susceptible Microorganisms	Infants 0–4 weeks of age BW <1,200 gm	Infants <1 week of age BW 1,200–2,000 gm	Infants <1 week of age BW >2,000 gm	Infants ≥1 week of age BW 1,200–2,000 gm	Infants ≥1 week of age BW >2,000 gm	Comments
Imipenem/ cilastatin[5] IV (preferred): Infuse over 30–60 minutes. IM: (painful, use only if necessary) **(Different formulations for IV and IM use, do not use IM formulation for IV administration.)**	*Bacteroides fragilis, E. coli, Haemophilus influenzae, Pseudomonas aeruginosa, Listeria monocytogenes,* Enterobacter, enterococci, Serratia species, streptococci, *S. aureus, S. epidermidis* including penicillinase producing strains; methicillin-resistant staphylococci are resistant)	25 mg/kg/dose every 12 hours	25 mg/kg/dose every 12 hours	25 mg/kg/dose every 12 hours	25 mg/kg/dose every 8 hours	25 mg/kg/dose every 8 hours	Reduce dose in renal dysfunction. May cause seizures.
Metronidazole[5] IV: Infuse over 1 hour	Reserved for treatment of meningitis	7.5 mg/kg/dose every 24–48 hours	7.5 mg/kg/dose every 24 hours	7.5 mg/kg/dose every 12 hours	7.5 mg/kg/dose every 12 hours	15 mg/kg/dose every 12 hours	Seizures; peripheral neuropathy; **Discontinue if abnormal neurologic signs appear**, GI upset; overgrowth of Candida; mild, reversible neutropenia; rash. *Note: This drug has shown carcinogenic potential in experimental animal data. Use is usually reserved to resistant infections for this reason.*

(continued on next page)

Antibiotic Route	Susceptible Microorganisms	Dose				Comments
		Infants 0–4 weeks of age BW <1,200 gm	Infants <1 week of age BW 1,200–2,000 gm	Infants <1 week of age BW >2,000 gm	Infants ≥1 week of age BW 1,200–2,000 gm / BW >2,000 gm	
Nafcillin[3] IV (preferred): Slow push over 5–10 minutes, but infusion over 30–60 minutes preferred.	Penicillinase-producing staphylococci	25 mg/kg/dose every 12 hours	25 mg/kg/dose every 12 hours	25 mg/kg/dose every 8 hours	25 mg/kg/dose every 8 hours / 25–35 mg/kg/dose every 6 hours	Rarely used today. Better penetration into CSF than other antistaphylococcal penicillins. Metabolized by liver. May cause agranulocytopenia. Blunting of peak aminoglycoside levels. May cause phlebitis. Monitor IV site carefully; can cause severe tissue damage with extravasation. Monitor CBC, liver function tests, and sodium levels (contains 2.9 mEq of sodium/gm). Decrease the dose in combined renal and hepatic dysfunction. Synergistic effect with aminoglycosides but **physically and chemically incompatible: do not combine or administer together.**

(continued on next page)

INFECTION IN THE NEONATE

Antibiotic Route	Susceptible Microorganisms	Dose					Comments
		Infants 0–4 weeks of age BW <1,200 gm	Infants <1 week of age BW 1,200–2,000 gm	Infants <1 week of age BW >2,000 gm	Infants ≥1 week of age BW 1,200–2,000 gm	Infants ≥1 week of age BW >2,000 gm	
Oxacillin[3] IV: Slow push.	Penicillinase-producing staphylococci	25 mg/kg/dose every 12 hours	25–50 mg/kg/dose every 12 hours	25–50 mg/kg/dose every 8 hours	25–50 mg/kg/dose every 8 hours	25–50 mg/kg/dose every 6 hours	Poor CSF penetration, good penetration in pleural, pericardial, and synovial fluid. Interstitial nephritis with hematuria. Bone marrow depression. Rash. Monitor CBC and urinalysis. Irritating to veins and tissues, watch for phlebitis/extravasation. Incompatible with aminoglycosides.
Penicillin G,[3] aqueous IV: Infuse over 30 minutes.	Group A Streptococcus, nonenterococcal Group D Streptococcus, Group B Streptococcus, S. pneumoniae, Listeria monocytogenes, Neisseria meningitidis, N. gonorrhoeae, Clostridium, Treponema pallidum	25,000–50,000 units/kg/dose every 12 hours	25,000–50,000 units/kg/dose every 12 hours	25,000–50,000 units/kg/dose every 8 hours	25,000–50,000 units/kg/dose every 8 hours	25,000–50,000 units/kg/dose every 6 hours	Inactivated by penicillinase. Poor CSF penetration. Renal excretion. Ampicillin, not penicillin, is preferred for use against Listeria. Follow Na$^+$ and K$^+$ levels and CBC.

(continued on next page)

Antibiotic Route	Susceptible Microorganisms	Dose					Comments
		Infants 0–4 weeks of age BW <1,200 gm	Infants <1 week of age BW 1,200–2,000 gm	Infants <1 week of age BW >2,000 gm	Infants ≥1 week of age BW 1,200–2,000 gm	Infants ≥1 week of age BW >2,000 gm	
Ticarcillin[6] *IV: Infuse over 30 minutes.*	P. aeruginosa, Proteus, E. coli	75 mg/kg/dose every 12 hours	75 mg/kg/dose every 12 hours	75 mg/kg/dose every 8 hours	75 mg/kg/dose every 8 hours	75 mg/kg/dose every 6 hours	Hypernatremia (5.2 mEq of sodium per gm). Hypokalemia resulting from tubular excretion of potassium. Monitor for bleeding caused by decreased platelet aggregation. Do not administer in the same solution as gentamicin or tobramycin. Monitor therapeutic levels: *Peak:* 125–150 µg/ml *Trough:* 25–50 µg/ml
Tobramycin[1,2] *IV: Infuse over 30 minutes.*	Pseudomonas, Klebsiella, E. coli, Enterobacter, Proteus, Serratia	2.5 mg/kg/dose every 18–24 hours	2.5 mg/kg/dose every 12 hours	2.5 mg/kg/dose every 12 hours	2.5 mg/kg/dose every 8–12 hours	2.5 mg/kg/dose every 8 hours	***Potential curare-like effect on neuromuscular function; use with caution especially in newborns whose mothers have received magnesium sulfate.*** Reduce dose in renal impairment; renal toxicity uncommon in neonates. Potential ototoxicity. Monitor therapeutic levels: *Peak:* 4–10 µg/ml *Trough:* 0.5–2 µg/ml

(continued on next page)

Antibiotic Route	Susceptible Microorganisms	Dose						Comments
		Infants 0–4 weeks of age BW <1,200 gm	Infants <1 week of age BW 1,200–2,000 gm	Infants <1 week of age BW >2,000 gm	Infants ≥1 week of age BW 1,200–2,000 gm	Infants ≥1 week of age BW >2,000 gm		
Vancomycin[1] *IV: Infuse over 1 hour.*	*Staphylococcus epidermidis,* methicillin-resistant *S. aureus, Clostridium difficile*	15 mg/kg/dose every 24 hours	10–15 mg/kg/dose every 12–18 hours	10–15 mg/kg/dose every 8–12 hours	10–15 mg/kg/dose every 8–12 hours	10–15 mg/kg/dose every 6–8 hours		Monitor therapeutic levels: *Peak:* 25–40 µg/ml *Trough:* 5–10 µg/ml Low CSF penetration. Neutropenia, phlebitis. Nephro/neuro/ototoxicity. Administer slowly, monitoring heart rate and blood pressure. Reduce dose in renal impairment.

BW = birth weight; IV = intravenous; IM = intramuscular; PO = oral.

[1] Optimal dosage should be based on determination of serum concentrations, especially in low birth weight (<1,500 gm) infants.
[2] Dosages for aminoglycosides may differ from those recommended by the manufacturer in the package insert.
[3] For meningitis, the larger dosage is recommended. Some experts recommend even larger dosages for group B streptococcal meningitis.
[4] Drug should not be administered to hyperbilirubinemic neonates, especially infants born prematurely.
[5] Safety in infants and children has not been established. Meropenem is preferred if a carbapenem is to be used in newborn infants.
[6] Same dosage for ticarcillin and clavulanate potassium.

Compiled from: American Academy of Pediatrics. 2003. *Red Book: Report of the Committee on Infectious Diseases,* 26th ed., Pickering L, ed. Elk Grove Village, Illinois: American Academy of Pediatrics; Young TE, and Mangum B. 2003. *Neofax.* 16th ed. Raleigh, North Carolina: Acorn; and Zenk KE, Sills JH, and Koeppel RM. 2003. *Neonatal Medications & Nutrition: A Comprehensive Guide,* 3rd ed. Santa Rosa, California: NICU Ink.

Appendix D

APPENDIX E

Recommendations for Immunizations for Communicable Diseases

From: American Academy of Pediatrics, Committee on Infectious Diseases. 2004. Recommended childhood and adolescent immunization schedule—United States, January–June 2004. *Pediatrics* 113(1 part 1): 143–146.

Recommended Childhood and Adolescent Immunization Schedule — United States, January – June 2004

Vaccine ▼ / Age ▶	Birth	1 mo	2 mo	4 mo	6 mo	12 mo	15 mo	18 mo	24 mo	4-6 y	11-12 y	13-18 y
Hepatitis B[1]	HepB #1	only if mother HBsAg (−)	HepB #2			HepB #3					HepB series	
Diphtheria, Tetanus, Pertussis[2]			DTaP	DTaP	DTaP		DTaP			DTaP	Td	Td
Haemophilus influenzae Type b[3]			Hib	Hib	Hib[3]	Hib						
Inactivated Poliovirus			IPV	IPV		IPV				IPV		
Measles, Mumps, Rubella[4]						MMR #1				MMR #2		MMR #2
Varicella[5]						Varicella					Varicella	
Pneumococcal[6]			PCV	PCV	PCV	PCV			PCV	PPV		
Hepatitis A[7]									Hepatitis A series			
Influenza[8]						Influenza (yearly)						

Range of Recommended Ages · Catch-up Immunization · Preadolescent Assessment

Vaccines below this line are for selected populations

INFECTION IN THE NEONATE

This schedule indicates the recommended ages for routine administration of currently licensed childhood vaccines, as of December 1, 2003, for children through age 18 years. Any dose not given at the recommended age should be given at any subsequent visit when indicated and feasible. ■ Indicates age groups that warrant special effort to administer those vaccines not previously given. Additional vaccines may be licensed and recommended during the year. Licensed combination vaccines may be used whenever any components of the combination are indicated and the vaccine's other components are not contraindicated. Providers should consult the manufacturers' package inserts for detailed recommendations. Clinically significant adverse events that follow immunization should be reported to the Vaccine Adverse Event Reporting System (VAERS). Guidance about how to obtain and complete a VAERS form can be found on the Internet: http://www.vaers.org/ or by calling 1-800-822-7967.

1. Hepatitis B (HepB) vaccine. All infants should receive the first dose of hepatitis B vaccine soon after birth and before hospital discharge; the first dose may also be given by age 2 months if the infant's mother is hepatitis B surface antigen (HBsAg) negative. Only monovalent HepB can be used for the birth dose. Monovalent or combination vaccine containing HepB may be used to complete the series. Four doses of vaccine may be administered when a birth dose is given. The second dose should be given at least 4 weeks after the first dose, except for combination vaccines which cannot be administered before age 6 weeks. The third dose should be given at least 16 weeks after the first dose and at least 8 weeks after the second dose. The last dose in the vaccination series (third or fourth dose) should not be administered before age 24 weeks.

Infants born to HBsAg-positive mothers should receive HepB and 0.5 mL of Hepatitis B Immune Globulin (HBIG) within 12 hours of birth at separate sites. The second dose is recommended at age 1 to 2 months. The last dose in the immunization series should not be administered before age 24 weeks. These infants should be tested for HBsAg and antibody to HBsAg (anti-HBs) at age 9 to 15 months.

Infants born to mothers whose HBsAg status is unknown should receive the first dose of the HepB series within 12 hours of birth. Maternal blood should be drawn as soon as possible to determine the mother's HBsAg status; if the HBsAg test is positive, the infant should receive HBIG as soon as possible (no later than age 1 week). The second dose is recommended at age 1 to 2 months. The last dose in the immunization series should not be administered before age 24 weeks.

2. Diphtheria and tetanus toxoids and acellular pertussis (DTaP) vaccine. The fourth dose of DTaP may be administered as early as age 12 months, provided 6 months have elapsed since the third dose and the child is unlikely to return at age 15 to 18 months. The final dose in the series should be given at age ≥4 years. Tetanus and diphtheria toxoids (Td) is recommended at age 11 to 12 years if at least 5 years have elapsed since the last dose of tetanus and diphtheria toxoid-containing vaccine. Subsequent routine Td boosters are recommended every 10 years.

3. Haemophilus influenzae type b (Hib) conjugate vaccine. Three Hib conjugate vaccines are licensed for infant use. If PRP-OMP (PedvaxHIB or ComVax [Merck]) is administered at ages 2 and 4 months, a dose at age 6 months is not required. DTaP/Hib combination products should not be used for primary immunization in infants at ages 2, 4 or 6 months but can be used as boosters following any Hib vaccine. The final dose in the series should be given at age ≥12 months.

4. Measles, mumps, and rubella vaccine (MMR). The second dose of MMR is recommended routinely at age 4 to 6 years but may be administered during any visit, provided at least 4 weeks have elapsed since the first dose and both doses are administered beginning at or after age 12 months. Those who have not previously received the second dose should complete the schedule by the 11- to 12-year-old visit.

5. Varicella vaccine. Varicella vaccine is recommended at any visit at or after age 12 months for susceptible children (i.e., those who lack a reliable history of chickenpox). Susceptible persons age ≥13 years should receive 2 doses, given at least 4 weeks apart.

6. Pneumococcal vaccine. The heptavalent pneumococcal conjugate vaccine (PCV) is recommended for all children age 2 to 23 months. It is also recommended for certain children age 24 to 59 months. The final dose in the series should be given at age ≥12 months. Pneumococcal polysaccharide vaccine (PPV) is recommended in addition to PCV for certain high-risk groups. See MMWR 2000;49(RR-9):1-38.

7. Hepatitis A vaccine. Hepatitis A vaccine is recommended for children and adolescents in selected states and regions and for certain high-risk groups; consult your local public health authority. Children and adolescents in these states, regions, and high-risk groups who have not been immunized against hepatitis A can begin the hepatitis A immunization series during any visit. The 2 doses in the series should be administered at least 6 months apart. See MMWR 1999;48(RR-12):1-37.

8. Influenza vaccine. Influenza vaccine is recommended annually for children age ≥6 months with certain risk factors (including but not limited to children with asthma, cardiac disease, sickle cell disease, human immunodeficiency virus infection, and diabetes; and household members of persons in high-risk groups [see MMWR 2003;52(RR-8):1-36]) and can be administered to all others wishing to obtain immunity. In addition, healthy children age 6 to 23 months are encouraged to receive influenza vaccine if feasible, because children in this age group are at substantially increased risk of influenza-related hospitalizations. For healthy persons age 5 to 49 years, the intranasally administered live-attenuated influenza vaccine (LAIV) is an acceptable alternative to the intramuscular trivalent inactivated influenza vaccine (TIV). See MMWR 2003;52(RR-13):1-8. Children receiving TIV should be administered a dosage appropriate for their age (0.25 mL if age 6 to 35 months or 0.5 mL if age ≥3 years). Children age ≤8 years who are receiving influenza vaccine for the first time should receive 2 doses (separated by at least 4 weeks for TIV and at least 6 weeks for LAIV).

For additional information about vaccines, including precautions and contraindications for immunization and vaccine shortages, please visit the National Immunization Program Web site at www.cdc.gov/nip/ or call the National Immunization Information Hotline at 800-232-2522 (English) or 800-232-0233 (Spanish).

Approved by the Advisory Committee on Immunization Practices (www.cdc.gov/nip/acip), the American Academy of Pediatrics (www.aap.org), and the American Academy of Family Physicians (www.aafp.org).

Appendix F

Therapeutic Serum Peak and Trough Levels for Antibicrobial Agents

Drug	Peak Level (µg/ml)	Trough Level (µg/ml)
Amikacin	20–30	3–5
Flucytosine	50–75	*
Gentamicin	4–10	0.5–2.0
Tobramycin	4–10	0.5–2.0
Piperacillin	150	15–50
Ticarcillin	125–150	25–50
Vancomycin	25–40	5–10

*Appropriate therapy does not require following trough levels for this drug.

Adapted from: Zenk KE, Sills JH, and Koeppel RM. 2003. *Neonatal Medications & Nutrition: A Comprehensive Guide,* 3rd. ed. Santa Rosa, California: NICU Ink.

Appendix F

Appendix G

Calculations for Evaluating White Blood Cell Count

The results of a sample white blood cell (WBC) count with differential are listed below. These laboratory results are used to demonstrate the calculations explained in this appendix.

WBC count	16.6×10^3
Platelet count	217×10^3
Segmented neutrophils (segs)	48%
Bands	23%
Metamyelocytes	4%
Myelocytes	1%
Lymphocytes	16%
Monocytes	7%
Eosinophils	1%
Nucleated red blood cells	20

Corrected WBC Count

Nucleated red blood cells (NRBCs) are often counted by automated analyzers as WBCs because they are similar in size. This artificially elevates the WBC count. Corrected WBC counts are routinely done by the laboratory, but health care providers can calculate a corrected WBC count themselves, to avoid delay. Here is the formula:

$$\text{Corrected WBC count} = \frac{\text{total WBCs} \times 100}{\text{number of NRBCs} + 100}$$

The sample lab values list 20 NRBCs. To correct the WBC count for the hypothetical infant, the calculation would be:

$$\text{Corrected WBC count} = \frac{16.6 \times 100}{20 + 100}$$

$$= \frac{1,660}{120}$$

$$= 13.8 \times 10^3 \text{ or } 13,800$$

Absolute Neutrophil Count

To calculate the absolute neutrophil count (ANC) in the total WBC count, use this formula:

ANC = (% segs + % immature cells [bands, metamyelocytes, myelocytes]) × WBCs

The ANC of the hypothetical infant would be:

$$ANC = [48\% + (23\% + 4\% + 1\%)] \times (16.6 \times 10^3)$$
$$= (.48 + .23 + .04 + .01) \times (16.6 \times 10^3) = 0.76 \times 16{,}600$$
$$= 12{,}616$$

The normal range for ANC is 1,800–14,400, but the number varies according to the infant's age.[1,2] (See Chapter 6, Table 6-5, for values from birth to ≥120 hours of age.)

Immature-to-Total Neutrophil Ratio

The following calculation is used to determine the ratio of immature neutrophils to total neutrophils (I:T ratio) in a peripheral smear. The upper limit of normal for the I:T ratio in uninfected neonates is 0.16 in the first 24 hours of life. The upper limit of normal for neonates ≤32 weeks gestation is 0.20. An I:T ratio of >0.20 is suspicious for infection.[1,2]

$$\text{I:T ratio} = \frac{\% \text{ immature neutrophils (bands + metamyelocytes + myelocytes)}}{\% \text{ mature neutrophils} + \% \text{ immature neutrophils}}$$

The I:T ratio of the hypothetical infant is:

$$\text{I:T ratio} = \frac{23 + 4 + 1}{48 + 28} = \frac{28}{76}$$

$$= 0.368, \text{ which rounds to } 0.37$$

Immature-to-Mature Ratio

Another ratio used in the comparison of neutrophil forms is the immature-to-mature (I:M) neutrophil ratio. A value of >0.3 is suspicious for infection. Here is the formula, as well as the calculation for the hypothetical infant:

$$\text{I:M ratio} = \frac{\% \text{ immature neutrophils (bands + metamyelocytes + myelocytes)}}{\% \text{ mature neutrophils (segmented neutrophils)}}$$

$$\text{I:M ratio} = \frac{23 + 4 + 1}{48} = \frac{28}{48}$$

$$= 0.58$$

Band-to-Seg Ratio

Like the I:M ratio, the band-to-seg (B:S) calculation compares immature to mature neutrophils, but it includes only bands in the immature category. The metamyelocytes and myelocytes are not counted in this calculation. A ratio >0.3 is suspicious for infection.

$$\text{B:S ratio} = \frac{\text{bands}}{\text{segmented neutrophils}} \quad \frac{\text{(immature)}}{\text{(mature)}}$$

$$\text{B:S ratio} = \frac{23}{48}$$

$$= 0.479, \text{ which rounds to } 0.48$$

References

1. Edwards MS. 2002. Postnatal bacterial infections, Part 2. In *Neonatal-Perinatal Medicine: Diseases of the Fetus and Infant*, 7th ed., Fanaroff AA, and Martin RJ, eds. Philadelphia: Mosby-Year Book, 706–745, 788–790.
2. Manroe BL, et al. 1979. The neonatal blood count in health and disease. Part I: Reference values for neutrophil cells. *Journal of Pediatrics* 95(1): 89–98.

Glossary

Acellular: Not made up of or containing cells.

Acid-fast stain: A staining technique that distinguishes bacteria that stain red (acid-fast bacteria) from those that do not stain red (non–acid-fast bacteria); used most commonly in the diagnosis of tuberculosis.

Acidophile: An organism that prefers an acidic environment.

Aerobe: An organism that lives and grows in the presence of oxygen.

Agglutination: The clumping of particles (e.g., red blood cells in solution).

Agranulocyte: A white blood cell without granules in its cytoplasm.

Anaerobe: An organism that lives and grows in the absence of oxygen.

Antibiotic: A chemical substance produced by a microorganism that inhibits or destroys bacteria.

Antibody: An immunoglobulin molecule that has the ability to adhere to and interact with a stimulus known as an antigen; often protective.

Antigen: A substance, usually foreign, that induces a specific immune response.

Antimicrobial agent: A drug, disinfectant, or other substance that kills or suppresses the growth of microorganisms.

Antiseptic: Usually refers to a chemical disinfectant that is safe to use on living tissues.

Arthropod: Includes insects such as flies, mosquitoes, fleas, lice, and arachnids such as mites and ticks.

Asepsis: A state of sterility, the absence of life.

Aseptic technique: A measure taken to ensure that pathogens are absent.

Attenuated: Usually describes certain microorganisms that are weakened or less pathogenic.

Attenuated vaccine: A vaccine prepared from an attenuated microorganism.

Autoimmune disease: A disease resulting from the production by the body of antibodies directed against its own tissues.

B cell, B lymphocyte: A lymphocyte that recognizes specific antigens and differentiates into plasma cells.

Bacillus (pl. bacilli): A rod-shaped bacterium; or a genus named *Bacillus*, made up of aerobic, Gram-positive, spore-forming bacilli.

Bacteremia: The presence of bacteria in the bloodstream.

Glossary

Bacteriocidal agent: A chemical agent that kills bacteria.

Bacteriostatic agent: A chemical agent that stops bacterial growth.

Bacterium (pl. bacteria): A single-cell, prokaryotic microorganism that reproduces by asexual division.

Bacteriuria: The presence of bacteria in the urine.

Basophil: A granulocyte found in blood; one type of white blood cell whose granules contain substances such as histamine.

Candidiasis: Infection caused by a yeast in the genus *Candida*—usually *Candida albicans*; also known as *moniliasis*.

Capsid: The shell of protein protecting the nucleic acid of a virus.

Capsomere: The protein that makes up the capsid of some virions.

Capsule: A layer of glycocalyx found on the outer surface of some bacterial cell walls. (Some yeasts are also encapsulated.)

Carrier: An asymptomatic individual with a microorganism that can be transmitted to other susceptible individuals.

Cell membrane: The wall of all cells.

Chemotactic agent: A chemical substance that attracts white blood cells.

Chemotaxis: The movement of leukocytes in response to chemicals formed in immunologic reactions (e.g., the attraction of phagocytes to an area of injury).

Coagulase: An enzyme that causes blood to clot.

Coccus (pl. cocci): A round-shaped bacterium.

Commensalism: A relationship in which one party derives benefit and the other party is unaffected in any way. (Most members of the indigenous microflora are commensals.)

Complement: A protein complex found in blood; involved in inflammation, chemotaxis, phagocytosis, and lysis of bacteria.

Cytokines: A protein or peptide that is released by certain cells on contact with antigens and serves to regulate the intensity and duration of the immune response.

Dimorphism: A phenomenon whereby an organism can exist in two shapes or forms (e.g., dimorphic fungi can exist either as yeasts or molds).

Diplococci: Cocci arranged in pairs.

Disinfect: Using a chemical agent to destroy pathogens or inhibit their growth activity; usually refers to a chemical agent used on nonliving materials.

DNA polymerase: An enzyme necessary for DNA replication.

Electron microscope: A type of microscope that uses electrons as a source of illumination.

Encephalitis: Inflammation or infection of the brain.

Endospore: A thick-walled body formed within a bacterial cell for the purpose of survival.

Enterotoxin: A bacterial exotoxin that has specific action on the cells of the intestinal mucosa.

Enzyme: A protein molecule that causes or enhances biochemical reactions.

Eosinophil: A type of granulocyte or white blood cell found in blood.

Epidemic disease: A disease occurring at a higher than normal rate of cases in a population during a given time interval.

Epidemiology: The study of relationships between the various factors that determine the frequency and distribution of diseases.

Episome: An extrachromosomal plasmid that either integrates into the host bacterium's chromosome or replicates and functions stably when physically separated from the chromosome.

Erythema: Red discoloration of the skin. (A reddened area of skin is described as being *erythematous*.)

Erythrocyte: A red blood cell.

Eucaryotic cell: A cell containing a true nucleus. (Organisms having such cells are referred to as *eukaryotes*.)

Exotoxin: A toxin that is released from the cell.

Exudate: Any fluid that oozes from tissue, often as a result of injury, infection, or inflammation.

Facultative anaerobe: An organism that can exist in either the presence or absence of oxygen.

Fastidious bacterium: A bacterium that is difficult to isolate from specimens and grow in the laboratory due to its complex nutritional requirements.

Fibronectin: A glycoprotein involved in hemostasis, vascular integrity, and wound healing that augments the performance of phagocytic cells.

Flagellum (pl. flagella): Whiplike structure providing an organism with motility.

Fomite: An inanimate object such as linen or a utensil or a substance such as soap capable of absorbing and transmitting a pathogen.

Frontal bossing: An unusually prominent forehead.

Fungicidal agent: A chemical agent or drug that kills fungi.

Fungus (pl. fungi): A eucaryotic, nonphotosynthetic microorganism that is saprophytic or parasitic.

Gene: A functional unit of heredity located on a chromosome.

Genotype: The complete genetic constitution of an individual (i.e., all of that individual's genes).

Genus (pl. genera): The first name in binomial nomenclature; contains closely related species.

Glycocalyx: A polysaccharide or glycoprotein covering on a cell surface. In bacterial cells, this covering forms masses of fibers that help the cell adhere to surfaces.

Golgi complex: Also know as Golgi apparatus or Golgi body, a membranous system found in the cytoplasm of a eukaryotic cell whose function is the transport and packaging of secretory proteins.

Gram's stain: A staining procedure that differentiates bacteria into those that stain blue to purple (Gram-positive) and those that stain pink to red (Gram-negative).

Granulocyte: A granular white blood cell. (Neutrophiles, eosinophils, and basophils are types of granulocytes.)

Growth curve: The change in size of a bacterial population over a period of time; includes a lag phase, a log phase, a stationary phase, and a death phase.

Hemoglobin: A protein carried by red blood cells that transports oxygen from the lungs to body tissues.

Hemolysin: A bacterial enzyme capable of breaking down erythrocytes, causing release of hemoglobin.

Hemolysis: Destruction of red blood cells (erythrocytes) in such a manner that hemoglobin is liberated.

Hemostasis: The process of arresting blood flow.

Histamine: A potent chemical released from cells (e.g., basophils and mast cells) during some immune reactions resulting in constriction of bronchial smooth muscles and vasodilation.

Host: The organism on or in which a parasite lives.

Hyaluronidase: A bacterial enzyme that breaks down hyaluronic acid, enabling bacteria to invade deeper into tissue.

Immune: Resistant to acquiring a particular infectious disease.

Immunity: Being immune or resistant.

Immunocompetent: Able to mount a normal immune response.

Immunoglobulin: A class of proteins, which includes antibodies that respond to antigens.

In vitro: In an artificial environment, as in a laboratory setting.

In vivo: In a living organism.

Inactivated vaccine: A vaccine prepared from killed microorganisms.

Inclusion body: A distinctive structure frequently formed in the nucleus and/or cytoplasm of cells infected with certain viruses.

Infection: The presence and multiplication of pathogens in or on the body.

Infectious disease: Any disease caused by a microorganism.

Inflammation: A nonspecific pathologic process consisting of cytologic and histologic reactions that occur in response to an injury or abnormal stimulation by a physical, chemical, or biologic agent.

Interferons: A group of proteins produced and excreted by virally infected cells; first lines of defense against viral infection, warning healthy cells of a potential infection.

Interleukins: A group of cytokines produced by T cells, macrophages, or tissue cells. (Interleukin-1 is produced by monocytes; interleukin-2 is produced by lymphocytes.)

Latent infection: An asymptomatic infection capable of manifesting symptoms when activated.

Leukocidin: A bacterial toxin capable of destroying leukocytes.

Leukocyte: A white blood cell.

Leukopenia: A reduced number of leukocytes in the blood.

Lymphokines: A group of cytokines released by sensitized lymphocytes (e.g., chemotactic factors and interleukins).

Lysis: Dissolution or destruction of a cell by a specific agent.

Lysosomes: A membrane-bound vesicle, found in the cytoplasm of eucaryotic cells, that contains a variety of digestive enzymes, including lysozyme.

Lysozyme: A digestive enzyme, found in body fluids, that is destructive to bacterial cell walls.

Macrophage: A large phagocytic cell that arises from a monocyte.

Mast cell: A cell found in a variety of tissues, closely resembling a basophil.

Meninges: Membranes that surround the brain and spinal cord.

Microorganism: A microscopic organism, also called a *microbe*. (These include algae, bacteria, fungi, protozoa, and viruses.)

Mitochondrion (pl. mitochondria): The structure responsible for energy production in eucaryotic cells.

Monocyte: A mononuclear, phagocytic leukocyte; transported to tissues such as liver and lung and develop into macrophages.

Motile: Possessing the ability to move.

Mycosis (pl. mycoses): Disease caused by a fungus.

Natural killer (NK) cell: A type of lymphocyte that has a function similar to a macrophage and T cells; identifies and destroys virus-infected and tumor cells.

Neurotoxin: A bacterial toxin that attacks the tissues of the nervous system.

Neutrophil: A type of granulocyte or white blood cell; also called a *polymorphonuclear cell*, *poly*, or *PMN*.

Nosocomial infection: Any infection acquired in the hospital.

Nucleic acid: High-density nucleotide polymer (i.e., RNA, DNA).

Obligate aerobe: An organism that requires oxygen to survive.

Obligate anaerobe: An organism that cannot survive in oxygen.

Obligate parasite: An organism incapable of a free-living existence.

Opportunistic pathogen: A microbe that has the potential to cause disease in susceptible persons with lowered resistance, but not under ordinary circumstances; also called an *opportunist*.

Opsonin: A substance (such as an antibody or complement component) that enhances phagocytosis.

Opsonization: The process by which bacteria are altered to be more easily engulfed by phagocytes; often involves coating the bacteria with antibodies and/or complement.

Pandemic disease: A disease in epidemic proportions worldwide.

Parasite: An organism that lives on or in another living organism.

Passive acquired immunity: Immunity or resistance resulting from the receipt of antibodies produced by another person or by an animal.

Pathogen: A microorganism that causes disease.

Peptide: A low molecular weight compound that on hydrolysis yields two or more amino acids.

Phagocyte: A cell capable of ingesting bacteria, yeasts, and other particulate matter by phagocytosis.

Phagocytosis: Ingestion of cellular matter using pseudopodia to surround the matter.

Phenotype: Manifestation of a genotype; all of the attributes or characteristics of an individual.

Pilus (pl. pili): A hairlike surface projection possessed by some bacteria.

Pinocytosis: A process similar to phagocytosis, but used to engulf and ingest liquids rather than solid matter.

Plasma: The fluid portion of blood.

Plasmid: A molecule of DNA that can stably function and replicate while physically separate from the bacterial chromosome.

Pleomorphism: Existing in more than one form; also known as *polymorphism*.

Prion: An infectious agent consisting of a minimum of one protein, but no nucleic acid.

Prokaryotic cells: A cell that lacks a true nucleus. (Organisms having such cells are referred to as *prokaryotes*.)

Protoplasm: The semifluid matter within living cells, two types of which are *cytoplasm* and *nucleoplasm*.

Protozoa: A type of eucaryotic microorganism frequently found in water and soil.

Pseudopodium (pl. pseudopodia): A temporary projection from the cell used for feeding or mobility.

Pyogenic: Causing the production of pus.

Pyrogen: An agent that causes a rise in body temperature.

Reticuloendothelial system (RES): Phagocytic cells that include macrophages and cells that line the sinusoids of the spleen, lymph nodes, and bone marrow.

Rhagades: Fissures or cracks in the skin, especially around the lips or anus.

Ribosome: The site of protein synthesis in both prokaryotic and eucaryotic cells.

Glossary

Saprophyte: An organism that lives on dead or decaying organic matter.

Sepsis: The presence of pathogens and/or their toxins in the bloodstream.

Septic shock: A type of shock resulting from sepsis or septicemia; often occurs as the result of the effects of toxins released by microorganisms.

Septicemia: A serious illness often with chills and fever when pathogens and/or their toxins are present in the blood.

Slime layer: A loosely formed, nonattached layer of glycocalyx coating a bacterial cell.

Species: A specific member of a given genus (e.g., *Escherichia coli* is a species in the genus *Escherichia*). (The name of a particular species consists of two parts—the generic name and the specific epithet.)

Staphylococcus: A coccus that grows in clusters, such as in the genus *Staphylococcus*.

Streptococcus: A coccus that grows in chains of varying lengths, such as in the genus *Streptococcus*.

Streptokinase: An enzyme produced by streptococci that interferes with blood clotting.

Superinfection: An overgrowth of one or more microorganisms.

Symbiosis: The living together or close association of two organisms.

T cell, T lymphocyte: A type of agranulocyte (white blood cell) that plays important roles in the immune system.

Toxin: A poison substance of high molecular weight produced by higher plants, certain animals, and pathogenic bacteria in their metabolic processes that stimulate the production of antitoxins in the body.

Vector: An animal, usually an arthropod such as a tick, mite, mosquito, or flea, capable of transmitting pathogens from one host to another.

Virion: An infectious viral particle.

Virulence: A measure of pathogenicity of a microorganism.

Virulence factor: A characteristic of a microorganism that contributes to its virulence or pathogenicity.

Virus: An acellular infectious microorganism, smaller than a bacterium, that replicates using the biochemical mechanisms of a host cell.

Index

Page numbers followed by *f* refer to figures, and those followed by *t* refer to tables. Page numbers 209–214 refer to the Glossary.

A

Abdominal distention, with infection, 73, 78, 92, 133
Abscess(es)
  brain, 75
  with pneumonia, 145
  scalp, 67, 70, 77
  staphylococcal, 70
Absolute neutrophil count (ANC), 136, 206
Absorption, in antimicrobial pharmacokinetics, 166
Acellular, defined, 209
Acid-base balance. *See* acidosis; alkalosis
Acid-fast stain, 2
  defined, 209
Acidophile, defined, 209
Acidosis
  with pneumonia, 146–147
  with sepsis, 71
  in septic shock, 154–155, 158, 160
Acute-phase proteins, 14, 33–34, 138–139
Acyclovir, 53, 55, 91, 174
Acylampicillins, 170
Adaptive immunity, 13, 15–16
Adenosine triphosphate (ATP), for cellular energy, 154–155
Adjunctive tests, for sepsis, 138–139
Adjunctive therapies, for neonatal sepsis, 176–178
Aerobe, defined, 209
  obligate, 3
  defined, 213
Aerobic metabolism, in septic shock, 154–155
Afterload, cardiac output and, 157, 159
Agglutination, 6
  defined, 209
Agranulocytes, 20–26
  defined, 209
AIDS Clinical Trial Group (ACTG) Protocol, for zidovudine in HIV prevention, 99, 102–103
AIDS-defining illness
  in neonates, 94, 97–98, 100–101
  tuberculosis prevention with, 105–106
Airborne transmission, of microorganisms, 11, 75, 78

viral, 4, 83–84, 88–91
D-Alanine, cell wall synthesis and, 164
D-Alanine transpeptidase-carboxypeptidases, 164
Alanine aminotransferase (ALT), 108–109, 112–116, 121
Aldosterone, in septic shock, 156
Alkalosis, respiratory, in septic shock, 158
α-hemolytic Streptococcus infections, 61, 63–64, 170
Amantadine, for influenza, 89
Amikacin, 168–169, 190
Aminoglycosides, 72, 75, 148, 151, 168–171
Amniocentesis, detection of intrauterine infections, 38–39, 45–46
Amniotic fluid, transmission of infection, 117, 130–131
  by aspiration, 64, 130, 132, 145
  bacterial infection, 61–62, 78
  meconium stained, 72, 144
Amphotericin B, 120–121, 172–173
  colloidal complex, 173
  lipid complex, 173
Ampicillin
  administration guidelines for, 190
  indications for, 66, 73, 148, 150, 170–171
Anaerobes, defined, 209
  facultative, 3
    defined, 211
  infections from, 75–76, 152
  obligate, 3
    defined, 213
Anaerobic metabolism, in septic shock, 154–155
Anemia, aplastic, with human Parvovirus, 55–56
Angiogenesis, 25
Angiotensin I and II, septic shock impact on, 156–157
Anomalies, congenital, 47, 131, 149
Antepartum transmission, of infection, 130
Anti-HGV-E2 antibody, 117
Antibiotics, 163
  administration guidelines for, 189–197
  basic mechanisms of action, 164–165
  blood culture results and, 134–135
  defined, 209
  overgrowth infection from widespread use of, 132
  pharmacokinetic principles of, 166–168

prophylactic. *See* chemoprophylaxis
resistance to. *See* drug resistance
selection of, 168–172
therapeutic peak and trough levels for, 203
Antibody(ies). *See also* immunoglobulin (Ig)
  classes of, 22, 27
  defined, 209
  diagnostic detection of. *See* immunoassays
  in immune response, 16, 26–27, 29
    complement activation, 29–30
  monoclonal, 22, 86–88
  neonate production of, 23
  structure of, 26–27
  in utero synthesis of, 22, 33–34
Antibody-dependent cell-mediated cytotoxicity (ADCC), 27
Antibody titers, for protozoa identification, 8
Antifungal agents, 7, 172–174
Antigen(s), defined, 209
  hepatitis B, 107, 109–111, 114–115
  hepatitis D, 114
  in immune response, 13, 15–16, 27, 29
    B cell development and, 22–23, 27
    complement activation, 29–30
    natural killer cells and, 25
    opsonization and, 19, 27, 30, 213
    T cell development and, 23–24, 27
Antigen-presenting cells (APCs), 24, 27
Antigenic drift, in influenza subtypes, 88
Antimicrobial agents
  administration guidelines for, 189–197
  basic mechanisms of action, 164–165
  defined, 209
  ideal properties of, 163–164
  patient assessment for use of, 143–145
  pharmacokinetic principles of, 166–168
  therapeutic peak and trough levels for, 203
Antiretroviral therapy
  for HIV-infected infants, 100–101
  for HIV vertical transmission prevention, 98–100, 175
    ACTG Protocol for, 99, 102–103
    during breastfeeding, 101
    during labor and delivery, 99
    in neonate, 99
    during pregnancy, 98–99
Antiseptic, defined, 209
Antiviral agents, 91, 174–175
  for human immunodeficiency virus. *See* antiretroviral therapy

INDEX

for respiratory syncytial virus, 85–88
Apgar score, infection impact on, 144–145
Aplastic anemia, with human Parvovirus, 55–56
Apnea, with infection, 65, 71, 73, 84, 133
Arrhythmias, with septic shock, 160
Arterial blood gas monitoring, 85, 146–147, 158, 160
Arterial tone, with septic shock, 155–157
Arthritis. *See* septic arthritis
Arthropod, defined, 209
Ascending transmission, of infection, 61, 130
Asepsis, defined, 209
Aseptic technique, 122, 134
  defined, 209
Aspartate transaminase (AST), 108, 121
Asphyxia, perinatal, as infection risk, 131, 145
Aspirate cultures, 84–85, 135, 151
Aspiration, as infection risk, 64, 130, 132, 145
Asymptomatic infants, evaluation for treatment, 144–145, 149
Atmospheric requirements, for bacteria, 3
Attenuated, defined, 209
Attenuated vaccine, defined, 209
Autoimmune disease, defined, 209
Autonomic nervous system (ANS), septic shock and, 156
Autoregulation mechanism, with septic shock, 155–157
Azlocillin, indications for, 170

B

B cell/B lymphocyte
  defined, 209
  development of, 22–23, 27, 34
  differences in neonates, 22–23
  immune function of, 18, 22–24
    memory as, 27, 29
Bacilli, 2
  defined, 209
Bacteremia, 147
  defined, 209
Bacteria
  defined, 210
  fastidious, 211
  flagellated, 2–3
  laboratory identification of, 2–3
  microbiology of, 1–4
    atmospheric requirements, 3
    biochemical activities, 3
    cellular reproduction, 1–2
    genetic composition, 1–2, 4
    growth, 3
    metabolic activities, 3
    morphology (shape), 2
    movement, 3
    nutrient requirements, 3
    pathogenicity, 3–4

protein sequencing, 4
staining, 2
peptidoglycan layer of cell wall, 164
Bacterial infections, 61–79. *See also* specific infection
  early-onset *versus* late-onset, 62–63
  streptococcal, 64–66
  emerging patterns of, 79. *See also* drug resistance
  historical patterns of, 61–63
  incidence of, 61, 78–79
  with influenza, 88–89
  risk factors for, 62, 78
  specific agents causing, 63–78
    anaerobic, 75–76
    Chlamydia, 78
    Gram-negative, 72–75
    Gram-positive, 63–67, 72
    Listeria, 72
    Mycobacterium, 77–78
    Mycoplasma, 77
    Neisseria, 76
    spirochetes, 76–77
    Staphylococcus, 68–72
    Streptococcus, 63–68
  transmission routes of, 10–11, 61, 130
Bacterial meningitis, 164
  enterococcal, 73–75
  listeriosis, 72
  management of, 148, 168, 170
  staphylococcal, 71
  streptococcal, 64–65, 67–68
Bacteriocidal agents, 164
  defined, 210
Bacteriostatic agents, 164
  defined, 210
Bacteriuria, 149
  defined, 210
Bacteroides fragilis, 170–171
Bacteroides infections, 75, 170–171
Band-to-seg ratio (B:S), 137, 207
Bartonella infection, with HIV infection, 104–105
Basophils, 20, 27, 136
  defined, 210
Behavior alterations, with sepsis, 133
β-hemolytic Streptococcus infections, 63–67, 147. *See also* Group B Streptococcus (GBS)
β-lactam antibiotics, 72, 77, 169 171
Biochemical activities, of bacteria, 3
Biopsy, for detection of intrauterine infections, 39
Biotransformation, of antimicrobials, 167
Birth canal
  HIV transmission in, 37, 56, 94–96
  prevention strategies for, 98–100
  microorganisms in, 10–11

transmission of, 61, 64, 76, 130
Blindness
  from herpes simplex virus, 51–52
  from intrauterine toxoplasmosis, 41–43
Blood-borne viral infections, 83, 94–116
  hepatitis A as, 106–107
  hepatitis B as, 107–111
  hepatitis C as, 111–114
  hepatitis D as, 114–115
  hepatitis E as, 115–116
  hepatitis G as, 116–117
  human immunodeficiency virus as, 94–106
Blood cells, developmental timetable for, 16–17, 22–23, 25
Blood cultures, 71, 134–135
Blood flow, in septic shock, 155–157
  organ-specific, 158
  restoration of, 159–160
Blood glucose
  in high-risk neonates without meningitis, 182
  in sepsis, 71
Blood product transfusions
  for enteroviral hepatitis, 93
  hepatitis transmission by, 106–107, 111, 114, 116
  intrauterine, for hydrops, 56
  for septic shock, 159
Blot tests, for virus identification, 6, 95, 100
Body composition, in antimicrobial pharmacokinetics, 167
Body fluid transmission, of microorganisms, 4, 10–11, 107, 111
Body temperature
  in innate immunity, 14
  instability, with sepsis, 65, 71, 133
Bone marrow, hematopoiesis role of, 17, 19, 23, 137
Borrelia infections, 76
Bradycardia, with sepsis, 71
Brain, septic shock effects on, 155–156
Brain abscess, 75
Breastfeeding, transmission of viruses during, 94, 101, 111–112, 116
Bronchiolitis, respiratory syncytial virus and, 83–84
Bronchodilators, for respiratory syncytial virus, 86
Bronchopulmonary dysplasia (BPD), 77, 84–85
Budding yeast, 6, 120
Bullous impetigo, 69, 152

C

C-reactive protein (CRP), 34, 133, 138–139
Campylobacter infection, with HIV infection, 103, 105

216

Candida albicans, 117–119
Candida glabrata, 117
Candida guilliermondii, 117
Candida infections, 117–121
   antimicrobials for, 173–174
   clinical manifestations of, 118–120, 150
   defined, 210
   diagnosis of, 120
   epidemiology of, 117–119
   etiology of, 117–119
   immunosuppression and, 7, 11
   in late-onset sepsis, 131
   prevention of, 121
   treatment of, 120–121
Candida parapsilosis, 117–119
Candida tropicalis, 117
Candidiasis, defined, 210
Capsid, 4
   defined, 210
Capsomere, defined, 210
Capsule, 4, 9
   defined, 210
Carbapenems, 171
Carbon, bacterial pathogenicity and, 3
Carboxypenicillins, 170
Cardiac output
   four variables of, 159
   septic shock impact on, 156, 158–159
Cardiogenic shock, 153, 158
Cardiovascular dysfunction
   with pneumonia, 145–146
   with sepsis, 132–133
   with septic shock, 153, 155–158
Carrier, defined, 210
Cataracts, in congenital rubella syndrome, 47
Catecholamines, in septic shock, 154
CD cells, development of, 22–23
$CD4^+$ T-lymphocyte count
   in HIV infection classification, 94, 98–99
   PCP pneumonia prophylaxis and, 101
Cefazolin, 66
Cefotaxime, 73, 75, 190
Ceftazidime, 191
Ceftriaxone, 75, 191
Cell(s)
   bacterial, 1–3
   energy sources for, 154–155
   fungal, 7
Cell membrane, 164
   defined, 210
Cell multiplication
   bacterial factors, 3
   viral factors, 4–5
Cell wall
   antimicrobial inhibition of synthesis, 164
   damage in septic shock, 154–155
Cellular lysis, 6, 30
   defined, 212

Cellular mediators, of immunity, 13–14, 18
   components of, 18–27
Centers for Disease Control and Prevention (CDC)
   immunization recommendations of
     for communicable diseases, 89, 92, 199–201
     for hepatitis, 107, 110–111, 113–115, 117
     for HIV-infected infant, 106
   intrapartum GBS prophylaxis guidelines of, 65–66, 144–145
Central nervous system (CNS) disease. *See also* neurodevelopmental sequelae
   with enteroviruses, 92–93
   with herpes simplex virus, 51–52
   with varicella-zoster virus, 54–55, 90–91
Central venous catheters (CVCs)
   blood cultures from, 135
   as infection risk, 67, 71, 121, 131
   removal indications for, 71, 121–122
Cephalosporins, 72–75, 118, 148, 171
Cerebral atrophy, from herpes simplex virus, 51
Cerebral calcifications, from toxoplasmosis, 41, 43
Cerebrospinal fluid (CSF)
   antimicrobials effectiveness in, 164
   diagnostic debate about, 135
   findings in high-risk neonates without meningitis, 182
   findings in preterm infants, 182
   findings in term infants, 183
     in first 24 hours, 182
     on first and seventh day, 182
   findings in very low birth weight infants, 183
   in meningitis diagnosis, 53, 147–148
CHAST LOVER, 37
CHEAP TORCHES, 37
Chemical mediators, of immune response, 14–15
Chemoprophylaxis
   for Candida infections, 121
   for hepatitis infections, 107, 110–111, 113–115, 117
   for influenza, 89
   intrapartum
     drug resistance and, 72–73
     for Group B Streptococcus, 65–68, 144–145
   for *Pneumocystis carinii* pneumonia, 101, 103
   for respiratory syncytial virus, 86–88
   for tuberculosis exposure, 105–106
   for varicella-zoster virus, 91–92
Chemotactic agent, 15
   defined, 210

Chemotaxis, 30
   defined, 210
   development of, 15, 19–20
Chest x-ray, 45, 65, 133
   of disseminated varicella-zoster virus, 90–91
   pneumonia, 91*f*
   of influenza, 89
   of pneumonia, 145, 146*f*
   of RSV pneumonia, 84*f*
   for tuberculosis exposure, 105
Chickenpox, neonatal, 90–92. *See also* varicella-zoster virus (VZV)
Chlamydia trachomatis, 78, 153
Chorioamnionitis, as neonatal infection risk, 62, 73, 77, 131, 144
Chorioretinitis, 41, 43, 51, 54
Chronic lung disease (CLD), 77
   with influenza, 88
   respiratory syncytial virus and, 85–87
Cilia, protozoal, 8
Citrobacter diversus, 75
Citrobacter infections, 74–75
Clavulinic acid, 170
Clindamycin, 171, 191
Clinical evaluation. *See* evaluation of infection
Clinical management. *See* management of infection
Clinical presentations. *See* presentations of infection
Clostridium botulinum, 75–76
Clostridium difficile, 76
Clostridium infections, 9, 75–76
Clostridium perfringens, 9, 76
Clostridium tetani, 76
Clot formation, in DIC, 160
Coagulase, 9
   defined, 210
Coagulase-negative Staphylococcus (CoNS), 69–72, 131. *See also Staphylococcus epidermidis*
Coagulase-positive Staphylococcus, 68. *See also Staphylococcus aureus*
Coagulation factors, in innate immunity, 14
Coagulopathy, in DIC, 4, 10, 155, 160
Cocci, 2
   defined, 210
Coccidioides, antimicrobials for, 174
Coccoid bacteria, 2
Colitis, with sepsis, 74
   necrotizing. *See* necrotizing enterocolitis
Collaboration, in immune response, 16
Collagenase, bacterial virulence and, 9
Colonization, by microorganisms
   Candida, 117–118, 121
   Gram-negative enteric bacilli, 72–75
   in infant, 131–132
   as infection risk, 8, 10–11, 145
   in maternal genital tract, 10, 130–131, 144

Index

Mycoplasma, 77
Staphylococcus, 68–69
Streptococcus, 64–65
Colony-stimulating factors
  in immune response, 26, 32
  for treatment of neonatal sepsis, 177–178
  with sepsis, 65
Commensalism, in human body, 6
  defined, 210
  nonpathogenic, 10–11
  pathogenic, 8–9, 11
Communicable diseases, immunizations for
  CDC recommendations for, 89, 92, 199–201
  for hepatitis, 107, 110–111, 113–115, 117
  for HIV-infected infant, 106
Complement system, in immune response, 15–16
  cascade pathways, 29–30, 34
  cellular functions, 19, 26–27
  defined, 210
  differences in neonates, 30
  as innate, 14–15
Complete blood count (CBC)
  diagnostic applications of, 89, 121, 133, 137
  for monitoring HIV exposures, 106
Computerized tomography (CT) scan, for intrauterine infections, 41–42, 46
Congenital anomalies, 47, 131, 149
Congenital heart disease (CHD), respiratory syncytial virus and, 84–85
Congenital rubella syndrome (CRS), 46–48
Congenital varicella syndrome, 54–55
Conjunctivitis, 70, 78, 150, 153
Contact precautions, for viral infections, 91, 93, 105, 107
Contact transmission, of microorganisms, 4, 10–11, 90–92
Core antigen, hepatitis B (HBcAg), 107, 114
Corticosteroids, for respiratory syncytial virus, 86
Coxsackieviruses, 92–93
Cristispira infections, 76
Cryptosporidium infections, with HIV infection, 103, 105
Crystal violet stain, for bacteria, 2
Culture media, 69, 78, 134
Cultures, 133–135, 139
  anaerobic, 75
  aspirate, 84–85, 135, 151
  blood, 71, 134–135
  for bone infections, 151
  for eye infections, 153
  intrapartum, 65–66, 77
  with intrauterine infections, 39, 45–47, 53
  nasopharyngeal, 84–85, 88–89
  for pneumonia, 84, 146
  postpartum, 143–144

for septic shock, 158–159
for skin infections, 90, 152
stool, 93, 115
surface/swab, 64, 135
for urinary tract infections, 135, 149–150
viral, 84–85, 88–90, 93, 106
Curved bacteria, 2
Cutaneous infections. *See* skin infections
Cyanosis, with infections, 65, 84
Cyst transmission, of protozoa, 8
Cytokines, in immune response, 16, 24
  defined, 210
  diagnostic applications of, 139
  functions of, 31–32
  reduced in neonates, 24–26
  sources of, 31–32
Cytology, for detection of intrauterine infections, 39
Cytomegalovirus (CMV)
  antimicrobials for, 174–175
  as intrauterine infection, 43–46
    clinical manifestations of, 44–45
    consequences of maternal infection, 44
    diagnosis of, 44–45
    incidence of, 43–44
    transmission of, 37–38, 43–45
Cytopathology, of viruses, 5–6
Cytotoxicity, in immune response, 23, 25–27

D

Deafness, neonatal, from intrauterine infections, 45, 47, 50
Defense function, of immune response, 13
Defensins, 19
Delta protein antigen, hepatitis D (HDAg), 114
Dendritic cell, 18, 26–27
Dermatophytes, antimicrobials for, 174
Developmental immunology, 33–35
Diapedesis, in innate immunity, 15, 19
Diarrhea, with infection, 73–74, 76, 103
Differential white blood cell count, in premature infants, 185
Dimorphism, 6–7
  defined, 210
Diphtheria, immunization recommendations for, 106, 200–201
Diplococci, defined, 210
Disinfect, defined, 210
Disseminated disease
  with enteroviruses, 92–93
  with herpes simplex virus, 52–54
  with varicella-zoster virus, 90–91
Disseminated intravascular coagulation (DIC), 4, 10, 155, 160
Distribution, in antimicrobial pharmacokinetics, 166–167

Diversity, in adaptive immunity, 16
DNA
  analysis of, 135
  antiviral agents impact on, 174
  in bacterial cells, 1, 4
  protein-synthesis and, 165
  in viruses, 4–6, 43, 46, 54–55, 107
DNA polymerase, defined, 210
DNA probes, diagnostic applications of, 4, 109
Dohle bodies, in neutrophils, 137
Droplet precautions, indications for, 11, 75, 78
  with viral infections, 4, 83–84, 88–90
Drug delivery route, in antimicrobial pharmacokinetics, 166
Drug resistance,
  to antibiotics, 2
  bacterial infections and, 62, 71, 79
  intrapartum prophylaxis impact on, 72–73
  management principles for, 165, 169, 171–172

E

E antigen, hepatitis B (HBeAg), 107, 109
Ear infections, 150
Early-onset sepsis
  clinical evaluation of, 136, 139
  late-onset *versus*
    bacterial, 62–63
    streptococcal, 64–66
  maternal risk factors for, 62, 64, 130–131
Echoviruses, 92
Edema, interstitial, with pneumonia, 146
Effector function, of immunoglobulins, 27
Effusions
  pericardial, 77
  pleural, 146
  subdural, 147
Electron microscope
  defined, 210
  for detection of intrauterine infections, 39, 56
  virus identification by, 6, 115
Encephalitis, defined, 210
Encephalopathy, noninfectious, 147
Endocarditis, 71, 75
Endospore, defined, 210
Endotoxins
  as a bacterial byproduct, 3–4
  complement activation, 29–30
  in septic shock, 153–154
  as a virulence factor, 9–10
Enterobacter cloacae, 171
Enterobacter infections, 145, 171
Enterococcus infections, 67, 71, 149
  antimicrobials for, 169–171
  in late-onset sepsis, 63, 131

maternal transmission of, 130
Enterocolitis, necrotizing, 71, 73, 76, 171
Enterotoxin, 9
  defined, 210
Enteroviruses
  clinical manifestations of, 92–93
  diagnosis of, 93
  epidemiology of, 92
  etiology of, 92
  intrauterine transmission of, 37, 56
  nonpoliovirus species, 92
  prevention of, 93–94
  treatment of, 93
Enveloped viruses, 4
Enzyme(s)
  in antimicrobial pharmacokinetics, 164, 166–167
  bacterial virulence and, 3, 9
  defined, 210
  in immune response, 19, 26
  lysosomal, in septic shock, 154–155, 158
  proteolytic, DIC and, 160
Enzyme-linked immunosorbent assay (ELISA)
  for human immunodeficiency virus, 95, 98, 100
  for intrauterine infections, 42, 46, 54
  for viral infections, 84, 88
Eosinophils, 20, 27, 136
  defined, 210
  fluconazole impact on, 121
Epidemic disease, 88
  defined, 210
Epidemiology, defined, 210
Epinephrine, in septic shock, 156
Epiphysial plate, osteomyelitis and, 150–152
Episome, defined, 210
Erythema, 152
  defined, 211
Erythrocyte, defined, 211
Erythromycin, 78, 153, 192
Escherichia coli
  antimicrobials for, 73, 168, 191*t*
  infections from, 73, 145, 147, 149–150, 152
  maternal transmission of, 130
  in sepsis, 62–63, 131
  stress and, 20
Ethnicity, as hepatitis factor, 106–108, 111, 114–115
Eucaryotic cell, defined, 211
Evaluation of infection, 129–133
  as basis for management, 143–145
  incidence awareness, 129–130
  laboratory diagnosis, 2–3, 5–6, 133–139
  obstacles to, 129, 139–140
  predisposing factor identification, 131–132
  presentation assessment, 132–133

transmission routes and, 130–131
Excretion, in antimicrobial pharmacokinetics, 167–168
Exocytosis, 26
Exotoxins, 9, 152, 154
  defined, 211
Extracellular fluid volume, in antimicrobial pharmacokinetics, 166
Extracorporeal membrane oxygenation (ECMO), 143, 147
Exudate, defined, 211
Eye disorders, from toxoplasmosis, 41–43
Eye infections, 51–53, 76, 153

F

Facultative anaerobe, 3
  defined, 211
Family support, for HIV-infected infant, 106
Fasciitis, necrotizing, 76, 152–153
Fastidious bacterium, defined, 211
Fecal-oral transmission, of microorganisms, 4, 74, 106, 115
Feeding, poor
  with sepsis, 65, 71, 133
  with viral infections, 84, 92
Fetal distress, with *in utero* infection, 132–133, 135
Fetal infections. *See also* intrauterine infections
  with placental infection, 39
  without placental infection, 38
Fever
  maternal, as infection risk, 62, 64, 131
  neonatal
    with sepsis, 71, 73–74, 78
    with viral infections, 84, 92–93
Fibrin, bacterial virulence and, 9
Fibrinogen, in immune response, 26
Fibrinolysis, for homeostasis in DIC, 160
Fibronectins (Fns), in immune response, 32–33
  defined, 211
Fifth disease, 55
Filling volume, cardiac output and, 157, 159
Flagella
  bacterial, 2–3, 9
  defined, 211
  protozoal, 8
Fluconazole, 120–121, 174
Flucytosine, 173–174
Fluid resuscitation, for septic shock, 159
Folinic acid (Leucovorin), in toxoplasmosis therapy, 43
Fomite, 11
  defined, 211
Food preparation, HIV-infected infant and, 105

Food transmission, of microorganisms, 11, 105
Foreign agent/bodies
  immune response to, 13–16, 29–30
  as infection risk, 131
Free fatty acids (FFAs), in septic shock, 154
Free radicals, in immune response, 19
Frontal bossing, defined, 211
Functional residual capacity ($V_{MAX}FRC$), respiratory syncytial virus and, 86
Fungal infections. *See also* specific infection
  Candida as, 117–121, 131, 150, 210
  Malassezia as, 121–122
Fungi
  defined, 211
  laboratory identification of, 8
  microbiology of, 6–8
    classifications, 6–8
    in diagnosing, 8
    reproduction mechanisms, 7
Fungicidal agents, 172–174
  defined, 211

G

Galactosemia, as infection risk, 132
Ganciclovir, 46, 175
Gastric emptying time, in antimicrobial pharmacokinetics, 166
Gastrointestinal tract
  colonization by microorganisms, 10–11, 72–75
  septic shock effects on, 158
Gender, as infection risk, 131–132, 147
Gene, defined, 211
Genetic composition
  of bacterial cells, 1–2, 4
  of viruses, 4–6
Genitalia, colonization by microorganisms, 10–11, 130–131, 144
Genotype, defined, 211
Gentamicin
  administration guidelines for, 192
  indications for, 66, 71, 150, 153, 168–170
Genus (genera), defined, 211
Gerdes and Polin screening criteria, for sepsis, 138
Gestational age, hematopoiesis timetable based on, 16–17, 22–23, 25
Giardiasis, with HIV infection, 105
Giemsa smear, for herpes simplex virus, 53
Glomerular filtration rate (GFR), in antimicrobial pharmacokinetics, 167–168
Glucagon, in septic shock, 154
Glucose
  cerebrospinal fluid values for, 182–183
  serum level of. *See* blood glucose

INDEX

Glucose metabolism, in septic shock, 154–155
Glucuronidation, of antimicrobials, 167
Glycocalyx, defined, 211
Golgi bodies, 1, 6–7
Golgi complex, defined, 211
Gonococcal infections, 76, 169–170
Graft-versus-host reactivity, T cell development and, 23
Gram-negative bacteria, 2, 164
   antimicrobials for, 168–171
   blood culture techniques for, 134–135
   infections from, 72–75
   maternal transmission of, 130
   in septic shock, 153–154
   toxins produced by, 9–10
Gram-negative sepsis, 4, 10
Gram-positive bacteria, 2, 164
   antimicrobials for, 168–172, 191*t*
   blood culture techniques for, 134–135
   infections from, 63–67, 72
   in septic shock, 154
Gram's stain
   defined, 211
   diagnostic applications of, 134–135
   for specific infections, 2, 146, 148–149, 151–153
Granulocyte colony-stimulating factor (G-CSF), 26, 32, 177–178
Granulocyte-monocyte colony-stimulating factor (GM-CSF), 26, 32, 177–178
Granulocytes, 18–20
   defined, 211
   transfusions, for neonatal sepsis, 177–178
Gray baby syndrome, 167
Group A Coxsackievirus, 92
Group A Streptococcus
   antimicrobials for, 170
   infections from, 63–64, 152
   in late-onset sepsis, 63
Group B Coxsackievirus, 92–93
Group B Streptococcus (GBS)
   antimicrobials for, 168, 170
   human reservoir for, 64
   infections from, 145, 147, 149–150, 152
      early-onset *versus* late-onset, 64–66
      historical patterns of, 61–62
      management of, 66–68
      intrapartum antibiotic prophylaxis for
         CDC guidelines for, 65–66
         neonate algorithm for, 67–68, 144–145
         screening algorithm for, 67
   maternal transmission of, 64–65, 130
   screening panels for, 66–67
   stress and, 20
Group D Streptococcus, 67
Growth curve, defined, 211
Growth factors, regulation of hematopoiesis, 17–18

Growth plate, osteomyelitis and, 150–152
Grunting, with sepsis, 65

H

Haemophilus influenzae (Hib), 75, 145, 150, 153, 191*t*
Haemophilus influenzae type b
   immunization recommendations for, 106, 200–201
   maternal transmission of, 62, 130
Handwashing, 145, 149
   bacterial infections and, 61, 69–70, 72, 74
   fungal infections and, 118–119, 121–122
   viral infections and, 84, 89, 94, 104, 107
Health care workers
   hepatitis A risks for, 106–107
   hepatitis B risks for, 111
   hepatitis C risks for, 113–114
   transmission of Candida, 118–119
   treatment of RSV with ribavirin, concerns for 85
Hearing loss, from intrauterine infections, 45, 47, 50
Heart, septic shock impact on, 156, 158–159
Heart rate, cardiac output and, 159
Hemagglutination, 6
   defined, 209
   influenza subtypes based on, 88
Hematocrit, normal values for, 181
Hematopoiesis
   regulation of, 18–19, 137
   timetable for development of, 16–17, 22–23, 25
Hematopoietic stem cells (HSCs)
   in immune system, 16–17
   pluripotent, 17–18
Hemodynamic monitoring, during sepsis, 153, 155–158, 160
Hemoglobin, 181
   defined, 211
Hemolysin, 9
   defined, 211
Hemolysis
   defined, 211
   in Streptococcus classification, 63–64
Hemorrhage, pulmonary, with pneumonia, 146–147
Hemostasis, defined, 211
Hepatic disease, with viral infections, 92–93, 95
Hepatitis A (HAV)
   clinical manifestations of, 106–107
   diagnosis of, 107
   epidemiology of, 106
   etiology of, 106
   immunization recommendations for, 107, 200–201
   prevention of, 107

   treatment of, 107
Hepatitis B (HBV), 107–111
   clinical manifestations of, 109
   diagnosis of, 109
   epidemiology of, 107–109
   etiology of, 107
   four stages of, 108–109
   immunization recommendations for, 106, 110, 200–201
   intrauterine transmission of, 37
   prevention of, 110
   treatment of, 109–111
Hepatitis B core antigen (HBcAg), 107, 114
Hepatitis B e antigen (HBeAg), 107, 109
Hepatitis B surface antigen (HBsAg), 107, 109–111, 114–115
Hepatitis C (HCV), 111–114
   clinical manifestations of, 112
   diagnosis of, 112–113
   epidemiology of, 111–112
   etiology of, 111
   prevention of, 113–114
   treatment of, 113
Hepatitis D (HDV)
   clinical manifestations of, 114
   diagnosis of, 114–115
   epidemiology of, 114
   etiology of, 114
   prevention of, 115
   treatment of, 115
Hepatitis D delta protein antigen (HDAg), 114
Hepatitis E (HEV)
   clinical manifestations of, 115
   diagnosis of, 115
   epidemiology of, 115
   etiology of, 115
   prevention of, 115–116
   treatment of, 115
Hepatitis G (HGV)
   clinical manifestations of, 116
   diagnosis of, 116–117
   epidemiology of, 116
   etiology of, 116
   prevention of, 117
   treatment of, 117
Herpes simplex virus (HSV)
   antimicrobials for, 174–175
   diagnosis of, 53
   incidence of, 50, 53
   incubation period for, 50
   as intrauterine infection, 50–54
      central nervous system disease, 52
      clinical presentations of, 51–54
      disseminated disease, 52–54
      risk percentages, 51
      skin, eye, and mouth disease, 51–52
      transmission of, 37, 51, 53

lesion characteristics, 50–51
  prevention of, 53
  treatment of, 53–54
Histamine, 14, 34, 155
  defined, 211
Histamine₂ blockers, Candida infection with, 118
Homeostasis
  fibrinolysis in DIC and, 160
  immune response and, 13
Host, 11
  antimicrobials impact on, 163–164
  defense deficiencies predisposing to infection, 132
  defined, 211
Host cell
  protozoa interactions with, 8
  virulence and, 9
  virus interactions with, 4–6
Human immunodeficiency virus (HIV), 94–106
  AIDS-defining illness criteria for, 94, 97–98, 100–101
  antiretroviral protocol for, 174–175
    infected infants, 100–101
    vertical transmission prevention, 98–100
      ACTG Protocol for, 99, 102–103
      during breastfeeding, 101
      during labor and delivery, 99
      in neonate, 99
      during pregnancy, 98–99
  clinical manifestations of, 95, 97–98
  diagnosis of, 95, 98, 100–101
  epidemiology of, 94–96
  etiology of, 94
  family support for, 106
  hematologic monitoring of exposures, 106
  immunization recommendations and, 106
  immunologic monitoring of exposures, 106
  intrauterine transmission of, 37, 56, 94–96
  opportunistic infections with, 101–106
    PCP as, 95, 101, 103
    prevention of, 103–105
    tuberculosis as, 77–78, 105–106
  pediatric infection classifications of, 95, 97–99
    based on clinical status, 95, 97–98
    based on immunologic status, 95, 98–99
    based on infection status, 95, 99
  prevention strategies for, 98
  treatment of, 98–106
    antiretroviral protocol for, 98–103, 174–175
    opportunistic infections, 101–106
Human Parvovirus (HPV) B19
  clinical presentations of, 55
  incidence of, 55
  as intrauterine infection, 55–56
  transmission of, 37–38, 55
Humoral mediators, of immunity, 13–14, 18, 26
  components of, 18, 27–33
  other factors, 33–34
Hyaline membranes, pneumonia impact on, 145–146
Hyaluronidase, 9
  defined, 212
Hydrocephalus, 41, 43, 77, 147
Hydrogen, bacterial pathogenicity and, 3
Hydrops fetalis, with human Parvovirus, 55–56
Hypocalcemia, in septic shock, 160
Hyperbaric oxygen therapy, 153
Hyperbilirubinemia, with septic shock, 158
Hyperglycemia, with sepsis, 71
Hypertension, pulmonary, with pneumonia, 146–147
Hyphae, 6
Hypotension
  with sepsis, 65, 133
  in septic shock, 153–154, 159
Hypotonia, with sepsis, 65, 133, 158
Hypoxemia
  with pneumonia, 146–147
  in septic shock, 153–154, 158

I

Imipenem, 171
Imipenem/cilastatin, 193
Immature-to-mature neutrophil ratio (I:M), 206
Immature-to-total neutrophil ratio (I:T), 136–138, 206
Immune globulin (HBIG), for hepatitis, 110, 115–116
  postexposure, 107
Immune system
  components of, 13, 18–34
    cellular, 13–14, 18–27
    defined, 212
    soluble, 13–14, 18, 27–34
  development of, 13, 16–18
    summary of, 22, 33–34
    timetable for, 16–17, 22–23, 25
  functional phases of response, 13–16
  host functions of, 13, 132
  mediators of, 13–15, 18
  neonatal deficiencies of, 34–35, 132
  white blood count and, 136
Immunity, 13
  adaptive (specific), 13, 15–16
  defined, 212
  innate (nonspecific), 13–15
Immunizations, for communicable diseases
  CDC recommendations for, 89, 92, 199–201
  for hepatitis, 107, 110–111, 113–115, 117
  for the HIV-infected infant, 106
Immunoassays
  for acute-phase reactants, 138
  for detection of intrauterine infections, 39, 41–42, 45–46, 53–56
  for hepatitis, 107
  for human immunodeficiency virus, 95, 98, 106
  for viral infections, 84, 88, 90
Immunocompetent, defined, 212
Immunocompromised infants
  Candida albicans and, 7, 11, 118
  Listeria infections and, 72
  respiratory syncytial virus (RSV) and, 84–85
Immunoglobulin (Ig)
  in B lymphocyte development, 22–23, 27
  classes of, 27–29
  defined, 212
  immune function of, 6, 19, 27, 29
  as intrauterine infection marker, 39, 41–42, 45–46, 53–56
  intravenous immunoprophylaxis
    for enteroviruses, 94
    for hepatitis, 107, 110, 115–116
    for infection 176–177
  intravenous
    for hydrops, 56
    for neonatal sepsis, 176–177
Immunoglobulin A (IgA), 27–28, 145
Immunoglobulin D (IgD), 28–29
Immunoglobulin E (IgE), 28–29
Immunoglobulin G (IgG)
  functions of, 27–29
  in hepatitis infection, 107, 112, 114–115
  intravenous, for neonatal sepsis, 56, 94, 176–177
Immunoglobulin M (IgM), 28–29, 107, 114
Immunology, developmental, 33–35
Immunoprophylaxis
  for hepatitis infections, 107, 110–111, 113–115, 117
  for respiratory syncytial virus, 86–88
  for varicella-zoster virus, 91–92
Immunosorbent agglutination assay (ISAGA), for toxoplasmosis, 42
Immunotherapy, for respiratory syncytial virus, 86
Impetigo, bullous, 69, 152
In utero
  antibody synthesis as, 22, 33–34
  infection transmission. *See* vertical transmission
  ribavirin exposure cautions, 85
In vitro, 169
  defined, 212
In vivo, defined, 212

INDEX

Inactivated vaccine
　defined, 212
　for polio, 106
Incidence, of infection, 129–130. *See also* specific infection
Inclusion body, 6
　defined, 212
Incubation time, for cultures, 134
Infant risk factors, for neonatal infection, 10–11, 131–132
Infection(s)
　defined, 212
　impact on phagocytosis, 20
　in infants. *See* neonatal infection
　opportunistic with HIV infection, 95, 101–106
　　PCP as, 101, 103
　　prevention of, 103–105
　　tuberculosis as, 77–78, 105–106
Infectious disease, defined, 212
Inflammation
　defined, 212
　in innate immunity, 14–15
　with meningitis, 147
　of middle ear, 150
　with pneumonia, 145–146
　white blood count and, 136
Influenza
　antigenic types of, 88
　clinical manifestations of, 88
　diagnosis of, 88–89
　epidemiology of, 88
　etiology of, 88
　immunity to, 88
　immunization recommendations for, 89, 200–201
　prevention of, 89
　treatment of, 89
Influenza A, 88
Influenza B, 88
Influenza C, 88
Influenza vaccine, CDC recommendations for, 89, 200–201
Innate immunity, 13–15
Inotropic drugs, for septic shock, 160
Interferon (IFN), in immune response, 14, 24–25
　defined, 212
　functions of, 31–32
　sources of, 31
Interleukin-6 (IL-6), in early-onset sepsis, 139
Interleukins (IL), in immune response, 24–26, 31–32, 139
　defined, 212
Internalin, 9
Interstitial edema, with pneumonia, 146
Intestinal transit time, in antimicrobial pharmacokinetics, 166

Intestines, septic shock effects on, 158
Intracellular parasite, obligate, 4
Intracranial calcifications, from toxoplasmosis, 41, 43
Intrapartum antibiotic prophylaxis (IAP)
　drug resistance increases with, 72–73
　for Group B Streptococcus
　　CDC guidelines for, 65–66
　　neonate algorithm for, 67–68, 144–145
　　screening algorithm for, 67
Intrapartum transmission, of infection, 62, 130
Intrauterine infections, 37–57
　detection of, 39–40
　general effects of, 37–38
　historical trends, 37, 56–57, 61–63
　incidence of, 38
　organisms causing, 37–39
　　cytomegalovirus, 43–46
　　enterovirus, 56
　　herpes simplex virus, 50–54
　　human immunodeficiency virus, 37, 56, 94–96
　　human Parvovirus, 55–56
　　rubella, 46–48
　　Toxoplasma gondii, 40–43
　　Treponema pallidum, 48–50
　　varicella-zoster virus, 54–55
　outcomes of maternal infection, 38–39
　serology interpretation with, 38
Intrauterine transfusions, for hydrops, 56
Intravenous drug use, as infection risk, 106–107, 111
Intravenous fluids, for septic shock, 159
Intravenous immunoglobulin G (IGIV)
　for enterovirus infections, 94
　for hydrops, 56
　for neonatal sepsis, 176–177
Intrinsic factors, in DIC, 160
Invasive nosocomial candidiasis, 119–121
Invasive procedures, as infection risk, 71, 75, 121, 131, 145, 149
Irritability, with infection, 84, 92, 147–148, 158
Isolation, for varicella-zoster virus, 91
Isoniazid (INH), for tuberculosis, 78, 106

J

Jaundice, with viral infections, 92, 109, 115
Joint infections. *See* septic arthritis

K

Keratin, as fungal byproduct, 7
Kidney function
　in antimicrobial pharmacokinetics, 167–168
　septic shock effects on, 155–156, 158
Kinases, bacterial virulence and, 9

Kinins, in innate immunity, 14, 34
Klebsiella infections, 73–74, 145, 149–150
Klebsiella pneumoniae, in late-onset sepsis, 63, 131
Krebs cycle, of cellular energy, 154–155

L

Labor and delivery, HIV transmission during, 37, 56, 94–96
　antiviral drug prevention protocol for, 99
Laboratory tests. *See also* specific test
　accuracy and reliability of, 133–134
　adjunctive, 138–139
　for bacteria, 2–3
　for bone infections, 151
　on cerebrospinal fluid, 182–183
　　findings in very low birth weight infants, 183
　　in high-risk neonates without meningitis, 182
　　in preterm infants, 182
　　in term infants, 182–183
　cultures as, 71, 134–135, 139
　for fungal infections, 120–121
　for hepatitis, 107–109, 112–117
　for HIV exposures, 106
　for intrauterine infections, 38, 42–43, 45–47, 50, 53–56
　for meningitis, 90, 135, 148
　normal values for, 136, 181–183, 185, 187
　platelet count as, 137–138
　for pneumonia, 84, 146
　predictive values of, 133–134
　screening panels as, 138
　　for Group B Streptococcus, 66–67
　for urinary tract infections, 149–150
　for viruses, 5–6, 84, 88–90, 92–93, 98
　white blood cell count as, 133, 135–137
Lactate, cerebrospinal fluid values for, 183
Lactic acid, in septic shock, 154–155
Lactoferrin, in immune response, 19, 34
Lag time, in bacterial growth, 3
Langerhans' cell, 18, 26–27
Late-onset sepsis, 130–131
　early-onset *versus*
　　bacterial, 62–63
　　streptococcal, 64–67
Latent infection, defined, 212
Latent syphilis, 48–49
Latex agglutination, 54, 84, 135
Left shift, in white blood cell count, 137
Left-sided heart failure, in septic shock, 158
Leptospira infections, 76
Lethargy
　with meningitis, 147–148
　with sepsis, 65, 71, 73, 158
　with tuberculosis, 78
　with viral infections, 84, 92

Leucovorin. *See* folinic acid
Leukocidin, 9
    defined, 212
Leukocyte, defined, 212
Leukocyte count, 135–137, 187. *See also* white blood cell count
Leukopenia, 89
    defined, 212
Limb hypoplasia, from varicella-zoster virus, 54
Lipid transfusions, fungal infections with, 118, 121–122
Lipopolysaccharide (LPS), 9–10
Liposomal amphotericin B, 120–121, 173
Listeria monocytogenes
    antimicrobials for, 168–171
    maternal transmission of, 62, 130
Listeriosis, 72, 105, 147
Liver function
    in antimicrobial pharmacokinetics, 167
    hematopoiesis as, 16–17, 23, 25
    septic shock effects on, 158
Long bone infection. *See* osteomyelitis
low birth weight (LBW) infants, sepsis risk in, 62, 73, 131
Lumbar puncture (LP), 90, 135
Lung disease. *See* chronic lung disease (CLD)
Lungs, septic shock effects on, 158
Lyme disease, intrauterine transmission of, 37
Lymph nodes, hematopoiesis role of, 17, 26
Lymphadenopathy, with human immunodeficiency virus, 95
Lymphocytes, in immune system, 21–25
    B cells, 22–23
        defined, 209
    diagnostic applications of, 136
    T cells, 23–25
        defined, 214
    types of, 18, 21–22
    natural killer cells, 25
        defined, 212
Lymphoid stem cells, in immune system, 17–18
Lymphokines, defined, 212
Lysis, cellular, 6, 30
    defined, 212
Lysosomes
    defined, 212
    in septic shock, 154–155, 158
Lysozyme, 14, 19
    defined, 212

M

M protein, bacterial virulence and, 9
Macrophage, 16, 25–26, 145
    defined, 212
Malassezia furfur, 121–122

Malassezia infections, 121–122
    clinical manifestations of, 121
    diagnosis of, 121
    epidemiology of, 121
    etiology of, 121
    prevention of, 122
    treatment of, 121–122
Malassezia pachydermatis, 121–122
Malnutrition, maternal, as infection risk, 62, 131
Management of infection, 143–161
    collateral care in, 143
    for complications, 153–160
    evaluation for, 143–145
    pharmacologic, 163–178
    primary principle of, 143
    specific pathogen guidelines, 145–153
Margination, in innate immunity, 15, 19
Mast cells, 20, 27
    defined, 212
Maternal genital tract. *See also* birth canal
    colonization by microorganisms, 10–11, 130–131, 144
Maternal risk factors, for neonatal infection, 10–11, 62, 131, 144
Measles, immunization recommendations for, 200–201
Mechanical ventilation
    Candida infection with, 117–118
    indications for, 143, 150
        with influenza, 89
        with pneumonia, 146–147
        with respiratory syncytial virus, 85, 87
        with septic shock, 159
Meconium, in amniotic fluid, 72, 144
Mediators, of immune response, 13–14, 18
Membrane attack complex (MAC), 30
Memory, in adaptive immunity, 16, 22, 25, 27, 29
Meninges, defined, 212
Meningitis, 147–149
    antimicrobials for, 168, 170, 173–174
    bacterial. *See* bacterial meningitis
    candidal, 173
    clinical manifestations of, 147–148, 182
    clostridial, 76
    cryptococcal, 173
    diagnosis of, 148
    enterococcal, 73–75
    enteroviral, 93
    gonococcal, 76
    herpes, 52–53
    incidence of, 147
    listeriosis, 72
    management of, 148
    Mycoplasma, 77
    pathology of, 147
    predisposing factors for, 147

prognosis with, 148–149
staphylococcal, 71
streptococcal, 64–65, 67–68
varicella-zoster, 90
Metabolic acidosis
    with pneumonia, 146–147
    with sepsis, 71
    in septic shock, 154–155, 158, 160
Metabolism
    aerobic *versus* anaerobic, in septic shock, 154–155, 158
    in antimicrobial pharmacokinetics, 167
    bacterial activities in, 3
Methicillin-resistant *Staphylococcus aureus* (MRSA), 62, 69
Metronidazole, 193
Mezlocillin, 170
Microbiology
    of bacteria, 1–4
    of fungi, 6–8
    of viruses, 4–6
Microcephaly
    from cytomegalovirus, 46
    from herpes simplex virus, 51–52
    from toxoplasmosis, 41, 43
    from varicella-zoster virus, 54
Microorganism(s)
    classifications of, 1
    colonization by, 8, 10–11
    defined, 212
    enzymes facilitating invasion by, 9
    as normal flora, 6, 8–11, 153, 210
    as pathogenic, 8–9
    structural factors of, 9
    toxins secreted by, 9–10
    virulence factors of, 9
Middle ear infection, 150
Mitochondrion
    defined, 212
    in fungi, 6–7
Molds, 6
Monitoring guidelines
    for HIV exposures, 106
    for pneumonia, 146–147, 158, 160
    for respiratory syncytial virus, 85
    for sepsis, 153, 155–158, 160
Monoclonal antibodies
    diagnostic applications of. *See* immunoassays
    nomenclature system for, 22
    for respiratory syncytial virus, 86–88
Monocyte colony-stimulating factor (M-CSF), 26, 32
Monocytes
    defined, 212
    diagnostic applications of, 136
    in immune response, 16, 23, 25–26
Mononuclear phagocyte system, 25–26

INDEX

Motile, 9
  defined, 212
Mucocutaneous Candida infection, 118–120
Mucous membranes, in innate immunity, 14, 27
Multiple births, as infection risk, 131
Mumps, immunization recommendations for, 200–201
Mushrooms, 6
Mycobacterium infections, 77–78, 104–105
Mycobacterium marinum, with HIV infection, 104–105
Mycobacterium tuberculosis, 77–78
Mycoplasma infections, 2, 77
Mycosis(es), defined, 212
Myeloid stem cells, in immune system, 17–18
Myelomeningocele, as infection risk, 149
Myocardial contractility, cardiac output and, 159
Myocardial perfusion, in septic shock, 155–157, 159

N

Nafcillin, 153, 170, 194
Nasopharynx
  colonization by microorganisms, 10–11, 68–70, 78
  viral cultures of, 84–85, 88–89
Natural killer (NK) cell, 25, 27
  defined, 212
Necrotizing enterocolitis, 71, 73, 76, 171
Necrotizing fasciitis, 76, 152–153
Needle aspiration, for bone infections, 151–152
Needlesticks, hepatitis transmission by, 107
Negative predictive value (NPV), of laboratory tests, 133–134
Neisseria gonorrhoeae, 76, 153, 191*t*
  antimicrobials for, 169–170
Neisseria meningitidis, 76, 191*t*
Neonatal infection(s)
  evaluation of
    clinical signs and symptoms, 129–133
    laboratory tests for, 2–6, 133–139, 181–183
  incidence of, 61, 129–130
  latent, defined, 212
  management of
    for complications, 153–160
    pharmacologic, 163–178
    principles for, 143–145
    specific infection guidelines, 145–153
  risk factors for, 10–11, 62, 129, 131–132, 144
  signs and symptoms of. *See* presentations of infection
  transmission of, 4, 8, 10–11, 130–131

Neural tube defects, as infection risk, 149
Neuraminidase subtypes, of influenza, 88
Neurodevelopmental sequelae
  of congenital rubella syndrome, 47
  of herpes simplex virus, 51–52
  of intrauterine cytomegalovirus, 46
  of intrauterine toxoplasmosis, 41, 43
  of meningitis, 148–149
  of sepsis, 132
Neurogenic urinary bladder, as infection risk, 149
Neurotoxin, 9
  defined, 212
Neutropenia, 19–20, 65, 137
Neutrophil count
  diagnostic applications of, 71, 136–137, 206
  immune response impact on, 19–20
  normal values for, 136, 187
Neutrophilia, 19, 137
Neutrophils, in immune system, 18–20
  defined, 213
  development stages of, 136–137
  as innate, 14–15, 34
  morphologic changes in, 137
Nitric oxide, indications for, 143, 147
Nitrogen, bacterial pathogenicity and, 3
Nonspecific immunity, 13–15
Nontreponemal tests, for syphilis, 50
Norepinephrine, in septic shock, 156
Normal flora
  Candida as, 11, 117–118
  defined, 210
  microorganisms as, 8–11, 153
Nosocomial candidiasis, 117–119
  invasive, 119–121
Nosocomial infections, 61, 63, 89, 106, 132
  defined, 213
Nosocomial pneumonia, 145
Nucleic acid. *See also* DNA; RNA
  defined, 213
  antimicrobial inhibition of synthesis, 165, 174
Nursery environment, as infection risk, 132
Nutrition
  parenteral, as infection risk, 131
  requirements, for microorganisms, 3, 11
Nystatin, for Candida infection, 120

O

Obligate aerobe, 3
  defined, 213
Obligate anaerobe, 3
  defined, 213
Obligate parasite
  defined, 213
  intracellular, 4
Oliguria, with sepsis, 133

Omphalitis, 63, 73, 76, 152
Opacity-associated proteins (Opa), 9
Ophthalmic infections, 76, 153
  of herpes simplex virus, 51–53
Opportunistic infections, with HIV infection, 101–106
  PCP as, 95, 101, 103
  prevention of, 103–105
  tuberculosis as, 77–78, 105–106
Opportunistic pathogen, defined, 213
Opsonin
  defined, 213
  in innate immunity, 15, 27, 30
Opsonization, 19, 27, 30
  defined, 213
Oral candidiasis, 118–119
Oseltamivir, 89
Osteomyelitis, 150–152
  causes of, 69, 74–75, 150
  defined, 150
  diagnosis of, 151
  management of, 151–152
  prognosis with, 152
Otitis media, 150
Oxacillin, 170, 195
Oxygen
  bacterial pathogenicity and, 3, 19
  as cellular energy source, 154–155
  decreased perfusion in septic shock, 155–159
  increased requirements with sepsis, 71, 85
Oxygen free radicals, 19
Oxygen tension, in innate immunity, 14
Oxygen therapy, 143, 150
  hyperbaric, 153
  for influenza, 89
  for pneumonia, 146–147
  for respiratory syncytial virus, 85, 87

P

Palivizumab (Synagis), for respiratory syncytial virus, 86–87
Pancreatic enzymes, in antimicrobial pharmacokinetics, 166
Pandemic disease, defined, 213
Parasites. *See also* protozoa
  classifications of, 8, 40
  defined, 213
  laboratory identification of, 8
  obligate, 4, 213
Parenteral nutrition, as infection risk, 131
Parvovirus. *See* human Parvovirus (HPV) B19
Passive acquired immunity, defined, 213
Pathogen(s)
  antimicrobials selective action against, 163–164
  defined, 8–9, 11, 213
  resistant. *See* drug resistance

Pathogenicity. *See* virulence
Peak therapeutic level, for antimicrobial agents, 203
Penicillin(s), 50, 66, 71, 75, 169–171
Penicillin-binding proteins (PBPs), cell wall synthesis and, 164, 169–170
Penicillin G aqueous, 195
Peptide, defined, 213
Peptidoglycan layer, of bacterial cell wall, 164
Pericardial effusions, 77
Peripartum infection, as infection risk, 131
Peritonitis, 73
Persistent pulmonary hypertension (PPHN), 147
Pertussis, immunization recommendations for, 106, 200–201
Pets, cautions with
  for HIV-infected infants, 103–105
  Malassezia infections, 121
  Toxoplasma gondii, 40
pH
  in antimicrobial pharmacokinetics, 166
  bacterial pathogenicity and, 3
  in innate immunity, 14
  septic shock effects on, 155–156
Phagocytes, 14–15
  defined, 213
  mononuclear, 25–26
Phagocytosis
  defined, 213
  development of, 19–20, 26, 30
  stress impact on, 20, 33
Pharmacokinetics, of antimicrobials, 166–168
Pharmacologic management, 163–178. *See also* specific class or agent
  adjunctive therapies, 176–178
  antimicrobial selection, 168–175
  basic mechanisms of action, 164–165
  ideal properties of agents, 163–164
  intrapartum, for Group B Streptococcus, 65–68
  principles of, 163, 166–168, 178
    absorption as, 166
    distribution as, 166–167
    excretion as, 167–168
    metabolism as, 167
  resistance to. *See* drug resistance
Pharyngitis, 63, 84
Phenotype, defined, 213
Pili, 3, 9
  defined, 213
Pinocytosis, defined, 213
Piperacillin, 170
Placental infections. *See also* intrauterine infections
  with fetal infection, 39
  without fetal infection, 38–39

Plasma, defined, 213
Plasma cells, in B lymphocyte development, 22
Plasma proteins, in antimicrobial pharmacokinetics, 167
Plasmalemma, 7
Plasmid, 2
  defined, 213
Platelet count, 137–138, 181
Platelets, in immune system, 26
Pleomorphism, defined, 213
Pleural effusions, with pneumonia, 146
Pneumococcal vaccine, recommendations for, 200–201
Pneumococcus infections, 68, 170
Pneumocystis carinii pneumonia (PCP), 95, 101, 103
Pneumonia, 145–147
  chlamydial, 78
  clinical manifestations of, 146
  diagnosis of, 146
  enterococcal, 73–75
  enteroviruses and, 92
  management of, 146–147
  Mycoplasma, 77
  pathology of, 145–146
  Pneumocystis carinii, 95, 101, 103
  respiratory syncytial virus and, 83–84
  risk factors for, 145
  staphylococcal, 70–71
  streptococcal, 64–65, 67
Pneumonitis, with intrauterine cytomegalovirus, 45
Polio, immunization recommendations for, 106, 200
Polymerase chain reaction (PCR)
  for hepatitis, 109, 112–113, 115, 117
  for intrauterine infections, 38–39, 42, 45, 47, 53, 56
  for monitoring HIV exposures, 106
  organism identification by, 135
  virus identification by, 6, 84, 93, 100
Polymorphonuclear leukocytes (PMNs), in immune system, 18–20, 34
  diagnostic applications of, 136–137
  in innate immunity, 14–15
Polyvinyl chloride (PVC) tubing, 70
Positive predictive value (PPV), of laboratory tests, 133–134
Postexposure immune globulin, for hepatitis B, 107
Postpartum transmission, of infection, 131
Potassium-sodium pump, in septic shock, 154
Poverty, as infection risk, 62, 131
Predictive values, of laboratory tests, 133–134
Pregnancy
  antiviral protocol for HIV transmission prevention, 98–100

infection transmission during, 37, 61, 130. *See also* intrauterine infections
  rubella immunization and, 47
  termination with toxoplasmosis, 43
Preload, cardiac output and, 157, 159
Prematurity. *See also* preterm infants
  as infection risk, 62, 64, 131
Prenatal care, lack of, as infection risk, 62, 131
Presentations of infection
  in eyes, 153
  generalized, 65, 71, 73–74, 78, 132–133, 135, 144
  in long bones, 151
  with meningitis, 147–148
  with otitis media, 150
  in respiratory tract, 146
  with sepsis, 65, 71, 73
  with shock, 153–158
  of skin, 152–153
  in urinary tract, 149
Preservatives, in hepatitis vaccines, 110
Preterm infants, laboratory values in
  cerebrospinal fluid, 182
  for leukocytes, 187
  for neutrophils, 187
  for red blood cells, 181
  for white blood cells and differential, 185
Primary syphilis, 48
Prion, defined, 213
Progenitor stem cells, 17–20
Prokaryotic cell, 1–2
  defined, 213
Prolonged rupture of membranes (PROM), as infection risk, 51, 62, 64, 131, 144
Prostacyclin, in septic shock, 155
Proteases, in immune response, 19
Protein(s)
  antimicrobial inhibition of synthesis, 165
  bacterial virulence and, 4, 9
  cerebrospinal fluid values for, 182–183
  in immune response. *See* complement system
  in viruses, 4, 6
Proteolytic enzymes, DIC and, 160
Proteus infections, 63, 74, 170
Protoplasm, defined, 213
Protozoa, 8, 40
  defined, 213
Pseudomonas aeruginosa, 75, 131, 153, 170–171
Pseudomonas infections, 75, 145, 150, 153
  antimicrobials for, 75, 168, 170–171
  in late-onset sepsis, 63, 131
Pseudopodium, defined, 213
Pulmonary edema, in septic shock, 158
Pulmonary function tests, for respiratory syncytial virus, 86
Pulmonary hemorrhage, with pneumonia, 146–147

225

Index

Pulmonary hypertension, with pneumonia, 146–147
Pulmonary vascular resistance, in septic shock, 157–159
Pyogenic, defined, 213
Pyrimethamine, 43
Pyrogen, defined, 213

R

Radiography, chest. *See* chest x-ray
Rapid plasma reagin (RPR), for syphilis diagnosis, 50
Rash, with viral infections, 90, 92–93
Rectum, colonization by microorganisms, 10–11
Red blood cell (RBC), developmental timetable for, 16–17, 22–23, 25
Red blood cell count, 181
 in cerebrospinal fluid, 182–183
Renal function, in antimicrobial pharmacokinetics, 167–168
Renin-angiotensin feedback system, 156–157, 157f
Replication, of viruses, 5, 174–175
Reservoir, 11
Resistance, to antibiotics. *See* drug resistance
RespiGam
 prophylactic use of, 86–88
 therapeutic use of, 86, 177
Respiratory acidosis
 with pneumonia, 146–147
 in septic shock, 158
Respiratory alkalosis, in septic shock, 158
Respiratory distress
 with respiratory syncytial virus, 84–85
 with sepsis, 132–133, 135
  evaluation for management of, 143
  Mycoplasma, 77
  staphylococcal, 71
  streptococcal, 65
  tuberculosis, 78
 in septic shock, 158–160
Respiratory distress syndrome (RDS), impact on phagocytosis, 20, 33
Respiratory support, 143
 for pneumonia, 146–147
Respiratory syncytial virus (RSV), 83–88
 clinical manifestations of, 84
 diagnosis of, 84–85
 epidemiology of, 83–84
 etiology of, 83–84
 immunity to, 84
 prevention of, 86–88
 risk factors for, 84–85
 transmission of, 83–84
 treatment of, 85–86

Respiratory syncytial virus immune globulin (RSV-IGIV)
 prophylactic use of, 86–88
 therapeutic use of, 86, 177
Respiratory tract infections, 145–147
 clinical manifestations of, 146, 153
 diagnosis of, 146
 with influenza, 88–89
 management of, 146–147
 pathology of, 145–146
 risk factors for, 145
Reticulocytes, 181
Reticuloendothelial system (RES), 154, 158
 defined, 213
Retroviruses, 94. *See also* human immunodeficiency virus (HIV)
Reverse-transcriptase polymerase chain reaction (RT-PCR), for rubella, 47
Rhagades, defined, 213
Rhinitis, respiratory syncytial virus and, 84
Ribavirin (Virazole), 85–86
 health care worker, concerns for, 85
Ribosome, 3, 7
 defined, 213
Rimantadine, 89
Risk factors, for neonatal infection, 10–11, 129
 infant, 131–132
 maternal, 10–11, 62, 131, 144
 nursery, 132
Ritter's disease, 152
RNA
 antiviral agents impact on, 85, 174
 protein-synthesis and, 165
 in viruses, 4–6, 46, 83, 92, 111–116
Rod shaped bacteria, 2
Rodwell screening criteria, for sepsis, 138
Rovamycine. *See* spiramycin
Rubella
 adult infections of, 46–47
 immunization recommendations for, 200–201
 effectiveness of, 46
 pregnancy and, 47–48
 as intrauterine infection
  clinical manifestations of, 47–48, 55
  exposure testing, 47
  prevention of, 47–48
  prognosis for, 47
  sequelae of, 47
  transmission of, 37, 46–47

S

Sabin-Feldman dye test, for toxoplasmosis, 42
Safrinin stain, for bacteria, 2
Salmonella infections, 74, 105
Saprobes, 6
Saprophyte, defined, 214

Scalded skin syndrome, 69, 152
Scalp abscesses, 67, 70, 77
Scarlatina, nonstreptococcal, 152
Screening panels
 for Group B Streptococcus, 66–67
 for sepsis, 138
Screening programs
 for hepatitis B, 114
 for influenza, 89
 for intrauterine infections, 39–40
Secondary syphilis, 48–49
Seizures, with sepsis, 65, 148
Selective toxicity, 164–165
Sensitivity, of laboratory tests, 133–134
Sepsis
 adjunctive tests for, 138–139
 antimicrobials for, 168–175
 clinical presentations of, 132–133
 defined, 214
 diagnosis of
  laboratory findings in, 133–139
  obstacles to, 129, 139–140
 early-onset
  clinical evaluation of, 136, 139
  versus late-onset, 62–63
  maternal risk factors for, 62, 64, 130–131
  streptococcal, 64–66
 Gram-negative, 4, 10
 impact on immune response, 24, 33–34
 incidence of, 129–130
 influenza and, 88
 late-onset, 62–63, 130–131
  streptococcal, 64–67
 management of
  adjunctive therapies for, 176–178
  for complications, 153–160
  principles for, 143–153
 risk factors for, 62, 131–132
 screening panels for, 138
 staphylococcal, 70
Septic arthritis, 150–152
 causes of, 69, 75, 150
 diagnosis of, 151
 management of, 151–152
 prognosis with, 152
Septic shock, 153–160
 clinical manifestations of, 24, 158
 defined, 214
 diagnosis of, 158–159
 etiology of, 65, 133, 153–154
 local metabolic effects of, 157
 local responses to, 155
 management of, 159–160
 monitoring during, 160
 pathology of, 154–155
 specific organ effects of, 157–158
 symptoms of, 154
 systemic responses to, 155–158

226

Septic shock syndrome, T cells and, 24
Septicemia, 149
　defined, 214
　streptococcal, 64–65
Serology
　for intrauterine infection, maternal *versus* fetal, 38, 42–43, 45–46, 53, 56
　for protozoa identification, 8
　for virus identification, 6
Serotonin, in immune response, 26
Serratia infections, 74–75, 145, 170
Serratia marcescens, 74–75, 145
Seven-point scoring system, for sepsis screening, 138
Sexual practices, as infection risk, 106–107, 111, 116
Shigella infections, 74
Shock. *See* septic shock
Silent syphilis, 49
Skin
　colonization by microorganisms, 10–11
　eye, and mouth disease, with herpes simplex virus, 51–52
　in innate immunity, 14, 27
Skin disorder, as infection risk, 132
Skin infections
　herpes simplex virus lesions, 51–53
　neonatal, 152–153
　varicella-zoster virus lesions, 90
"Slap-cheek" disease, 55
Slime layer, defined, 214
Social services, for HIV-infected infant, 106
Socioeconomic status, as infection risk, 44, 62, 92, 131
Sodium bicarbonate, for septic shock, 160
Soft tissue infection, with osteomyelitis, 150–151
Soluble mediators, of immunity, 13–14, 18, 26
　components of, 18, 27–33
　other factors, 33–34
Species, defined, 214
Specific immunity, 13, 15–16, 25
Specificity, of laboratory tests, 133–134
Spherical bacteria, 2
Spina bifida, as infection risk, 149
Spiral bacteria, 2
Spiramycin, 42–43
Spirochete infections, 76–77
Spleen, hematopoiesis in, 17
Stains and staining
　of bacteria, 2
　defined, 209
　Gram's iodine
　　defined, 211
　　diagnostic applications of, 134–135
　　for specific infections, 2, 146, 148–149, 151–153

Standard precautions, for Enterovirus infections, 93–94
Staphylococcus, 68
　coagulase classification of, 68–70
　colonization by, 68–70
　defined, 214
　in scalded skin syndrome, 69, 152
　virulence factors of, 9, 69, 131, 153
Staphylococcus aureus
　antimicrobials for, 168–170
　infections from, 69–70, 145, 150, 152
　　historical patterns of, 62
　in late-onset sepsis, 63
　methicillin-resistant, 62, 69
　virulence factors of, 9
Staphylococcus epidermidis
　antimicrobials for, 168, 170, 172
　infections from, 70–72
　　historical patterns of, 62
　in late-onset sepsis, 63
Staphylococcus haemolyticus, 70t
Staphylococcus warnerii, 70t
Stem cells
　hematopoietic, 16–18
　progenitor, 17–18
Stomach, septic shock effects on, 158
Stool cultures, 93, 115
Streptococcus
　colonization by, 64–65
　defined, 214
　virulence factors of, 9
Streptococcus infections, 63–68, 153
　antimicrobials for, 168, 170, 172
　Group A, 63–64, 152, 170
　Group B. *See* Group B Streptococcus (GBS)
　Group D, 67
Streptococcus pneumoniae, 68, 170
Streptococcus pyogenes, 61, 63–64
Streptococcus viridans, 68
Streptokinase, defined, 214
Stress, impact on phagocytosis, 20, 33
Subdural effusions, with meningitis, 147
Substance abuse, maternal, as infection risk, 62, 106–107, 111, 131
Sulfacetamide sodium eye ointment, 153
Sulfadiazine, 43
Superinfection, defined, 214
Supportive care, for influenza, 89
Suppressor T lymphocytes (T$_S$), 24
Surface antigen, hepatitis B (HBsAg), 107, 109–111, 114–115
Surface cultures, 64, 135
Surfactant production, sepsis impact on, 146, 158
Surfactant replacement, 147
Surveillance function, of immune response, 13
Survival rates, with sepsis
　early-onset, 62, 65

　late-onset, 63, 65, 130
Swab cultures, 64, 135
Symbiosis, 6
　defined, 214
Sympathetic nervous system (SNS), septic shock and, 156
Synovial infection. *See* septic arthritis
Syphilis
　adult infections of, 48–49
　antimicrobials for, 170
　as intrauterine infection
　　clinical manifestations of, 49–50
　　diagnosis of, 50
　　transmission of, 37, 48–49, 130
　　treatment algorithm for, 50–51
　neonatal, 76–77
Systemic perfusion, septic shock impact on, 153, 155–159
　restoration of, 159–160

T

T-cell antigen receptor (TCR), 21, 24
T cell/T lymphocyte
　CD4+ count in HIV infection, 94, 98–99, 101
　defined, 214
　development of, 18, 23, 35
　differences in neonates, 24–25
　immune function of, 16, 23–24
　memory as, 16, 22, 25
T cytotoxic (T$_C$) cells, 23, 25
T helper (T$_H$) cells, 23–25
T suppressor (T$_S$), 24
Tachycardia
　fetal, with sepsis, 65, 132–133, 144
　respiratory syncytial virus and, 84
Tachypnea, with sepsis, 65
Taxonomy, for microorganisms
　bacterial, 1
　fungal, 6–8
　viral, 4–5
Teratogen, ribavirin as, 85
Term infants, normal laboratory values in
　cerebrospinal fluid, 182–183
　red blood cell count, 181
Tertiary syphilis, 48–49
Tetanus
　immunization recommendations for, 106, 200–201
　neonatal, 76
Therapeutic levels, for antimicrobial agents
　peak, 203
　trough, 203
Thimerosal, in hepatitis vaccines, 110
Third-spacing, with septic shock, 155–158
Thrombin, DIC and, 160

INDEX

Thrombocytopenia, 71, 137–138
Thrombus formation, with central catheters, 121–122
Thrush, oral, 118–119
Thymus, hematopoiesis role of, 17, 23, 26
Ticarcillin, 170, 196
Tissue perfusion, septic shock impact on, 153, 155–159
  restoration of, 159–160
Tobramycin, 168–169, 196
TORCH, 37, 56
TORCH CLAP, 37
Total immature neutrophil count (INC), 136
Total leukocyte count, 136
Toxic epidermal necrolysis, 152
Toxic granules, in neutrophils, 137
Toxin(s), 19
  defined, 214
  in septic shock, 153–154
  staphylococcal, 69, 71
Toxoplasma gondii
  incidence of, 8, 40
  intrauterine transmission of, 37, 39–43
  life cycle of, 40
Toxoplasmosis
  with HIV infection, 104–105
  as intrauterine infection, 40–43
    clinical manifestations of, 40–41
    diagnosis of, 41–42
    drug therapy for, 42–43
    incidence of, 40
    prognosis for, 43
    screening programs for, 39
    termination of pregnancy for, 43
    transmission of, 37, 40
Trace metals, bacterial pathogenicity and, 3
Transfusions
  blood product
    for enteroviral hepatitis, 93
    hepatitis transmission by, 106–107, 111, 114, 116
    intrauterine, for hydrops, 56
    for septic shock, 159
    granulocyte, for neonatal sepsis, 177
    lipid, fungal infection with, 118, 121–122
Transmission, of pathogens. *See also* specific organism
  airborne, 4, 11, 75, 78, 83–84, 88–91
  body fluid, 4, 10–11, 107, 111
  contact, 4, 10–11, 90–92
  cystic, 8
  fecal-oral, 4, 74, 106, 115
  food and water, 11, 105
  nosocomial, 61, 63, 132
Transplacental, 37, 61, 130. *See also* intrauterine infections
  vertical, 37, 56, 61–62, 130–131, 145

Treponema pallidum, 76–77
  antimicrobials for, 170
  intrauterine transmission of, 37, 48–50, 130
Treponemal tests, for syphilis, 50
Trimethoprim/sulfamethoxazole (TMP-SMX), 101
Tromethamine (THAM), 160
Trough therapeutic level, for antimicrobial agents, 203
Tuberculosis (TB), with HIV infection, 77–78, 105–106
Tumor necrosis factor (TNF), in immune response, 24–26, 31
Tympanometry, 150
Tzanck smear, for herpes simplex virus, 53

U

Ultrasound, for detection of intrauterine infections, 38, 40, 42, 46, 54, 56
Umbilical cord care, 76
Umbilical vessels, blood cultures from, 135
Ureaplasma urealyticum, 77
Urinary bladder, neurogenic, 149
Urinary tract infections (UTIs)
  maternal, as neonatal infection risk, 62, 64, 131, 144
  neonatal, 149–150
    clinical manifestations of, 149
    diagnosis of, 149
    etiology of, 73, 149
    management of, 149–150
    pathophysiology of, 149
Urine cultures, 135, 149–150

V

Vaccines. *See also* immunizations
  attenuated, defined, 209
  inactivated, defined, 212
Vacuoles, in neutrophils, 137
Vaginal delivery, transmission of infection, 61, 64, 76, 130
  HIV and, 37, 56, 94–96, 98–100
Vancomycin, 71, 151, 171–172, 196
Varicella-zoster immune globulin (VZIG), 90–92
Varicella-zoster virus (VZV)
  antimicrobials for, 174–175
  clinical manifestations of, 90
  diagnosis of, 90
  epidemiology of, 90
  etiology of, 90
  immunization recommendations for, 200–201
  as intrauterine infection, 54–55
    clinical presentations of, 54
    diagnosis of, 54–55
    incidence of, 54
    transmission of, 37, 54

treatment of, 55
prevention of, 91–92
treatment of, 91
Vascular dysfunction, in septic shock, 155–158
Vasoconstriction, with septic shock, 155–157
Vasopressin, in septic shock, 156
VDRL slides, for syphilis diagnosis, 50
Vector, defined, 214
Venous stasis, DIC and, 160
Ventilation-perfusion mismatch, in septic shock, 158–159
Vertical transmission, of infection, 130–131, 145. *See also* intrauterine infections
  hepatitis viruses, 106, 109, 111–113
  HIV, 37, 56, 94–96
  prevention strategies for, 98–100
Very low birth weight (VLBW) infants
  incidence of infection in, 71, 129–131
  laboratory values in, 71, 183
  sepsis signs and symptoms in, 133
Vesicoureteral reflux, 149
Vidarabine, 174–175
Viral cultures, 90, 93
  for monitoring HIV exposures, 106
  nasopharyngeal, 84–85, 88–89
Viral infections, 83–117. *See also* specific infection
  blood-borne, 83, 94–116
  in conjunctivitis, 153
  neonate predisposition to, 24, 83
  specific agents causing, 83–117
    enteroviruses, 92–94
    hepatitis A, 106–107
    hepatitis B, 107–111
    hepatitis C, 111–114
    hepatitis D, 114–115
    hepatitis E, 115–116
    hepatitis G, 116–117
    human immunodeficiency virus, 94–106
    influenzavirus, 88–89
    respiratory syncytial virus, 83–88
    varicella-zoster virus, 90–92
  transmission routes of, 4, 130
Virion, defined, 214
Virulence, of microorganisms, 9–11
  bacterial, 3–4
  defined, 214
Virulence factor, 9
  defined, 214
Virus(es)
  defined, 214
  laboratory identification of, 5–6
    cultures for intrauterine infections, 39, 45–47
  microbiology of, 4–6
    cellular structure, 4
    classifications, 4–5

evaluation techniques, 5–6
replication, 5, 174–175
Vision deficits
in congenital rubella syndrome, 47
from herpes simplex virus, 51–52
from intrauterine toxoplasmosis, 41–43
Visitation restrictions, for influenza, 89
Vitamin K
DIC and, 160
microorganism production of, 11
Volume replacement, for septic shock, 159

W

Water, bacterial pathogenicity and, 3
Water transmission, of microorganisms, 11, 105
Western blot test, for human immunodeficiency virus, 95, 100
Wheezing, respiratory syncytial virus and, 84
White blood cell (WBC)
developmental timetable for, 16–17, 22–23, 25
in innate immunity, 14
White blood cell count
in cerebrospinal fluid of high-risk neonates without meningitis, 182
diagnostic applications of, 133, 135–137
calculations for, 205–207
scoring systems for, 138
normal values for, 187
in premature infants, 185
World Health Organization (WHO), eradication of hepatitis B, 110
Wound healing, 25

X

X antigen, 30
X-linked immunoregulatory genes, 132

Y

Yeasts. *See also* Candida infections
budding, 6, 120
Yolk sac, fetal, hematopoiesis in, 16, 23, 25

Z

Zanamivir, 89
Zidovudine (ZDV)
for HIV infected infants, 100–101
for HIV vertical transmission prevention, 98–100, 175
ACTG Protocol for, 99, 102–103
during breastfeeding, 101
during labor and delivery, 99
PCP chemoprophylaxis and, 103
in postnatal infant, 99
during pregnancy, 98–99

Index

Infection in the Neonate

Continuing Education Course
Test Directions

1. Please fill out the answer form and include all requested information. We are unable to issue a certificate without complete information.
2. All questions and answers are developed from the information provided in the book. Select the *one best answer* and fill in the corresponding circle on the answer form.
3. Mail the answer form to NICU Ink, 2270 Northpoint Parkway, Santa Rosa, CA 95407-7398 with a check for $50.00 (processing fee) made payable to NICU Ink. This fee is non-refundable.
4. Retain the test for your records.
5. You will be notified of your test results within 6–8 weeks.
6. If you pass the test (70%) you will earn 20 contact hours (2 CEUs) for the course. Provider, Neonatal Network, approved by the California Board of Registered Nursing, Provider #CEP 6261, for 20 contact hours; Iowa Board of Nursing, Provider #189; Alabama Board of Nursing, Provider #ABNP0169; and Florida Board of Nursing, Provider #FBN 3218, content code 2505. Neonatal Network, Provider #04-2567-A is an approved provider of continuing nursing education by the Texas Nurses Association, an accredited approver by the American Nurses Credentialing Center's Commission on Accreditation. This activity meets Type I criteria for mandatory continuing education requirements toward relicensure as established by the Board of Nurse Examiners for the State of Texas.
7. An answer key is available upon request with completion of the exam.

Course Objectives

After reading the book and taking the test, the participant will be able to:
1. Describe the characteristics used to identify bacteria, viruses, fungi, and protozoa.
2. Outline factors that determine the effects of microorganisms on the human body.
3. Identify common commensal organisms.
4. Define innate and adaptive immunities.
5. Outline the embryologic development of the immune system.
6. Discuss the role of each component of the immune system in the prevention and response to infection.
7. Outline methods used to detect intrauterine infection.
8. Discuss seven organisms responsible for intrauterine infections as to incidence and diagnosis.
9. Discuss seven organisms responsible for intrauterine infections as to maternal, fetal, and neonatal effects, and treatment of infection.
10. Identify historic trends in neonatal bacterial infections.
11. Outline risk factors for neonatal bacterial infections.
12. Discuss neonatal bacterial pathogens as to incidence, site of infection, and signs and symptoms.
13. For each of the following organisms—RSV, Influenzavirus, varicella, enteroviruses, HIV, hepatitis viruses, Candida, and Malassezia—outline the etiology and epidemiology.
14. For each of the following organisms—RSV, Influenzavirus, varicella, enteroviruses, HIV, hepatitis viruses, Candida, and Malassezia—describe the clinical manifestations and diagnosis of infection.
15. For each of the following organisms—RSV, Influenzavirus, varicella, enteroviruses, HIV, hepatitis viruses, Candida and Malassezia—discuss the treatment and prevention of infection with these pathogens.

---

1. Which of the following is an example of an epithet?
   a. coli
   b. Escherichia
   c. *Staphylococcus epidermidis*

2. Which of the following bacteria is arranged in chains?
   a. Neisseria
   b. staphylococci
   c. streptococci

3. Bacteria that grow with or without oxygen are referred to as:
   a. facultative anerobes
   b. obligate aerobes
   c. obligate anerobes

4. Endotoxins are produced by bacteria in which of the following families?
   a. Enterobacteriaceae
   b. Mycoplasma
   c. Streptococcus

5. Viruses with capsides are more likely to be transmitted by:
   a. airborne droplets
   b. blood and body fluids
   c. fecal-oral route

6. Which of the following is a characteristic of a DNA virus?
   a. assembly errors are more common
   b. genomes remain in the infected cell
   c. replication takes place in the cytoplasm

231

CONTINUING EDUCATION COURSE

7. Owl-eye inclusion bodies are characteristic of infections caused by:
   a. cytomegalovirus   c. rotavirus
   b. enterovirus

8. Hemagglutination is a feature of which type of virus?
   a. echovirus   c. varicella
   b. influenza

9. Which of following is an example of a dimorphic fungus?
   a. Candida   c. Ureaplasma
   b. Histoplasma

10. Most antifungal treatment is based on the fact that the inner cell wall in a fungus contains:
    a. cholesterol   c. triglycerides
    b. ergosterol

11. Most protozoa develop which of the following as a protective mechanism?
    a. cysts   c. spores
    b. slime layer

12. Laboratory diagnosis of an acute toxoplasmosis infection is made by measurement of:
    a. antibody titers   c. rapid antigen detection
    b. inclusion bodies

13. Commensals are also referred to as:
    a. normal flora   c. pathogens
    b. parasites

14. The ability of *E. coli* to cause cystitus is improved by the presence of:
    a. capsules   c. pili
    b. hyaluronidase

15. Which of the following proteins assists bacteria in penetrating host cells?
    a. hemolysin   c. leukocidin
    b. internalin

16. Bacterial secretion of kinase results in:
    a. breakdown of red blood cells
    b. dissolving of clots
    c. loosening of tissue bonds

17. Members of which bacterial family produce hemolysin?
    a. Escherichia   c. Streptococcus
    b. Staphylococcus

18. Lipopolysaccharide has been shown to cause which of the following?
    a. fever   c. vomiting
    b. hemorrhage

19. Factors that determine resident flora include:
    a. colonization with pathogens
    b. presence of transient organisms
    c. temperature

20. Normal flora in the gastrointestinal tract are responsible for the synthesis of vitamin:
    a. B_{12} c. K
    b. D

21. The site where bacteria reside prior to transferring to a host is known as the:
    a. fomite   c. vector
    b. reservoir

22. Which of the following is part of innate immunity?
    a. antibodies   c. lymphocytes
    b. skin pH

23. Which of following chemical mediators is released by white blood cells?
    a. acute-phase proteins   c. kinins
    b. histamine

24. In the early stages of inflammation, which phagocytic cell is most prevalent?
    a. lymphocyte
    b. monocyte
    c. polymorphonuclear leukocyte

25. The ability to squeeze between capillary endothelial cells is referred to as:
    a. chemotaxis   c. margination
    b. diapedesis

26. Which of the following cells is responsible for the immune system's ability to remember antigen exposures?
    a. B cells   c. T cells
    b. natural killer cells

27. Hematopoietic stem cells are first produced in the:
    a. bone marrow   c. yolk sac
    b. liver

28. The primary site of hematopoiesis between the 5th and 20th weeks of gestation is the:
    a. kidney   c. spleen
    b. liver

29. Granulocytes constitute what percentage of circulating leukocytes?
    a. 30–50   c. 70–90
    b. 50–70

30. The life span of granulocyte cells is _____ days.
    a. 2 to 3
    b. 5 to 7
    c. 10 to 12

31. PMNs remain in the circulating pool for _____ hours.
    a. 4
    b. 8
    c. 16

32. Which of the following is responsible for chemotaxis of PMNs?
    a. B cells
    b. interferon
    c. platelet-activating factor

33. Production and release of PMNs is regulated by:
    a. cytokines
    b. monocytes
    c. T cells

34. Eosinophils comprise what percentage of circulating leukocytes?
    a. 2–5
    b. 7–10
    c. 12–15

35. Eosinophils play an important role in infections caused by:
    a. bacteria
    b. parasites
    c. viruses

36. Mast cells are found in which of the following locations?
    a. blood
    b. muscle
    c. skin

37. Histamine is released from granules found in:
    a. basophils
    b. eosinophils
    c. PMNs

38. Where do T lymphocytes mature and differentiate?
    a. bone marrow
    b. liver
    c. thymus

39. In the fetus, circulating B cell levels reach adult equivalents by which week of gestation?
    a. 10
    b. 15
    c. 20

40. When stimulated by an antigen, B cells differentiate into:
    a. mast cells
    b. natural killer cells
    c. plasma cells

41. Placental transfer by IgG begins during which week of gestation?
    a. 17
    b. 21
    c. 25

42. What is the half-life of IgG (in days)?
    a. 7
    b. 14
    c. 21

43. In neonates, B cells preferentially synthesize:
    a. IgA
    b. IgG
    c. IgM

44. In addition to B cells, helper T cells interact with _____ to aid in pathogen destruction.
    a. basophils
    b. monocytes
    c. PMNs

45. Helper T cell function reaches adult levels by how many months of age?
    a. 6
    b. 12
    c. 18

46. In newborns, the most important deficiency in cell-mediated immunity is a shortage of which type of T cell?
    a. helper
    b. memory
    c. suppressor

47. Natural killer cells target and destroy which of the following?
    a. flagellated bacteria
    b. protozoa
    c. virus-infected cells

48. For how many hours do monocytes remain in the circulation?
    a. 8
    b. 16
    c. 24

49. Macrophages found in the liver are referred to as:
    a. histiocytes
    b. Kupffer cells
    c. mesangial cells

50. Which of the following is known to activate monocytes?
    a. cytokines
    b. mast cells
    c. platelet-activating factor

51. Which of the following interleukins is secreted by activated monocytes?
    a. 6
    b. 8
    c. 10

52. Which of the following is released by platelet granules?
    a. complement
    b. histamine
    c. serotonin

53. Where are Langerhans' cells found?
    a. cerebrospinal fluid
    b. connective tissues
    c. mucous membranes

Continuing Education Course

54. Which is the most abundant immunoglobulin in humans?
   a. IgA   c. IgM
   b. IgG

55. Which immunoglobulin is *most* efficient in activating the classical complement pathway?
   a. A   c. M
   b. G

56. The largest concentration of IgE is found in the gastrointestinal tract and the:
   a. cerebrospinal fluid   c. mucous membranes
   b. lungs

57. Allergic reactions and anaphylactic shock are mediated by which class of immunoglobulin?
   a. IgA   c. IgE
   b. IgD

58. Of the following, which immunoglobulin class predominates during a secondary exposure to an antigen?
   a. IgE   c. IgM
   b. IgG

59. Complement is synthesized by what organ?
   a. kidney   c. spleen
   b. liver

60. Complement activation via the classic pathway is most often initiated by the presence of:
   a. antigen-antibody complexes
   b. foreign molecules
   c. plasma cells

61. Which of the following cytokines serves as the first line of defense in a viral infection?
   a. interferons   c. tumor necrosis factor
   b. interleukins

62. Interleukins are produced by:
   a. B cells   c. T cells
   b. monocytes

63. What is the role of fibronectins in the immune response? They:
   a. augment phagocytosis
   b. convert B cells to plasma cells
   c. induce production of memory cells

64. An elevation in which of the following is a marker for infection in neonates?
   a. C-reactive protein   c. lactoferrin
   b. kinin

65. Viral nucleic acid sequences are identified by which of the following tests?
   a. cytology
   b. election microscopy
   c. polymerase chain reaction

66. The definitive host of *Toxoplasma gondii* is the:
   a. cat   c. pig
   b. dog

67. During acute infections, which stage of the parasite *T. gondii* predominates?
   a. bradyzoite   c. tachyzoite
   b. sporozoite

68. What percentage of the U.S. population is seropositive for *T. gondii*?
   a. 20   c. 40
   b. 30

69. Approximately 50 percent of infants with congenital *T. gondii* develop:
   a. chorioretinitis c. hydrocephalus
   b. congenital deafness

70. Diagnosis of congenital toxoplasmosis is confirmed by presence of which of the following in the cord blood?
   a. IgD   c. IgM
   b. IgG

71. Congenital toxoplasmosis is treated by three or four 21-day courses of:
   a. folinic acid   c. spiramycin
   b. pyrimethamine

72. CMV is a member of which family of viruses?
   a. Picornaviridae   c. Retroviridae
   b. Herpesviridae

73. Which of the following is the only known reservoir for CMV?
   a. cats   c. humans
   b. cows

74. In the U.S., what percentage of middle- to upper-socioeconomic class women develop a primary CMV infection each year?
   a. 2   c. 6
   b. 4

75. Five to fifteen percent of infants with asymptomatic CMV infection go on to develop learning disabilities or:
   a. blindness   c. mental retardation
   b. hearing loss

Infection in the Neonate

76. Newborn findings in CMV disease include:
    a. cataracts
    b. hydrocephalus
    c. thrombocytopenia

77. Which of the following drugs is used to treat CMV chorioretinitis in adults?
    a. acyclovir
    b. ganciclovir
    c. vidarabine

78. Prodromal symptoms of rubella infection include:
    a. conjunctivitis
    b. diarrhea
    c. myalgia

79. Congenital anomalies associated with congenital rubella syndrome include:
    a. anencephaly
    b. oomphalocele
    c. peripheral pulmonic stenosis

80. Syphillis is caused by a:
    a. Gram-positive cocci
    b. Gram-negative rod
    c. Gram-negative spirochete

81. The rash characteristic of secondary syphilis is typically found on the:
    a. face
    b. palms
    c. trunk

82. Early manifestations of congenital syphilis include:
    a. chorioretinitis
    b. deafness
    c. hydrops fetalis

83. Late findings characteristic of congenital syphilis include:
    a. leukemia
    b. mulberry molars
    c. rickets

84. Which of the following is the treatment of choice for syphilis?
    a. clindamycin
    b. penicillin
    c. tetracycline

85. What is the incubation period for HSV infection?
    a. three days
    b. one week
    c. two weeks

86. The risk of neonatal HSV infection following vaginal delivery in a mother with a reactivated infection is ____ percent.
    a. 0–5
    b. 5–10
    c. 10–15

87. Fetal findings in congenital HSV infection include which of the following?
    a. anencephaly
    b. limb atrophy
    c. vesicular skin lesions

88. In cases of SEM herpes disease, skin lesions usually appear in the first ____ days of life.
    a. 5
    b. 10
    c. 15

89. The mortality rate for disseminated HSV disease is ____ percent.
    a. 30
    b. 40
    c. 50

90. The recommended treatment for congenital HSV infection is:
    a. acyclovir
    b. ganciclovir
    c. vidarabine

91. Varicella virus is spread by which route?
    a. contaminated fomites
    b. fecal-oral
    c. respiratory droplets

92. A neonate whose mother develops varicella on delivery day should be given prophylactic:
    a. acyclovir
    b. varicella vaccine
    c. VZIG

93. Slap-cheek disease is caused by:
    a. Enterovirus
    b. human Parvovirus B19
    c. varicella-zoster virus

94. Congenital infection with Parvovirus is associated with:
    a. cutaneous lesions
    b. erythroblastosis fetalis
    c. nonimmune hydrops

95. Which of the following bacteria is known to cause transplacental infections in neonates?
    a. Group B β-hemolytic Streptococcus
    b. *Listeria monocytogenes*
    c. *Neisseria gonorrhoea*

96. What is the most important risk factor for neonatal sepsis?
    a. low birth weight
    b. maternal infection
    c. prolonged rupture of membranes

97. Organisms commonly responsible for early-onset neonatal infection include:
    a. *L. monocytogenes*
    c. *S. aureus*
    c. *S. edpidermidis*

98. The mortality rate for late-onset neonatal infections is ____ percent.
    a. 2–6
    b. 7–10
    c. 11–14

99. Group A Streptococcus commonly colonizes the:
    a. GI tract
    b. oropharynx
    c. skin

100. The most likely reservoir for Group B Streptococcus is:
    a. lower GI tract
    b. oropharynx
    c. urinary tract

101. What percentage of pregnant women are colonized with GBS?
    a. 5–10
    b. 15–20
    c. 25–30

102. Infants who are born to untreated GBS-positive women and who become colonized with GBS, have approximately what chance (percentage) of developing GBS sepsis?
    a. 1
    b. 7
    c. 10

103. What percentage of neonates with early-onset GBS are born to women with no risk factors?
    a. 25
    b. 35
    c. 45

104. Fifty percent of infants with late-onset GBS present with:
    a. meningitis
    b. pneumonia
    c. septicemia

105. The CDC guidelines recommend that pregnant women be screened for GBS at ____ weeks of gestation.
    a. 28 to 32
    b. 32 to 35
    c. 36 to 37

106. In infants, *Streptococcus viridans* forms part of the normal flora of the:
    a. ears
    b. mouth
    c. skin

107. The major source of colonization for *S. aureus* is:
    a. breast milk
    b. care provider's hands
    c. respiratory equipment

108. MRSA is commonly responsible for:
    a. meningitis
    b. pyelonephritis
    c. septic arthritis

109. *S. aureus* pneumonia is associated with the development of:
    a. pleural effusions
    b. pneumatoceles
    c. pulmonary interstitial emphysema

110. Risk factors for the development of CONs infection include:
    a. formula feeding
    b. presence of a central line
    c. prolonged hospital stay

111. *S. epidermidis* infections are usually treated with:
    a. cephalosporins
    b. gentamicin
    c. vancomycin

112. Reported epidemics of listeriosis are usually associated with:
    a. contaminated food
    b. parenteral nutrition
    c. tainted blood

113. The most common site for a Gram-negative infection is:
    a. lungs
    b. meninges
    c. urinary tract

114. The most common cause of Gram-negative sepsis is:
    a. *E. coli*
    b. *B. fragilis*
    c. *N. gonorrhoeae*

115. Shigella infections are usually limited to the:
    a. gastrointestinal tract
    b. lungs
    c. urinary tract

116. Citrobacter has been reported to cause:
    a. brain abscesses
    b. osteomyelitis
    c. pseudomembranous colitis

117. *H. influenzae* forms part of the normal flora of the:
    a. gastrointestinal tract
    b. skin
    c. upper respiratory tract

118. In infants, botulism has been associated with feeding of which of the following products?
    a. condensed milk
    b. corn syrup
    c. honey

119. *Clostridium perfringens* infection in neonates is associated with:
    a. cellulitis
    b. gastroenteritis
    c. pharyngitis

120. Gonococcal infections are more common in:
    a. autumn
    b. spring
    c. summer

121. Gonococcal ophthalmia neonatorum usually presents within how many days following delivery?
    a. 0–1
    b. 2–5
    c. 6–8

122. Low birth weight infants colonized with *Ureaplasma urealyticum* have an increased risk of developing:
    a. chronic lung disease
    b. necrotizing enterocolitis
    c. patent ductus arteriosus

123. Fetal tuberculosis acquired through the bloodstream results in infection of the lung or:
    a. heart
    b. kidney
    c. liver

124. Chlamydial infection in neonates presents as either conjunctivitis or:
    a. disseminated sepsis
    b. meningitis
    c. pneumonia

125. In North America, RSV season is typically:
    a. September–December
    b. October–April
    c. February–June

126. The incubation period for RSV is ____ days.
    a. 2 to 8
    b. 5 to 10
    c. 10 to 14

127. In the U.S., the only drug approved for the treatment of RSV is:
    a. palivizumab
    b. ribavirin
    c. RespiGam

128. The most significant complication of RSV-IVIG administration is:
    a. allergic reactions
    b. induction of bronchospasm
    c. volume overload

129. The recommended dose of palivizumab is ____ mg/kg.
    a. 10
    b. 15
    c. 20

130. A person who has contracted varicella is most contagious how many days prior to the rash appearing?
    a. 1–2
    b. 3–4
    c. 5–6

131. The recommended every 8 hour dose of acyclovir for treating varicella pneumonia is ____ mg/kg.
    a. 5
    b. 10
    c. 15

132. What is the minimum number of days of isolation required for neonates with varicella?
    a. 5
    b. 7
    c. 10

133. VZIG should be given within how many hours of exposure?
    a. 48
    b. 72
    c. 96

134. Enteroviruses spread by which of the following?
    a. fomites
    b. insect bites
    c. respiratory droplets

135. Factors which contribute to Enterovirus infection include:
    a. contaminated food
    b. poor hygiene
    c. winter season

136. Congenital Enterovirus infection has been implicated in the development of:
    a. diabetes
    b. heart disease
    c. systemic lupus erythematus

137. Which of the following cells are attacked by HIV?
    a. basophils
    b. monocytes
    c. neutrophils

138. Which of the following body fluids have been implicated in the spread of HIV?
    a. saliva
    b. semen
    c. urine

139. In cases of perinatal HIV infection, the median age of onset of symptoms is ____ year(s).
    a. 1
    b. 2
    c. 3

140. Presenting features of HIV infection during the first year of life include:
    a. leukemia
    b. oral candidiasis
    c. pulmonary tuberculosis

141. Which of the following is one of the preferred methods of testing infants born to an HIV-positive woman?
    a. ELISA
    b. PCR
    c. Western blot

142. Treatment of HIV-positive pregnant women with zidovudine reduces the risk of perinatal infection from 25 percent to ____ percent.
    a. 8
    b. 12
    c. 16

143. Which of the following side effects has been noted in infants treated with zidovudine?
   a. anemia
   b. neutropenia
   c. thrombocytopenia

144. The drug of choice for *Pneumocystis carinii* pneumonia prophylaxis in neonates is:
   a. doxycyclin
   b. metronidazole
   c. trimethoprim/sulfamethoxazole

145. For HIV-exposed neonates, the AAP recommends that a T cell profile be done at how many weeks of age?
   a. 2
   b. 4
   c. 6

146. Adults with hepatitis A can be expected to shed virus for:
   a. 4–7 days
   b. 2 weeks
   c. several months

147. Neonates with hepatitis A infection typically:
   a. become jaundiced
   b. develop fever and malaise
   c. show mild nonspecific symptoms

148. The hepatitis B virus can survive on counter tops for:
   a. several hours
   b. three or four days
   c. one week or more

149. In the majority of cases of neonatal hepatitis B infection, transmission occurs:
   a. at delivery
   b. during breastfeeding
   c. *in utero*

150. Features of fulminant neonatal hepatitis B infection include:
   a. elevated ALT
   b. liver cirrhosis
   c. renal failure

151. Term infants born to HbsAg-negative mothers should receive their first dose of hepatitis vaccine by _____ month(s) of age.
   a. one
   b. two
   c. three

152. Infants born to HBsAg-positive mothers should receive HBIG within how many hours after delivery?
   a. 12
   b. 24
   c. 48

153. In developed countries, the most common mode of transmission of hepatitis C (HCV) is:
   a. blood
   b. fecal-oral
   c. IV drug use

154. The average incubation period for HCV infection is _____ weeks.
   a. 2–3
   b. 4–5
   c. 6–7

155. Transmission of hepatitis E (HEV) is via:
   a. blood
   b. fecal-oral route
   c. sexual contact

156. HEV epidemics have been noted in:
   a. Alaska
   b. Mexico
   c. Puerto Rico

157. In healthy people, Candida species normally colonize the:
   a. GI tract
   b. nose
   c. urethra

158. Susceptibility to Candida infection is increased in neonates infected with:
   a. HIV
   b. HCV
   c. RSV

159. Cutaneous Candida infection is characterized by what type of lesion?
   a. macular
   b. satellite
   c. vesicular

160. Symptoms of systemic candidiasis include:
   a. hyperglycemia
   b. renal failure
   c. thrombocytopenia

161. The recommended initial dose of amphotericin B is _____ mg/kg given over 2–6 hours.
   a. 0.05–0.1
   b. 0.1–0.3
   c. 0.25–0.5

162. As an alternative to amphotericin, which of the following drugs is used to treat systemic candidiasis?
   a. fluconazole
   b. ketaconizole
   c. mycostatin

163. The portal of entry for Malassizia species is usually:
   a. intravenous catheters
   b. skin wounds
   c. surgical procedures

164. Treatment for *Malassizia furfur* infections includes:
   a. antifungal medication
   b. corticosteroids
   c. temporarily stopping lipids

165. The estimated rate of neonatal sepsis is _____ infants per 1,000 live births.
   a. 0.1–1
   b. 1–8
   c. 6–10

Infection in the Neonate

166. The predominant organisms responsible for early-onset neonatal sepsis include:
    a. *L. monocytogenes*
    b. Enterobacter
    c. *S. pneumoniae*

167. In addition to CONs, common causes of late-onset sepsis in neonates include:
    a. Enterococcus
    b. Haemophilus
    c. Streptococcus

168. Which of the following factors has been shown to be a key risk factor for neonatal sepsis?
    a. chorioamnionitis
    b. upper respiratory tract infection
    c. urinary tract infection

169. The most common neonatal risk factors for infection include:
    a. malpresentation
    b. meconium
    c. multiple births

170. Which metabolic disorder is associated with neonatal infection?
    a. congenital adrenal hyperplasia
    b. galactosemia
    c. tyrosinemia

171. The most common manifestation of sepsis in VLBW infants is:
    a. apnea
    b. feeding intolerance
    c. hypotension

172. Signs of septic shock in the neonate include:
    a. hypoglycemia
    b. oliguria
    c. seizures

173. Signs suggesting the need for a lumbar puncture as part of the sepsis workup include:
    a. neutrophilia
    b. persistent metabolic acidosis
    c. sustained tachycardia

174. Which of the following can cause a false elevation in WBC count?
    a. hemolysis
    b. Howell-Jolly bodies
    c. nucleated red blood cells

175. Which of the following factors influences normal WBC and differential counts?
    a. birth weight
    b. congenital heart disease
    c. maternal hypertension

176. Which of the following is associated with persistent neutropenia after birth?
    a. asphyxia
    b. hydrops fetalis
    c. postmaturity

177. The I:T ratio is most reliable in:
    a. early-onset infection
    b. late-onset infection
    c. both types of infection

178. In neonates, thrombocytopenia should be investigated any time the platelet count falls below ____/mm^3.
    a. 200,000
    b. 150,000
    c. 100,000

179. C-reactive protein (CRP) begins to rise how many hours after an inflammatory stimulus?
    a. 1–3
    b. 4–6
    c. 7–9

180. Which of the following can cause a false-positive elevation of CRP?
    a. asphyxia
    b. meconium aspiration
    c. transient tachypnea

181. For the most sensitive result, IL-6 should be drawn within how many hours after birth?
    a. 12
    b. 18
    c. 24

182. Pneumonia occurs in up to what percentage of NICU patients?
    a. 5
    b. 10
    c. 15

183. The *most common cause* of perinatally acquired pneumonia is:
    a. coagulase-negative Staphylococcus
    b. *E. coli*
    c. Group B Streptococcus

184. Organisms responsible for late-onset respiratory infections in NICU patients include:
    a. Haemophilus
    b. Klebsiella
    c. Shigella

185. Which of the following factors places neonates at increased risk of respiratory infection?
    a. absent cilia
    b. diminished lung macrophage activity
    c. reduced concentrations of IgM

186. Chest x-ray findings typical of neonatal pneumonia include:
    a. diffuse atelectasis
    b. hyperinflation of the alveoli
    c. pulmonary interstitial emphysema

187. Neonatal meningitis occurs at a rate of ____ per 1,000 live births.
    a. 0.4–1
    b. 1.2–1.6
    c. 1.8–2.2

188. What percentage of infants with a positive blood culture go on to develop meningitis?
    a. 15
    b. 20
    c. 25

189. Which of the following is among the organisms most commonly responsible for neonatal meningitis?
 a. Klebsiella
 b. Listeria
 c. *S. aureus*

190. In neonates, seizures may be more common in meningitis caused by:
 a. Gram-positive organisms
 b. Gram-negative organisms
 c. viruses

191. A CSF leukocyte count which exceeds ____/mm³, is indicative of meningitis.
 a. 12
 b. 22
 c. 32

192. Which of the following is the recommended initial therapy for suspected meningitis?
 a. ampicillin and an aminoglycoside
 b. ampicillin and a cephalosporin
 c. vancomycin and gentamicin

193. How many weeks should antibiotics be administered in cases of meningitis caused by a Gram-negative organism?
 a. two
 b. three
 c. four

194. Long-term complications of meningitis include:
 a. blindness
 b. microcephaly
 c. reading problems

195. Urinary tract infections are most often caused by:
 a. *E. coli*
 b. GBS
 c. Klebsiella

196. What definitive diagnostic test should be done to rule out a structural abnormality in neonates who have had a UTI?
 a. intravenous pyelogram
 b. nuclear scan
 c. voiding cystourethrogram

197. What percentage of neonates with a UTI also have septicemia?
 a. 5–15
 b. 15–30
 c. 30–45

198. In the first eight weeks of life, otitis media is estimated to occur in what percentage of term infants?
 a. 34
 b. 48
 c. 56

199. Approximately 50 percent of neonates with otitis media also have:
 a. conjunctivitis
 b. tonsillitis
 c. tympanic perforation

200. Organisms commonly responsible for osteomyelitis in the neonate include:
 a. Clostridium
 b. herpes
 c. *S. aureus*

201. Joint infections caused by Gram-negative organisms are usually treated with gentamicin or:
 a. cefotaxime
 b. erythromycin
 c. vancomycin

202. Omphalitis is usually caused by Staphylococcus or:
 a. *E. coli*
 b. Pseudomonas
 c. Streptococcus

203. Usual sites for scalded skin infection include the:
 a. buttocks
 b. neck
 c. toes

204. Which of the following may be used for the treatment of scalded skin infections?
 a. ampicillin
 b. gentamicin
 c. oxycillin

205. The *most* common cause of ophthalmia in neonates is:
 a. Chlamydia
 b. Haemophilus
 c. Streptococcus

206. Ophthalmia caused by Pseudomonas can result in the development of:
 a. brain abscess
 b. pneumonia
 c. renal failure

207. What substance is responsible for the development of septic shock?
 a. cytokines
 b. endotoxin
 c. histamine

208. In septic shock, the release of which of the following results in decreased vascular tone?
 a. aldosterone
 b. IL-6
 c. prostacyclin

209. During periods of moderate reduction in cardiac output, intense vasoconstriction may be experienced by which organ?
 a. bowel
 b. kidney
 c. skin

Infection in the Neonate

210. With septic shock, the initial effect on the heart is:
    a. a decrease in contractility
    b. a decrease in preload
    c. an increase in afterload

211. Which of the following would be an expected finding in early cardiogenic shock?
    a. hypertension
    b. respiratory acidosis
    c. warm, flushed skin

212. In septic shock, recurrent acidosis suggests a state of:
    a. cardiac decompensation
    b. hypoperfusion
    c. respiratory failure

213. THAM cannot be used for longer than ____ hours.
    a. 12
    b. 18
    c. 24

214. The most common mechanism by which antibiotics work is in the inhibition of ____ synthesis.
    a. cell wall
    b. nucleic acid
    c. protein

215. Drugs which inhibit cell wall synthesis include:
    a. clindamycin
    b. gentamycin
    c. vancomycin

216. Amphotericin works by which of the following mechanisms? Inhibition of:
    a. cell membrane function
    b. cell wall synthesis
    c. protein synthesis

217. Drugs that function by inhibiting nucleic acid synthesis include:
    a. ampicillin
    b. flucytosine
    c. imipenem

218. A newborn's ability to absorb oral antibiotics is diminished in part due to:
    a. acidic gastric pH
    b. decreased pancreatic enzyme activity
    c. rapid intestinal transit time

219. Compared with a term neonate, a premature neonate may require a higher dose of an aminoglycoside because of the presence of increased:
    a. extracellular fluid
    b. fat cells
    c. intracellular fluid

220. Which of the following antibiotics has been shown to significantly displace bilirubin from albumin-binding sites?
    a. amphotericin
    b. ceftriaxone
    c. vidarabine

221. The chief pathway for elimination of antibiotics in the neonate is via the:
    a. gut
    b. kidney
    c. lungs

222. Therapy to treat possible infection caused by anaerobic organisms is warranted in cases of:
    a. bowel perforation
    b. meningitis
    c. urinary tract infection

223. Among aminoglycosides, which drug is reserved for infections caused by multiply-resistant strains?
    a. amikacin
    b. gentamicin
    c. tobramycin

224. When combined with penicillins, aminoglycosides provide synergistic activity against:
    a. anerobic organisms
    b. enterococci
    c. Gram-negative bacilli

225. An effective choice for the treatment of *Treponema pallidum* is:
    a. gentamycin
    b. rifampin
    c. penicillin

226. Ampicillin is more effective than penicillin against most strains of:
    a. Group A Streptococcus
    b. *L. monocytogenes*
    c. Pneumococcus

227. Anti-staphylococcal penicillins include:
    a. nafcillin
    b. piperacillin
    c. ticarcillin

228. Compared to earlier penicillins, ticarcillin has increased activity against:
    a. *E. coli*
    b. Proteus
    c. Staphylococcus

229. Which of the following drugs is most active against *Pseudomonas aeruginosa*?
    a. azlocillin
    b. mezlocillin
    c. piperacillin

230. Third-generation cephalosporins are not suitable for single agent treatment of suspected sepsis because of their limited activity against:
    a. *E. coli*
    b. Klebsiella
    c. Listeria

231. The primary role of clindamycin in neonates is in the treatment of:
   a. Bacteroides
   b. Pseudomonas
   c. Serratia

232. Vancomycin is the drug of choice for the treatment of infections caused by:
   a. coagulase-negative Staphylococcus
   b. Enterococcus
   c. *S. aureus*

233. Rapid administration of IV amphotericin B may result in:
   a. respiratory arrest
   b. seizures
   c. systemic hypotension

234. The primary adverse effect of acyclovir is altered:
   a. hematologic profile
   b. liver function
   c. renal function

235. Which antiviral drug is currently being investigated for the treatment of congenital CMV?
   a. acyclovir
   b. ganciclovir
   c. vidarabine

INFECTION IN THE NEONATE

ANSWER FORM: Infection in the Neonate:
A Comprehensive Guide to Assessment, Management, and Nursing Care

Please completely fill in the circle of the **one best answer** using a dark pen.

Questions are numbered vertically.

1. a. ○ b. ○ c. ○
2. a. ○ b. ○ c. ○
3. a. ○ b. ○ c. ○
4. a. ○ b. ○ c. ○
5. a. ○ b. ○ c. ○
6. a. ○ b. ○ c. ○
7. a. ○ b. ○ c. ○
8. a. ○ b. ○ c. ○
9. a. ○ b. ○ c. ○
10. a. ○ b. ○ c. ○
11. a. ○ b. ○ c. ○
12. a. ○ b. ○ c. ○
13. a. ○ b. ○ c. ○
14. a. ○ b. ○ c. ○
15. a. ○ b. ○ c. ○
16. a. ○ b. ○ c. ○
17. a. ○ b. ○ c. ○
18. a. ○ b. ○ c. ○
19. a. ○ b. ○ c. ○
20. a. ○ b. ○ c. ○
21. a. ○ b. ○ c. ○
22. a. ○ b. ○ c. ○
23. a. ○ b. ○ c. ○
24. a. ○ b. ○ c. ○
25. a. ○ b. ○ c. ○
26. a. ○ b. ○ c. ○
27. a. ○ b. ○ c. ○
28. a. ○ b. ○ c. ○
29. a. ○ b. ○ c. ○
30. a. ○ b. ○ c. ○
31. a. ○ b. ○ c. ○
32. a. ○ b. ○ c. ○
33. a. ○ b. ○ c. ○
34. a. ○ b. ○ c. ○
35. a. ○ b. ○ c. ○
36. a. ○ b. ○ c. ○
37. a. ○ b. ○ c. ○
38. a. ○ b. ○ c. ○
39. a. ○ b. ○ c. ○
40. a. ○ b. ○ c. ○
41. a. ○ b. ○ c. ○
42. a. ○ b. ○ c. ○
43. a. ○ b. ○ c. ○
44. a. ○ b. ○ c. ○
45. a. ○ b. ○ c. ○
46. a. ○ b. ○ c. ○
47. a. ○ b. ○ c. ○
48. a. ○ b. ○ c. ○
49. a. ○ b. ○ c. ○
50. a. ○ b. ○ c. ○
51. a. ○ b. ○ c. ○
52. a. ○ b. ○ c. ○
53. a. ○ b. ○ c. ○
54. a. ○ b. ○ c. ○
55. a. ○ b. ○ c. ○
56. a. ○ b. ○ c. ○
57. a. ○ b. ○ c. ○
58. a. ○ b. ○ c. ○
59. a. ○ b. ○ c. ○
60. a. ○ b. ○ c. ○
61. a. ○ b. ○ c. ○
62. a. ○ b. ○ c. ○
63. a. ○ b. ○ c. ○
64. a. ○ b. ○ c. ○
65. a. ○ b. ○ c. ○
66. a. ○ b. ○ c. ○
67. a. ○ b. ○ c. ○
68. a. ○ b. ○ c. ○
69. a. ○ b. ○ c. ○
70. a. ○ b. ○ c. ○
71. a. ○ b. ○ c. ○
72. a. ○ b. ○ c. ○
73. a. ○ b. ○ c. ○
74. a. ○ b. ○ c. ○
75. a. ○ b. ○ c. ○
76. a. ○ b. ○ c. ○
77. a. ○ b. ○ c. ○
78. a. ○ b. ○ c. ○
79. a. ○ b. ○ c. ○
80. a. ○ b. ○ c. ○
81. a. ○ b. ○ c. ○
82. a. ○ b. ○ c. ○
83. a. ○ b. ○ c. ○
84. a. ○ b. ○ c. ○
85. a. ○ b. ○ c. ○
86. a. ○ b. ○ c. ○
87. a. ○ b. ○ c. ○
88. a. ○ b. ○ c. ○
89. a. ○ b. ○ c. ○
90. a. ○ b. ○ c. ○
91. a. ○ b. ○ c. ○
92. a. ○ b. ○ c. ○
93. a. ○ b. ○ c. ○
94. a. ○ b. ○ c. ○
95. a. ○ b. ○ c. ○
96. a. ○ b. ○ c. ○
97. a. ○ b. ○ c. ○
98. a. ○ b. ○ c. ○
99. a. ○ b. ○ c. ○
100. a. ○ b. ○ c. ○
101. a. ○ b. ○ c. ○
102. a. ○ b. ○ c. ○
103. a. ○ b. ○ c. ○
104. a. ○ b. ○ c. ○
105. a. ○ b. ○ c. ○
106. a. ○ b. ○ c. ○
107. a. ○ b. ○ c. ○
108. a. ○ b. ○ c. ○
109. a. ○ b. ○ c. ○
110. a. ○ b. ○ c. ○
111. a. ○ b. ○ c. ○
112. a. ○ b. ○ c. ○
113. a. ○ b. ○ c. ○
114. a. ○ b. ○ c. ○
115. a. ○ b. ○ c. ○
116. a. ○ b. ○ c. ○
117. a. ○ b. ○ c. ○
118. a. ○ b. ○ c. ○
119. a. ○ b. ○ c. ○
120. a. ○ b. ○ c. ○
121. a. ○ b. ○ c. ○
122. a. ○ b. ○ c. ○
123. a. ○ b. ○ c. ○
124. a. ○ b. ○ c. ○
125. a. ○ b. ○ c. ○
126. a. ○ b. ○ c. ○
127. a. ○ b. ○ c. ○
128. a. ○ b. ○ c. ○
129. a. ○ b. ○ c. ○
130. a. ○ b. ○ c. ○
131. a. ○ b. ○ c. ○
132. a. ○ b. ○ c. ○
133. a. ○ b. ○ c. ○
134. a. ○ b. ○ c. ○
135. a. ○ b. ○ c. ○
136. a. ○ b. ○ c. ○
137. a. ○ b. ○ c. ○
138. a. ○ b. ○ c. ○
139. a. ○ b. ○ c. ○
140. a. ○ b. ○ c. ○
141. a. ○ b. ○ c. ○
142. a. ○ b. ○ c. ○
143. a. ○ b. ○ c. ○
144. a. ○ b. ○ c. ○
145. a. ○ b. ○ c. ○
146. a. ○ b. ○ c. ○
147. a. ○ b. ○ c. ○
148. a. ○ b. ○ c. ○
149. a. ○ b. ○ c. ○
150. a. ○ b. ○ c. ○

Continuing Education Course

151. a. ○ b. ○ c. ○	160. a. ○ b. ○ c. ○	169. a. ○ b. ○ c. ○	178. a. ○ b. ○ c. ○	187. a. ○ b. ○ c. ○	196. a. ○ b. ○ c. ○	205. a. ○ b. ○ c. ○	214. a. ○ b. ○ c. ○	223. a. ○ b. ○ c. ○	232. a. ○ b. ○ c. ○
152. a. ○ b. ○ c. ○	161. a. ○ b. ○ c. ○	170. a. ○ b. ○ c. ○	179. a. ○ b. ○ c. ○	188. a. ○ b. ○ c. ○	197. a. ○ b. ○ c. ○	206. a. ○ b. ○ c. ○	215. a. ○ b. ○ c. ○	224. a. ○ b. ○ c. ○	233. a. ○ b. ○ c. ○
153. a. ○ b. ○ c. ○	162. a. ○ b. ○ c. ○	171. a. ○ b. ○ c. ○	180. a. ○ b. ○ c. ○	189. a. ○ b. ○ c. ○	198. a. ○ b. ○ c. ○	207. a. ○ b. ○ c. ○	216. a. ○ b. ○ c. ○	225. a. ○ b. ○ c. ○	234. a. ○ b. ○ c. ○
154. a. ○ b. ○ c. ○	163. a. ○ b. ○ c. ○	172. a. ○ b. ○ c. ○	181. a. ○ b. ○ c. ○	190. a. ○ b. ○ c. ○	199. a. ○ b. ○ c. ○	208. a. ○ b. ○ c. ○	217. a. ○ b. ○ c. ○	226. a. ○ b. ○ c. ○	235. a. ○ b. ○ c. ○
155. a. ○ b. ○ c. ○	164. a. ○ b. ○ c. ○	173. a. ○ b. ○ c. ○	182. a. ○ b. ○ c. ○	191. a. ○ b. ○ c. ○	200. a. ○ b. ○ c. ○	209. a. ○ b. ○ c. ○	218. a. ○ b. ○ c. ○	227. a. ○ b. ○ c. ○	
156. a. ○ b. ○ c. ○	165. a. ○ b. ○ c. ○	174. a. ○ b. ○ c. ○	183. a. ○ b. ○ c. ○	192. a. ○ b. ○ c. ○	201. a. ○ b. ○ c. ○	210. a. ○ b. ○ c. ○	219. a. ○ b. ○ c. ○	228. a. ○ b. ○ c. ○	
157. a. ○ b. ○ c. ○	166. a. ○ b. ○ c. ○	175. a. ○ b. ○ c. ○	184. a. ○ b. ○ c. ○	193. a. ○ b. ○ c. ○	202. a. ○ b. ○ c. ○	211. a. ○ b. ○ c. ○	220. a. ○ b. ○ c. ○	229. a. ○ b. ○ c. ○	
158. a. ○ b. ○ c. ○	167. a. ○ b. ○ c. ○	176. a. ○ b. ○ c. ○	185. a. ○ b. ○ c. ○	194. a. ○ b. ○ c. ○	203. a. ○ b. ○ c. ○	212. a. ○ b. ○ c. ○	221. a. ○ b. ○ c. ○	230. a. ○ b. ○ c. ○	
159. a. ○ b. ○ c. ○	168. a. ○ b. ○ c. ○	177. a. ○ b. ○ c. ○	186. a. ○ b. ○ c. ○	195. a. ○ b. ○ c. ○	204. a. ○ b. ○ c. ○	213. a. ○ b. ○ c. ○	222. a. ○ b. ○ c. ○	231. a. ○ b. ○ c. ○	

Evaluation Directions

Thank you for taking the time to assist us in evaluating the effectiveness of this course. Using the scale below, darken the circles corresponding to your responses. If an item is not applicable, leave it blank.

①	②	③	④	⑤
Strongly Disagree	Disagree	Neutral	Agree	Strongly Agree

Objectives:

I am able to:

1. Describe the characteristics used to identify bacteria, viruses, fungi, and protozoa. ① ② ③ ④ ⑤
2. Outline factors that determine the effects of microorganisms on the human body. ① ② ③ ④ ⑤
3. Identify common commensal organisms. ① ② ③ ④ ⑤
4. Define innate and adaptive immunities. ① ② ③ ④ ⑤
5. Outline the embryologic development of the immune system. ① ② ③ ④ ⑤
6. Discuss the role of each component of the immune system in the prevention and response to infection. ① ② ③ ④ ⑤
7. Outline methods used to detect intrauterine infection. ① ② ③ ④ ⑤
8. Discuss seven organisms responsible for intrauterine infections as to incidence and diagnosis. ① ② ③ ④ ⑤
9. Discuss seven organisms responsible for intrauterine infections as to maternal, fetal, and neonatal effects, and treatment of infection. ① ② ③ ④ ⑤
10. Identify historic trends in neonatal bacterial infections. ① ② ③ ④ ⑤

INFECTION IN THE NEONATE

11. Outline risk factors for neonatal bacterial infections. ① ② ③ ④ ⑤
12. Discuss neonatal bacterial pathogens as to incidence, site of infection, and signs and symptoms. ① ② ③ ④ ⑤
13. For each of the following organisms—RSV, Influenzavirus, varicella, enteroviruses, HIV, hepatitis viruses, Candida, and Malassezia—outline the etiology and epidemiology. ① ② ③ ④ ⑤
14. For each of the following organisms—RSV, Influenzavirus, varicella, enteroviruses, HIV, hepatitis viruses, Candida, and Malassezia—describe the clinical manifestations and diagnosis of infection. ① ② ③ ④ ⑤
15. For each of the following organisms—RSV, Influenzavirus, varicella, enteroviruses, HIV, hepatitis viruses, Candida and Malassezia—discuss the treatment and prevention of infection with these pathogens. ① ② ③ ④ ⑤

Presentation:

1. The material presented was relevant to my practice. ① ② ③ ④ ⑤
2. The questions on the test reflected the content of this book. ① ② ③ ④ ⑤
3. The content of the book was comprehensive. ① ② ③ ④ ⑤
4. The test directions were clear. ① ② ③ ④ ⑤
5. I perceive the education level of this course to be: 1 = Basic; 2 = Intermediate; 3 = Advanced ① ② ③
6. How long did it take you to complete the course? ____ hours ____ minutes
7. In what level unit do you practice? I___ II___ III___

What subjects would you like to see offered for CE courses? _____

Additional comments: _____

Iowa participants may submit a copy of this evaluation directly to the Iowa Board of Nursing, 400 SW 8th St., Ste. B, Des Moines, IA 50309-4685.

Print clearly

Name _____
Address _____
City _____
State _____ Zip _____
Phone (____) _____

E-mail _____
(to receive certificate via e-mail)

Nursing License # _____

State(s) of License _____

Academy (ANN) Membership # _____

━━━ Please complete the evaluation form beginning on the previous page. ━━━

| Test expires December 2010 | Mail with a $50.00 non-refundable processing fee for 20 contact hours to **2220 Northpoint Parkway, Santa Rosa, CA 95407**-7398. Please make check payable to NICU Ink. additional $10.00 for rush processing. International Participants: International Money Order drawn on U.S. bank only. |

--- FOR OFFICE USE ONLY ---
RECEIVED | CHECK | GRADE | CERTIFICATE ISSUED | REFERENCE #

Continuing Education Course